Color Atlas
OF
ENDODONTICS

Color Atlas
OF
ENDODONTICS

WILLIAM T. JOHNSON, DDS, MS

Professor
Department of Family Dentistry
and Dows Institute for Dental Research
The University of Iowa
College of Dentistry
Iowa City, Iowa

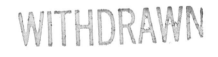
with 403 illustrations

W.B. SAUNDERS COMPANY
An Imprint of Elsevier Science
Philadelphia   London   New York   St. Louis   Sydney   Toronto

W.B. SAUNDERS COMPANY

The Curtis Center
Independence Square West
Philadelphia, Pennsylvania 19106

Library of Congress Cataloging in Publication Data

Color atlas of endodontics / [edited by] William T. Johnson—1st ed.

p.   cm.

Includes bibliographical references and index.

ISBN 0–7216–9030–0

1. Endodontics—Atlases,   I. Title.
    [DNLM: 1. Endodontics—Atlases.   WU 17 J71c 2002]

RK351 .J64 2002

617.6342—dc21   2001049986

Publishing Director: Linda L. Duncan
Senior Acquisitions Editor: Penny Rudolph
Developmental Editor: Jaime Pendill
Project Manager: Linda McKinley
Senior Production Editor: Jennifer Furey
Designer: Renée Duenow
Design Coordinator: Julia Dummitt

COLOR ATLAS OF ENDODONTICS   ISBN: 0–7216–9030–0

FIRST EDITION

Printed in the United States of America

Last digit is the print number: 9   8   7   6   5   4   3   2   1

CONTRIBUTORS

George A. Bruder, III, DMD
Harvard School of Dental Medicine
Boston, Massachusetts

G. Garo Chalian, DDS, MS, JD
Private Practice, Endodontics of Colorado LLC
Aurora, Colorado

Ty E. Erickson, DDS, MS
Assistant Clinical Professor, Department of
Endodontics
The University of Iowa
College of Dentistry
Iowa City, Iowa

Debra R. Haselton, DDS
Assistant Professor, Department of Family Dentistry
The University of Iowa
College of Dentistry
Iowa City, Iowa

David J. Holtzmann, DMD, MS
Private Practice
Endodontics of Colorado, LLC
Aurora, Colorado

William T. Johnson, DDS, MS
Professor, Department of Family Dentistry and Dows
Institute for Dental Research
The University of Iowa
College of Dentistry
Iowa City, Iowa

James L. Jostes, DDS, MS
Assistant Clinical Professor, Department of
Endodontics
The University of Iowa
College of Dentistry
Iowa City, Iowa

John A. Khademi, DDS, MS
Private Practice
Durango, Colorado

Keith V. Krell, DDS, MS, MA, FICD, FACD
Associate Clinical Professor, Department of
Endodontics
The University of Iowa
College of Dentistry
Iowa City, Iowa;
Diplomate, American Board of Endodontics

Frederick R. Liewehr, DDS, MS, FICD
Director, US Army Endodontic Residency Program
Assistant Clinical Professor, Department of
Endodontics
Assistant Adjunct Professor, Department of Oral
Biology and Maxillofacial Pathology
Medical College of Georgia
Augusta, Georgia;
Diplomate, American Board of Endodontics

Phillip J. Lumley, BDS, MSc, PhD, FDSRCPS
Department of Dental Prosthetics and Periodontics
University of Birmingham
The Dental School
Birmingham, England

Damien D. Walmsley, BDS, MSc, PhD, FDSRCPS
Department of Dental Prosthetics and Periodontics
University of Birmingham
The Dental School
Birmingham, England

Robert R. White, DMD
Director of Postdoctoral Endodontics
Harvard School of Dental Medicine
Boston, Massachusetts

PREFACE

Endodontics is the discipline of dentistry to which the responsibility for teaching the anatomy, morphology, histology, physiology, and pathology of the dental pulp and associated periradicular tissues is often delegated. Beyond an understanding of the basic sciences and their relationship to the dental pulp, the practice of endodontics requires great manual dexterity and the application of knowledge from other dental and medical disciplines. To be successful the endodontist must (1) integrate diagnostic and treatment planning skills; (2) apply knowledge of head and neck anatomy and morphology, pharmacology, microbiology, inflammation and immunology, systemic and oral pathology, pain, radiology, and biomaterials; (3) develop exceptional technical skills and expertise in performing surgical and nonsurgical procedures; and (4) manage a complex array of clinical problems. This must be accomplished in an environment characterized by an unprecedented increase in the knowledge base and an explosion in science and technology.

Unlike the "greatest generation" of World War II, today's patients expect to keep their natural dentition for the duration of their lives. As this dentate population ages, the demand for dental services will increase, as well as the complexity of treatment. This has created pressure on the dental profession to develop methods and materials to restore teeth that until recently would have been extracted.

To meet the needs and demands of the public and to ensure currency, the modern practitioner must be committed to lifelong learning. This process involves the transition from learning in a structured academic environment directed by experienced faculty and a set curriculum to self-instruction and exposure to new and varied philosophies. Direct benefits of lifelong learning include an increased knowledge base; the ability to evaluate new materials, techniques, and devices; and enhanced patient care. Indirect benefits are enthusiasm for the practice of endodontics, a challenge to continually improve, increased expectation of success, and confidence in the knowledge that the treatment being provided is based on sound biologic and scientific principles. Lifelong learning symbolizes an individual's commitment to pursue excellence. It is a professional requirement and an investment in the future.

The purpose of this atlas is to provide the clinician with current information on common clinical treatment techniques in the practice of endodontics. Emphasis is placed on presenting concepts that facilitate the process of applying existing knowledge to the unique clinical problems encountered in daily practice. Using a logical sequential approach, the atlas is designed to be an adjunct to the endodontic literature and serve as an educational resource for the clinician interested in lifelong learning and the specialty of endodontics.

William T. Johnson

ACKNOWLEDGMENTS

Through knowledge and experience come wisdom. With wisdom and a vision we can all contribute to the betterment of society. As Helen Keller stated "I long to accomplish a great and noble task, but it is my chief duty to accomplish small tasks as if they were great and noble." For the majority of us it is through the daily accomplishments of the common person that history is written. As Thomas Wolfe stated "So, then, to every man his chance—to every man, regardless of his birth, his shining golden opportunity—to every man his right to live, to work, to be himself, to become whatever his manhood and his vision can combine to make him—this, seeker, is the promise of America."

In every time and place there are friends and colleagues who influence an individual's life and career. With this in mind I would like to acknowledge the following individuals:

First and foremost, I would like recognize my parents, Alvah and Gaillard Johnson, for providing me the opportunity to fulfill my dreams. Their commitment to education and public service was a major influence on my choosing an academic career in dentistry.

I wish to thank Dr. Arne M. Bjorndal for accepting me into the specialty of endodontics and for serving as a friend and mentor.

I wish to thank Dr. Edward M. Osetek for teaching that those individuals who are privileged to participate in endodontics have obligations to the specialty.

I wish to thank Dr. Richard E. Walton for his commitment to scientific methodology and scholarship.

I wish to thank Dr. Patrick M. Lloyd for his support and encouragement in the development of this atlas.

I wish to thank the contributors to this atlas who dedicated their expertise, time, and talents to the cause of bettering the specialty of endodontics and advancing the oral health care delivered to the public.

And, last but not least, I would like to thank my wife, Georgia, and my two sons, Aaron and Jarod, for their support.

CONTENTS

Color Atlas
OF
ENDODONTICS

DIAGNOSIS OF PULPAL AND PERIRADICULAR PATHOSIS

WILLIAM T. JOHNSON

Diagnosis and treatment planning are common elements in all disciplines of dentistry. Although some clinicians may wish to limit their practice to certain procedures, diagnostic skills are a universal requirement.

The specialty of endodontics is unique among the dental specialties, requiring the successful clinician to integrate knowledge of anatomy and morphology, histopathology, pharmacology, microbiology, inflammation and immunology, pathology, pain, radiology, and biomaterials into the diagnostic and treatment planning process. The endodontist accomplishes this in an atmosphere characterized by unprecedented change in science and technology.

Although the majority of pulp and periradicular pathosis is asymptomatic, these disease processes can produce variable symptoms.[1] The astute clinician must be able to differentiate pulpal and periradicular problems from other pathologic entities.[2] Orofacial pain produced by trigeminal neuralgia, cluster headaches, temporal arteritis, atypical facial pain, acute maxillary sinusitis, cardiogenic jaw pain, herpes zoster, temporomandibular dysfunction (TMD), and facial pain resulting from malignant neoplasms may mimic pulpal pain. Furthermore, disorders such as cysts, periapical cementoosseous dysplasia, fibroosseous lesions, benign and malignant tumors, and periodontal disease can be confused with periradicular disease.

The development of a systematic approach to pulpal and periradicular diagnosis is the first step in developing treatment options and a definitive treatment plan. To ensure a correct diagnosis, the clinician must collect an accurate database. This involves obtaining a medical and dental history, performing a clinical examination and relevant tests, and making and interpreting appropriate radiographs. The process is the same for the asymptomatic, urgent, or emergent patient.

After the collection of a complete database, the diagnostic process requires correlation and interpretation of the information obtained. The experienced clinician realizes that arriving at a clinical diagnosis is often difficult because of a lack of sensitive and specific tests. The discriminating power of a test is defined by its sensitivity and specificity. *Sensitivity* is the rate or proportion of persons with a disease who test positive for it. *Specificity* is defined as the proportion of persons without a disease who nevertheless test positive for it.

In evaluating a patient, the clinician evaluates information from the history and clinical findings; this information may suggest a clinical diagnosis. This intuitive pre-test probability plays a significant role in the establishment of a correct diagnosis. The purpose of clinical testing is to confirm or exclude the presence of pulpal or periradicular disease. The clinician must be convinced that the probability the patient has pathosis exceeds the threshold for initiating treatment or that the information gathered excludes the potential of pulpal and periradicular pathosis. Clinical tests either convince the clinician that the threshold for treatment has been met or eliminate the possibility that the disease is of pulpal or periradicular origin. Experience in test result interpretation is important because pulp tests and radiographic interpretation are not always accurate. The interpretation and clinical usefulness of these tests depend on preexisting probability; the result of any test does not confirm a diagnosis.[3]

For example, two patients are evaluated. The first is a 28-year-old woman who is asymptomatic but exhibits a large carious lesion associated with her mandibular right first molar. Clinical examination reveals a draining sinus tract on the buccal mucosa opposite this tooth, as well as a periapical radiolucent area. From this information the clinician can make a tentative diagnosis of pulp necrosis and chronic periradicular abscess. Pulp testing reveals that the mandibular right second premolar and second molar respond to pulp testing, but the first molar is not responsive. This supports the diagnosis of pulp necrosis. The second patient is a 75-year-old man who is also asymptomatic. Examination reveals that he has all his teeth except the third molars and has no restorations. Radiographic examination indicates incipient enamel caries on the mesial aspect of the mandibular right first molar and considerable calcification of the pulp chambers in the posterior teeth. A tentative diagnosis of reversible pulpitis is established. Pulp testing reveals that none of the posterior teeth in the quadrant is responsive. In this case, clinical information and previous knowledge play a significant role in diagnosis. The lack of a distinct etiology, the fact that calcified teeth may not respond to testing, the decreased innervation of the pulp with age, and the knowledge that pulp tests are subjective (requiring interpretation by the patient) lead the practitioner to place less emphasis on test results.

Because spontaneous pulp necrosis does not occur and inflammatory periradicular pathosis occurs as a sequela of pulp necrosis, etiology is a major diagnostic consideration. Therefore identification of the etiology should be an important aspect in establishing a diagnosis. Although bacterial invasion of the pulp is a major etiologic category, restorative treatment, traumatic injury, nonendodontic pathosis, and radiation therapy should also be considered.

ACQUIRING A DIAGNOSTIC DATABASE

A fundamental principle in establishing a diagnosis is gathering information relevant to the disease process. The clinician must complete the database before beginning the interpretive and decision making process. The database begins with the patient's medical history.

Medical History

Obtaining a comprehensive written medical history is mandatory and should precede the examination and treatment of all patients. The medical history provides information regarding the patient's overall health and susceptibility to disease and indicates the potential for adverse reactions to treatment procedures. Information regarding current medications, allergies, and diseases, as well as the patient's emotional and psychologic status, can be assessed as it relates to the clinical problem. This information is important in diagnosis because the patient may have a systemic disease with oral manifestations. Moreover, a systemic disease may present initially as an oral lesion.

Dental History

The taking of a dental history allows the clinician to build rapport with the patient and is often more impor-

tant than the examination and testing procedures. The dental history almost always contributes to the establishment of a diagnosis.

The dental history should include the chief complaint and a history of the present illness if the patient has signs and/or symptoms of disease. The clinician should question the patient regarding the inception, location, type, frequency, intensity, duration, and cause of any pain or discomfort to develop a differential and definitive diagnosis. The process of information gathering may provide the clinician with a tentative diagnosis and guide the examination and testing process.

Pain is a complex physiologic and psychologic phenomenon and often cannot be used to differentiate endodontic problems from nonendodontic pathosis. Although most endodontic pathosis is asymptomatic, pulpal and periradicular pathosis is a leading cause of oral facial pain.[4] Identifying the source of a patient's pain may be routine or complex. In cases that are difficult to diagnose, a complete history and database become even more important.

Inflammation and pain in the dental pulp are often difficult to localize and may be referred to a tooth in the opposing quadrant or to the preauricular region. Pain intensity has been shown to affect the reporting of referred pain significantly, whereas duration and quality have little influence on its incidence.[5] Vertical referral patterns are common but not diagnostic because of horizontal overlap.

Information on previous traumatic injury, a previous pulp cap or "nerve treatment," or a cracked tooth can be instrumental in a diagnosis. A history of previous pain from a symptomatic tooth is also an important finding.[1] Reviewing entries in the chronologic record of treatment and viewing historical radiographs of the area are often helpful practices.

Clinical Examination

Visual inspection of the soft tissues should include an assessment of color, contour, and consistency. Localized redness, edema, swelling, or a sinus tract can indicate inflammatory disease. Examination of the hard structures may reveal clinical findings such as developmental defects, caries, abrasion, attrition, erosion, defective restorations, fractured cusps, cracked teeth, and tooth discoloration (Figure 1-1).

Diagnostic Testing

PULP TESTING.   Pulp tests are an assessment of the patient's response to stimuli and as such are subjective. They are designed to assess responsiveness and localize symptomatic teeth by reproducing the patient's symptoms. A positive response to pulp testing does not indicate vitality, only sensory perception of the stimuli. Pulp testing is essential in establishing a clinical diagnosis. Testing ensures the identification of the offending tooth or teeth and is

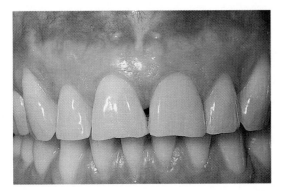

FIGURE 1-1   A 32-year-old woman presents for treatment of spontaneous pain that keeps her awake at night. She relates a history of orthodontics and a frenectomy as an adolescent, as well as traumatic injury to the maxillary anterior area during a basketball game. Clinical examination reveals normal-appearing soft tissues, scar formation consistent with location of the suture placed after the frenectomy, and discoloration of the maxillary left central incisor, tooth #9.

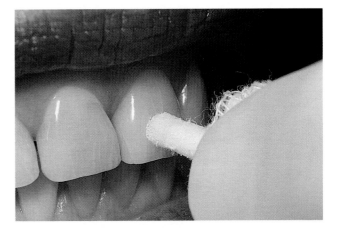

FIGURE 1-3 CO_2 snow application to tooth #9, which is non-responsive.

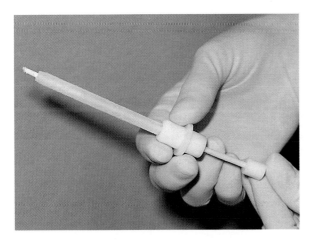

FIGURE 1-2 CO_2 snow is an excellent method of thermal testing because it provides a temperature of $-50°$ C and transforms from a solid to a gaseous state, eliminating the potential for stimulation of adjacent teeth.

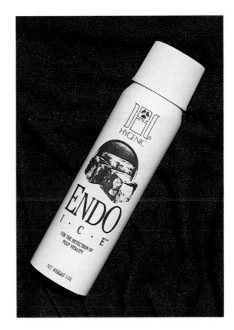

FIGURE 1-4   Dichlorodifluoromethane is also an effective method of cold testing. The material can be sprayed on a cotton pellet or cotton-tip applicator for use. As with CO_2 snow, it has no liquid state.

part of the methodology in the differential diagnosis of diseases of nonodontogenic origin. Electrical and thermal testing procedures have been shown to produce reliable results.[6,7]

THERMAL TESTING.   Thermal sensitivity is a common chief complaint in pulp pathosis. Testing with hot and cold identifies the tooth and is instrumental in determining whether the pulp is normal or inflamed.

Cold testing is usually performed first. Carbon dioxide, or CO_2 (Figures 1-2 and 1-3), ethyl chloride, dichlorodifluoromethane (Figure 1-4), and ice sticks (Figure 1-5) are frequently used to apply cold to teeth. These tests have been shown to be safe and do not cause damage to the pulp[8,9] or enamel.[10] Patients should be advised of the testing method and expected sensations. The testing should begin on a normal "control" tooth (usually of the same tooth group or type) to educate the patient regarding what to expect from the test, determine whether the test will provoke a response (validating the use of the

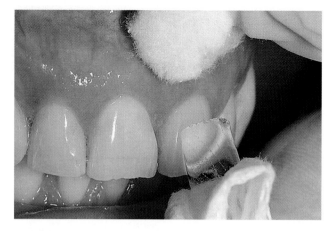

FIGURE 1-5 Ice may also be used to assess vitality. However, because it has a liquid state it may stimulate adjacent teeth. When ice is used the most posterior teeth should be tested first.

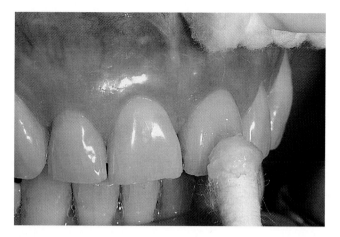

FIGURE 1-6 When pulp testing with heat, temporary gutta-percha stopping can be used. The material is heated over an alcohol torch and applied to the tooth surface. Petroleum jelly should be applied to the tooth surface before testing to prevent the temporary stopping from sticking to the tooth surface.

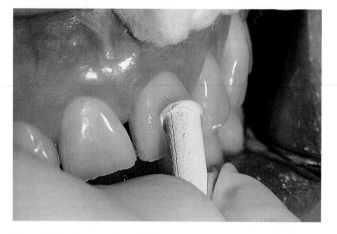

FIGURE 1-7 After applying the petroleum jelly, the clinician can apply the heated temporary stopping. As with CO_2 testing, tooth #9 is nonresponsive.

test), and allow the clinician to observe the patient's reaction to the stimulus.

Pulpal pain occurs as a result of tissue damage, and often the response to thermal stimulation is altered. In the normal pulp, perception of thermal stimulation is sharp and immediate but disappears with the removal of the stimulus. This dentinal pain is conducted by myelinated A-delta nerve fibers and is the result of fluid movement in the dentinal tubules (hydrodynamic theory).[11] Dentinal pain is a warning sign and does not necessarily indicate tissue damage. During pulp testing only the A-delta nerve fibers are stimulated. C nerve fibers do not respond to thermal or electric pulp testing because of their high stimulation threshold.[12,13]

During injury to the pulp tissue, inflammatory mediators are released and the inflammatory process stimu-

lates unmyelinated C nerve fibers, producing pain that is not well localized. This pain is often spontaneous and is described as burning and radiating. It begins without stimulus and frequently alters the patient's lifestyle. Prolonged pain after thermal stimulation is often the first indication that irreversible pulp damage has occurred. The spontaneous, radiating pain that keeps patients awake or awakens them at night results from C nerve fiber stimulation and indicates tissue damage and inflammation. C nerve fiber stimulation is also responsible for referred pain.

Thermal testing with heat is indicated when a patient complains of sensitivity to hot food or liquids.[14] It is performed by applying petroleum jelly to the tooth surface (Figure 1-6) and heating a stick of gutta-percha temporary stopping in an open flame. As the temporary

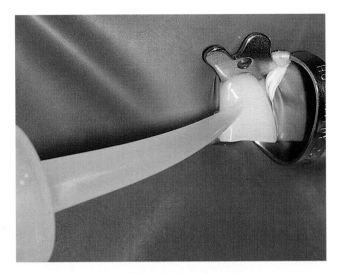

FIGURE 1-8 An alternative method of thermal testing involves isolating individual teeth with a rubber dam and flooding the tooth with the appropriate hot or cold liquid. This method is especially useful when a patient complains of thermal sensitivity and traditional testing does not reproduce the patient's symptoms.

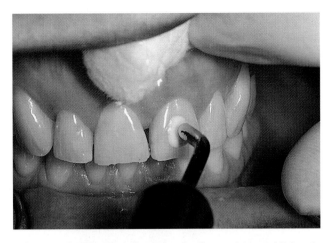

FIGURE 1-9 Electric pulp testing can be used to establish pulp vitality or confirm nonresponsiveness. In this case the failure of tooth #9 to respond confirms the results obtained with thermal testing.

stopping begins to soften, the clinician applies it to the lubricated tooth surface (Figure 1-7). A dry rubber prophylaxis cup can also be used to generate frictional heat. A more effective method of heat testing involves isolating individual teeth with a rubber dam and flooding the tooth with hot water (Figure 1-8). This method permits the application of a uniform temperature to each tooth and replicates the patient's normal activities. The technique is effective with full coverage restorations and can also be used with cold testing. Heat testing is the least valuable pulp test but is essential when the patient complains of sensitivity to heat.

ELECTRIC PULP TESTING. Electric pulp testing stimulates the A-delta nerve fibers. The electric pulp test (EPT) indicates only whether the pulp is responsive or unresponsive. It does not provide information regarding the health of the pulp, nor can it differentiate degrees of pulp pathosis other than to indicate necrosis when no response occurs.[15] It is often used to confirm the results of previous tests. The EPT requires an isolated dry field. Traditionally the electrode is coated with a conducting medium, usually toothpaste, and placed on the dry enamel labial or buccal surface of the tooth to be tested (Figure 1-9). Evidence indicates that the incisal edge is the optimal placement site for the electric pulp tester electrode to determine the lowest response threshold.[16] Contact with metallic restorations is to be avoided. The Analytical Technology (Analytic Endodontics, Sybron Dental Specialties, Orange, CA) pulp tester is recommended because it begins at zero current and increases the current gradually at a rate predetermined by the op-

erator.[17] Patients are instructed to place a hand on the metal handle to begin the test and release the handle when they perceive a tingling sensation to stop the test. Having control of the test is reassuring to the patient. As with other tests, the clinician should test a normal tooth first to familiarize the patient with the procedure and sensation.

All pulp tests have a potential for false positive and false negative results. A false positive can occur when a tooth with a necrotic pulp nevertheless responds to testing. This can result from stimulation of adjacent teeth or the attachment apparatus, the response of vital tissue in a multirooted tooth with pulp necrosis in one or more canals, and patient interpretation. Furthermore, the clinician must keep in mind that the cell bodies of the neurons innervating the pulp lie in the Gasserian ganglion. Only the axons enter the pulp, so the nervous tissue can maintain vitality in a mass of necrotic pulp tissue. Neural elements have been shown to be more resistant to necrosis[18] and C nerve fibers can function in a hypoxic environment.[19] Finally, pulp tests are not objective and require the patient to interpret the response, adding considerable subjectivity.

An example of a false negative in a pulp test is a tooth with a vital pulp that nevertheless does not respond to stimulation. False negatives can result from inadequate contact with the stimulus, tooth calcification, immature apical development, traumatic injury, and the subjective nature of the tests. They can also occur in elderly patients who have undergone regressive neural changes and in patients who have taken analgesics for pain. The neural elements develop after

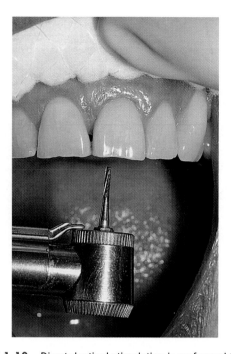

FIGURE 1-10 Direct dentinal stimulation is performed to eliminate the possibility of a false negative result with traditional testing. In this case no caries or restorations are present, leaving trauma as the only distinct etiology. Direct dentinal stimulation is employed when the clinician suspects that a tooth that does not respond is in fact vital.

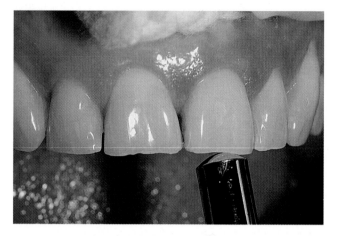

FIGURE 1-11 Percussion can be performed with digital pressure, a mirror handle, or the Tooth Slooth. If the patient is symptomatic and complains of sensitivity to biting pressure, digital pressure may be all that is required to identify the offending tooth. In other cases, percussion with a mirror handle may be required to assess the periapical status.

eruption of the tooth,[20] and the aging of the dental pulp produces structural and neurochemical regressive changes that affect pulp innervation.[21] Traumatic injury can damage the neural elements but leave the vascular supply to the tissue intact.[22]

DIRECT DENTINAL STIMULATION (TEST CAVITY). The test cavity is an invasive procedure that is often used to ensure that a negative response to previous pulp tests was accurate. Because this test is invasive and requires removal of tooth structure and/or restorative materials, it is used primarily to exclude false negative results. The test can be used in clinical cases in which a tooth does not respond to cold testing and EPT but lacks a distinct etiology for necrosis. In such cases direct dentinal stimulation can be used to reveal necrosis or establish vitality.

Direct dentinal stimulation involves removing enamel or restorative materials using a high-speed handpiece without local anesthesia (Figure 1-10). If the tooth is vital, the patient will experience a sharp, painful response when dentin is reached. Clinicians must caution patients that they will feel the sensations of vibration and pressure so that they can interpret the test correctly.

PERCUSSION. As pulp pathosis extends beyond the tooth into the supporting periodontal tissues and sur-

rounding bone, the patient's ability to localize the offending tooth increases. Proprioceptive fibers in the periodontal ligament are stimulated by force applied to the tooth and produce localized discomfort. Percussion is performed by applying force on the incisal or occlusal surface in an axial direction. This can be accomplished using digital pressure, tapping on the tooth with an instrument handle (Figure 1-11), or having the patient bite on a Tooth Slooth (Professional Results Inc., Laguna Niguel, CA) or cotton swab.

Although a positive response to percussion can indicate apical periodontitis secondary to pulp pathosis, other potential etiologies should also be considered. Tenderness to percussion can result from a variety of clinical problems such as a high restoration, traumatic injury, traumatic occlusion, a cracked tooth, a vertical root fracture, orthodontic treatment, a periodontal abscess, and maxillary sinusitis.

Clinicians can also use pressure to test for pulpal pathosis. Pressure can be applied by having the patient bite on a cotton swab or the Tooth Slooth (Figure 1-12), a device that permits the application of force to individual cusps and can be of value in the diagnosis of fractured or cracked teeth.

PALPATION. As periradicular inflammation extends through the cortical bone into the soft tissues, it can fre-

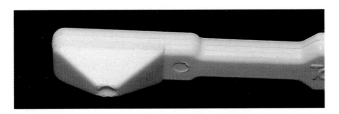

FIGURE 1-12   The Tooth Slooth can be used to assess cracked teeth and incomplete cuspal fractures. The unique design allows the patient to exert pressure on individual cusps.

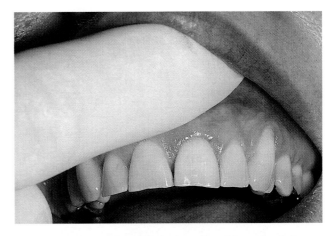

FIGURE 1-13   Palpation of the buccal and lingual soft tissues can detect areas of sensitivity and swelling, as well as determine the character of the swelling.

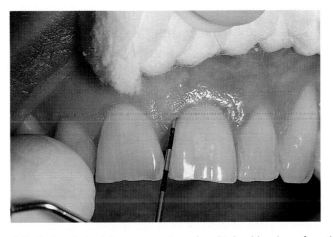

FIGURE 1-14   A limited periodontal assessment can be obtained by circumferential periodontal probing of the area. Often an isolated defect can be identified that is not otherwise apparent in the clinical and radiographic assessment.

quently be detected by digital palpation of the soft tissues over the apex of the root (Figure 1-13). When the mucoperiosteum is inflamed, the clinician will detect sensitivity in the involved area. As the inflammatory process progresses the operator may detect swelling of the soft tissues. The clinician should note the consistency of any swelling because not all swelling is the result of inflammatory disease. Palpation is not restricted to intraoral tissues. For example, palpation of extraoral structures can reveal lymphadenopathy.

MOBILITY.   Tooth mobility can be assessed by moving the tooth in a facial or buccal-lingual direction. Mobility can be assessed by placing an index finger on the lingual surface and applying lateral force with an instrument handle from the buccal surface. The Miller Index of Tooth Mobility is commonly used to interpret the clinical findings.[23] Class 1 is the first distinguishable sign of greater-than-normal movement, Class 2 is movement of the crown as much as 1 mm in any direction, and Class 3 is movement of the crown more than 1 mm in any direction and/or vertical depression or rotation of the crown in its socket. Common causes of tooth mobility include periodontal disease, bruxism, clenching, traumatic occlusion, improper partial denture design, root fractures, and periradicular inflammation caused by pulp necrosis.

PERIODONTAL PROBING.   Examination of the periodontal tissues is an essential component of the diagnostic process. Endodontic and periodontic lesions may mimic each other or occur concurrently. Because periodontal bone loss may not be detected radiographically and the gingival tissues may appear normal, probing is required (Figure 1-14). Keeping a record of the probing depths aids in determining the patient's periodontal health and

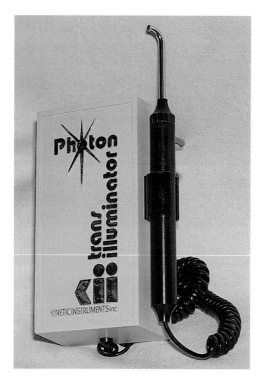

FIGURE 1-15 Transillumination is employed to evaluate teeth for fracture lines.

prognosis, and the pattern of probing also provides important information. To obtain adequate information when examining a specific tooth, the clinician should probe the entire circumference. Often a narrow probing defect can be detected with normal sulcular depths immediately adjacent to the defect. Common etiologies for isolated probing defects include periodontal disease, periapical pathosis forming a sinus-like trap through the periodontium, developmental defects such as a vertical groove defect, cracked teeth and vertical root fractures, and external root resorption.

TRANSILLUMINATION/DYE STAINING. The use of a fiberoptic light (Figure 1-15) is an excellent method of examining teeth for coronal cracks and vertical root fractures.[24] The tooth or root should be examined in the presence of minimal background lighting. The fiberoptic light is then placed on the varied surfaces of the coronal tooth structure or on the root after flap reflection. Fracture lines can be visually detected when light fails to traverse the fracture line. The fractured segment near the light appears brighter than the segment away from the light.

Application of dyes to the tooth can also demonstrate fractures as the dye penetrates the fracture line. An ancillary technique is the application of dye to the internal surfaces of a cavity preparation or access opening; the clinician leaves the dye in place for a week before reexamining the tooth.

SELECTIVE ANESTHESIA/ANESTHETIC TEST. Because pain of pulpal origin is not referred beyond the midline, the administration of local anesthesia can help localize pain to a specific area in cases where patients exhibit referred pain that cannot be localized by the patient or by testing. Administration of a mandibular inferior alveolar nerve block will determine whether the pain is from the maxillary or mandibular teeth on the affected side. The pain will cease if it is from a mandibular tooth and persist if it is from a maxillary tooth. Although some clinicians feel that pain from an individual tooth can be isolated by administering local anesthetic with a periodontal ligament (PDL) injection, evidence suggests that this is inappropriate. PDL injections have been shown to anesthetize teeth adjacent to the tooth being anesthetized.[25]

CARIES EXCAVATION. Caries excavation is a frequently used procedure to assess pulpal status. In patients exhibiting moderate to severe decay and normal responses to pulp testing, the clinician must remove the caries before deciding on a pulpal diagnosis. The initial response of the pulp to caries is chronic inflammation consisting of plasma cells and lymphocytes. This is a specific immune response to antigens leaching through the tubules. Excavation of caries and placement of a restoration remove the irritants and establish an environment for healing. As the dental pulp is exposed and bacteria invade, the existing chronic inflammatory response becomes acute as the host responds with polymorphonuclear leukocytes. This acute nonspecific inflammatory response results in the release of lysosomal enzymes and the destruction of host tissue as well as the invading bacteria. This is the crossover point from reversible to irreversible pulpitis.[26]

Radiographic Examination

Radiographic examination of the hard tissues can often provide valuable information regarding caries and existing restorations, calcifications, internal and external resorptions, tooth and pulpal morphology, root fractures, the relationship of anatomic structures, and the architecture of the osseous tissues (Figure 1-16). In addition, radiographs can be used to trace sinus tracts,[27] demonstrate periodontal defects, and diagnose resorptive lesions (Figure 1-17). However, they do have many limitations and are of little value in assessing pulpal status. Vital and necrotic pulps cast the same image. Moreover, radiographs are only two-dimensional images of three-dimensional structures.

Because radiography and some other imaging methods require ionizing radiation, during the clinical examination the clinician must prescribe the projection that will provide the most information at the lowest dose regarding the patient's problem. In most cases this is a periapical film or image, although bite-wing and extraoral films may be necessary.

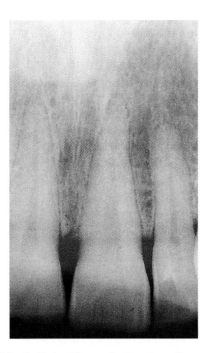

FIGURE 1-16   Radiographic examination generally requires a periapical projection, although bite-wings and pantomographic projections are often useful. In this case the periradicular tissues appear normal; however, a comparison of the root canal space of #8 and #9 reveals that the space in tooth #9 is considerably larger. This is consistent with the clinical presentation, symptoms, and diagnostic testing results, which indicate necrosis. The radiographic appearance of the root canal system is caused by the lack of secondary dentin formation over time.

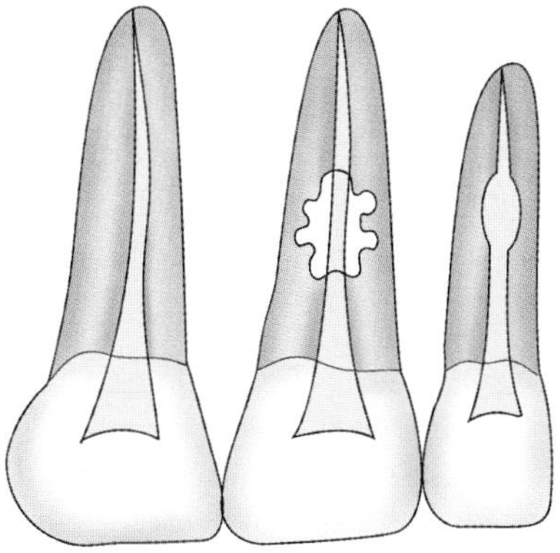

FIGURE 1-17   Radiographs are useful in diagnosis. External resorptive defects such as the one depicted in the maxillary left central incisor are often irregular, with the root canal coursing through the lesion. Internal resorption such as that depicted in the maxillary left lateral incisor is often symmetric and exhibits destruction of the canal wall. In addition, internal resorptive lesions remain centered on angled radiographs.

Periapical radiographs and other images should be exposed using a positioning device and a paralleling technique. This provides the most distortion-free image and accurate diagnostic information. Although great emphasis is often placed on the radiographic examination, it is an imperfect diagnostic aid because of the varied techniques and methods for obtaining the film or image and the variable ability of practitioners to interpret the information correctly.[28-30] Subtle and moderate changes are often difficult to detect early in the pulpal and periradicular disease process. As the disease progresses, lesions become more distinct and easier to detect. Evidence suggests that a periapical lesion must erode the cortical plate to be visible on the film or image.[31] Making a second film using an angled projection can increase the diagnostic accuracy.[32]

Periradicular lesions resulting from pulp necrosis have a characteristic appearance. The radiolucency exhibits a "hanging drop" appearance, with the lesion beginning on the lateral osseous surfaces of the root and extending apically into the osseous tissues. The lamina dura is absent, and the lesion does not move when angled films are taken. In general, a radiolucent lesion associated with a tooth with a vital pulp is not of endodontic origin.

Condensing osteitis is a proliferative response of bone to periradicular inflammation. It is characterized by a diffuse appearance without distinct borders.

Radiographs and digital images appear to be equal in their diagnostic ability, although the astute clinician will use the radiographic examination to confirm the clinical examination.[28-30]

DIAGNOSTIC CATEGORIES

The clinical diagnosis is based on the correlation of information. Because the information in the database is often incomplete or inconsistent, experience and the application of biologic principles allow for rational assessment.

Pulpal

NORMAL.   The category of *normal* is used for teeth that are asymptomatic, respond normally to pulp testing, and are free of caries, deficient restorations, developmental defects, and cracks. Radiographically the periradicular tissues appear normal with an intact lamina dura.

REVERSIBLE PULPITIS.   The category of *reversible pulpitis* is used for teeth that respond normally to pulp testing.

These teeth may be asymptomatic or have mild to moderate symptoms such as thermal sensitivity, sensitivity to sweets, pain to tactile stimulation, or pain when chewing. The pain generally subsides with removal of the irritant or stimulus, indicating A-delta nerve fiber activity. Common etiologies to consider are caries, deficient restorations, attrition, abrasion, erosion, cracks, or developmental defects that lead to exposed dentin. Dentinal hypersensitivity is a form of reversible pulpitis. Treatment may involve caries excavation, placing or replacing restorations, or sealing the dentin. If symptoms occur after a treatment procedure such as placement of a restoration or scaling and root planing, time may be required for symptoms to subside. The periradicular tissues appear normal.

IRREVERSIBLE PULPITIS. The etiologies for *irreversible pulpitis* are the same as those for reversible pulpitis, except that the symptoms are more severe and consistent with C nerve fiber activity. The tooth still responds to pulp testing. In general, the more intense the pain, the more likely that the pain is caused by irreversible pulpitis. Continuous or prolonged pain after a thermal stimulus is one of the first indications of irreversible pulpitis. Spontaneous pain is also associated with the condition. Pain that keeps the patient awake or awakens him or her is often indicative of irreversible pulpitis. A painful response to heat that is relieved by cold is a classic symptom. Root canal treatment, vital pulp therapy, or extraction is required. Generally the periradicular tissues appear normal, although in some cases the lamina dura appears widened or shows evidence of condensing osteitis.

NECROSIS. The positive response to cold and EPT occurs regardless of pulp status in normal, reversible, and irreversible pulpitis. *Necrotic* pulps do not respond. Teeth with necrotic pulps may or may not exhibit periradicular pathosis. Because teeth with necrotic pulps may exist within normal periradicular structures, the astute clinician performs pulp testing on all teeth before initiating restorative treatment. Pulp necrosis has two forms: dry and liquefactive. Dry necrosis is characterized by a root canal system devoid of tissue elements. This type of necrosis is most likely to produce periradicular pathosis. Liquefactive necrosis is characterized by pulp tissue with structure but lacking significant vascular elements. Liquefactive necrosis is more likely to produce symptoms and less likely to produce periradicular pathosis.

Periradicular

NORMAL. The category of *normal* is used to describe the periradicular status of teeth that are asymptomatic to percussion or palpation and exhibit normal-appearing osseous structures with an intact lamina dura.

ACUTE APICAL PERIODONTITIS. The category of *acute apical periodontitis* applies to teeth that exhibit normal periradicular structures but are painful to percussion because of the stimulation of proprioceptive fibers. The etiology can be pulp pathosis, but high restorations, traumatic occlusion, orthodontic treatment, cracked teeth and vertical root fractures, periodontal disease, and maxillary sinusitis may also produce this response. Treatment depends on the diagnostic findings. If pulp pathosis is the etiology, pulpectomy followed by root canal treatment or extraction is the most common treatment option.

CHRONIC APICAL PERIODONTITIS. *Chronic apical periodontitis* results from pulp necrosis and is characterized by the development of an asymptomatic periradicular lesion at the periapex and at the portal of exit in cases exhibiting lateral canals on the side of the root. Histologically this lesion is categorized as a granuloma or cyst. Root canal treatment or extraction are the treatment options.

CHRONIC PERIRADICULAR ABSCESS. *Chronic periradicular abscess* is similar to chronic apical periodontitis except that it is characterized by the presence of a draining sinus tract. The lesion is asymptomatic with an intermittent discharge of pus through the sinus tract. This lesion is also referred to as *chronic suppurative apical periodontitis*. Root canal treatment or extraction is required.

ACUTE PERIRADICULAR ABSCESS. *Acute periradicular abscess* is an inflammatory reaction resulting from pulp necrosis that is characterized by rapid onset, pain, and tenderness to percussion. Evidence of osseous destruction may or may not be present. A discharge of pus is evident, but swelling may or may not occur. The exudate can be confined to the alveolar bone, cause localized swelling of soft tissue, or extend into fascial spaces (cellulitis). The exacerbation of a previously asymptomatic chronic apical periodontitis has been termed a *phoenix abscess*.

The primary method of treating an acute periradicular abscess is to remove the irritants and provide drainage. This can be accomplished by initiating root canal treatment and débriding the radicular space or extracting the tooth. Antibiotics are not a substitute for definitive treatment procedures designed to remove the necrotic tissue and bacteria from the radicular space. Drainage can be accomplished through the tooth or through an incision of the involved soft tissues. This procedure relieves pressure, increases vascular flow, and evacuates the purulent exudate. In these cases, antibiotics serve a supportive role as adjuvants to treatment. Clinicians should prescribe antibiotics to medically compromised patients and patients with an increased temperature and systemic involvement.

CONDENSING OSTEITIS. *Condensing osteitis* is a proliferative inflammatory response to an irritant. The lesion is generally asymptomatic and is characterized radiographically by an increase in radiopacity.

SUMMARY

Clinicians must be knowledgeable and skilled in the process of diagnosis and treatment planning. They should be able to recognize that the patient has a problem, identify the etiology, establish a pulpal and periradicular diagnosis, and develop methods of treatment. Consultation with medical and dental specialists is often necessary during this process.

Pulpal and periradicular pathosis are inflammatory in nature. The accuracy of the clinical diagnosis is confirmed by resolution of the patient's signs and symptoms and healing of the involved tissues. Therefore periodic recall examination is an important part of the diagnostic process.

References

1. Bender IB: Pulpal pain diagnosis–a review, *J Endodon* 26:175, 2000.
2. Okeson JP, Falace DA: Nonodontogenic toothache, *Dent Clin North Am* 41:367, 1997.
3. Chang P: Evaluating imaging test performance: an introduction to Bayesian analysis for urologists, *Monogr Urology* 12:18, 1991.
4. Lipton JA, Ship JA, Larach-Robinson D: Estimated prevalence and distribution of reported orofacial pain in the United States, *J Am Dent Assoc* 124:115, 1993.
5. Falace DA, Reid K, Rayens MK: The influence of deep (odontogenic) pain intensity, quality, and duration on the incidence and characteristics of referred orofacial pain, *J Orofac Pain* 10:232, 1996.
6. Georgopoulou M, Kerani M: The reliability of electrical and thermal pulp tests. A clinical study, *Stomatologia* 46:317, 1989.
7. Peters DD, Baumgartner JC, Lorton L: Adult pulpal diagnosis. I. Evaluation of the positive and negative responses to cold and electrical pulp tests, *J Endodon* 20:506, 1994.
8. Rickoff B et al: Effects of thermal vitality tests on human dental pulp, *J Endodon* 14:482, 1988.
9. Dummer PM, Tanner M, McCarthy JP: A laboratory study of four electric pulp testers, *Inter Endo J* 19:161, 1986.
10. Peters DD, Mader CL, Donnelly JC: Evaluation of the effects of carbon dioxide used as a pulpal test. 3. In vivo effect on human enamel, *J Endodon* 12:13, 1986.
11. Ahlquist M et al: Dental pain evoked by hydrostatic pressures applied to exposed dentin in man: a test of the hydrodynamic theory of dentin sensitivity, *J Endodon* 20:130, 1994.
12. Narhi MV et al: The neurophysiological basis and the role of inflammatory reactions in dentine hypersensitivity, *Arch Oral Biol* 39(suppl):23S, 1994.
13. Hirvonen T, Narhi MV, Hakumaki MO: The excitability of dog pulp nerves in relation to the condition of dentin surface, *J Endodon* 10:294, 1984.
14. Rosenberg RJ: Using heat to assess pulp inflammation, *J Am Dent Assoc* 122(2):77, 1991.
15. Lado EA, Richmond AF, Marks RG: Reliability and validity of a digital pulp tester as a test standard for measuring sensory perception, *J Endodon* 14:352, 1988.
16. Bender IB et al: The optimum placement-site of the electrode in electric pulp testing of the 12 anterior teeth, *J Am Dent Assoc* 118:305, 1989.
17. Kleier DJ, Sexton JR, Averbach RE: Electronic and clinical comparison of pulp testers, *J Dent Res* 61:1413, 1982.
18. Torneck CD: Changes in the fine structure of the human dental pulp subsequent to carious exposure, *J Oral Pathol* 6:82, 1977.
19. Narhi MV et al: Role of intradental A- and C-type nerve fibres in dental pain mechanisms, *Proc Finn Dent Soc* 88(suppl 1):507, 1992.
20. Johnsen DC, Karlsson UL: Development of neural elements in apical portions of cat primary and permanent incisor pulps, *Anat Rec* 189:29, 1977.
21. Fried K: Aging of the dental pulp involves structural and neurochemical regressive changes in the innervation of the pulp, *Proc Finn Dent Soc* 88:517, 1992.
22. Bhaskar SN, Rappaport HM: Dental vitality tests and pulp status, *J Am Dent Assoc* 86:409, 1973.
23. Miller SC: *Textbook of periodontia*, ed 3, Philadelphia, 1950, Blackstone.
24. Schindler WG, Walker WA, III: Transillumination of the beveled root surface: an aid to periradicular surgery, *J Endodon* 20:408, 1994.
25. D'Souza JE, Walton RE, Peterson LC: Periodontal ligament injection: an evaluation of the extent of anesthesia and postinjection discomfort, *J Am Dent Assoc* 114:341, 1987.
26. Trowbridge HO: Pathogenesis of pulpitis resulting from dental caries, *J Endodon* 7:52, 1981.
27. Bonness BW, Taintor JF: The ectopic sinus tract: report of cases, *J Endodon* 6:614, 1980.
28. Goldman M, Pearson AH, Darzenta N: Reliability of radiographic interpretations, *Oral Surg Oral Med Oral Pathol Oral Radiol Endod* 38:287, 1974.
29. Gelfand M, Sunderman EJ, Goldman M: Reliability of radiographical interpretations, *J Endodon* 9:71, 1983.
30. Holtzmann DJ et al: Storage phosphor based computed radiography versus film based radiography in detection of pathologic periradicular bone loss in a cadaver model: an ROC study, *Oral Surg Oral Med Oral Pathol Oral Radiol Endod* 86:90, 1998.
31. Bender IB: Factors influencing the radiographic appearance of bony lesions, *J Endodon* 23:5, 1997.
32. Brynolf I: Roentgenologic periapical diagnosis. One, two or more roentgenograms? *Swed Dent J* 63:345, 1970.

ENDODONTIC ACCESS

JOHN A. KHADEMI

Traditional endodontic textbooks present "ideal" endodontic access concepts and techniques as though clinicians usually treat caries-free, unrestored teeth with large canals and visible, patent orifices. Unfortunately, endodontic treatment involves teeth exhibiting caries, extensive restorations, calcifications, or a combination of these factors.

The clinician performing endodontic treatment is almost invariably treating a tooth compromised by caries, restorations, a crown placed over one or more restorative materials that may have a base, or a combination of these factors. Access to the coronal surface of the tooth is compromised by the patient's ability to open the mouth, requiring the clinician to work in a restricted area. Visibility is compromised by inadequate light and poor position (teeth are in the mouth—a deep, dark hole). Canal orifices are frequently constricted because of calcific metamorphosis (calcification) and may be blocked by pulp stones and dentinal shelves. Include root caries, changes in tooth angulation and often position masked by the placement of a crown, and difficulty in isolation, and clinicians cannot be faulted for marveling that endodontics can be performed proficiently with predictable success. The ideal exists only in the mind. Clinically, complicating factors must be balanced with the pursuit of perfection.

GOALS OF ENDODONTIC ACCESS
First, Do No Harm

"Access preparation is the most important phase of the technical aspects of root canal treatment!"[1] The bulk of procedural errors and treatment difficulties are related to errors or problems in obtaining adequate access.

Endodontics has undergone tremendous change in the past decade, both in the number of procedures performed and in the development of new materials, instruments, and techniques. Mineral trioxide aggregate (MTA), Geri-store (Den-Mat, Santa Maria, CA), resorbable membranes, rotary nickel-titanium (NiTi) instruments, System B (Analytic Technology, Sybron Dental Specialties, Inc., Orange, CA), Thermafil (Dentsply Tulsa Dental, Tulsa, OK), and microscopes have done more than improve the way clinicians provide care—they permit treatment of more complex cases. However, despite these advances and other changes, the discipline has also emphasized a return to the fundamentals: débridement, shaping, and obturation of the radicular space. In some ways these advances, especially microscopic techniques, have instilled a new appreciation for the complex radicular anatomy of the pulp.

As the aging "baby boomer" population moves through its fourth, fifth and sixth decades of life, clinicians can expect a continued increase in the number of endodontic procedures over the next two decades. This generation has the dental knowledge, desire, motivation, and finances to seek the best in health care. As their 20- and 30-year-old amalgams fracture and their crowned teeth develop recurrent decay, prepared clinicians will witness a new golden age for endodontics. Endodontists cannot possibly perform all the endodontic procedures that will be needed in the coming years. General practitioners will need to review what many would say is the most challenging and stressful part of endodontic treatment: obtaining adequate access.

The ideals of endodontic access are as follows:

1. Complete removal of the chamber roof
2. Removal of coronal pulp
3. Straight-line access to facilitate placement of endodontic instruments

These ideals are balanced with the following constraints:

1. Conservation of tooth structure
2. Retention and esthetics of the final restoration

A great deal of frustration that many practitioners have with endodontic treatment stems from the difficulty of placing a 25-mm instrument in the mesiobuccal (MB) canal of a distally inclined maxillary second molar. Correct access design and straight-line access to facilitate instrument placement can greatly reduce frustration and dramatically decrease treatment time.

With the advent of hyperflexible NiTi instruments, clinicians might mistakenly conclude that minimizing instrument flexure is of lesser importance. In fact, straight-line access and minimizing of instrument flexure is of increased importance in the use of NiTi instruments. Conventional stainless steel files can be precurved and "hooked" into canals. If a rotary NiTi file is curved or bent, it is ruined and must be discarded. In addition, straight-line access and reduced instrument flexure improve the clinician's ability to use the instruments as feeler gauges and improve control over the instruments' cutting action.

Specialists are often referred cases in which the general practitioner cannot find the canals. Most of the time the canals are in the chamber, but the access preparation precludes the practitioner from locating the canals. The problem is usually too small an access preparation with improper location and suboptimal shape. After the access has been reshaped, the canals are easily located. This is of particular importance with posterior teeth whose canals can be easily missed, leading to periapical pathosis or continued symptoms.

Unroofing the Chamber

Unroofing the chamber and removing the coronal pulp facilitates the clinician's ability to visualize the chamber floor and aids in locating the canals. Complete removal of tissue and debris prevents discoloration and subsequent infection.

Unroofing the chamber and removing the coronal pulp (in vital cases) allow the clinician to see the pulpal floor. In cases of patent canals, most or all of the canal orifices may be easily located before the chamber is completely unroofed, but the clinician may nevertheless miss canals. In cases of calcification, performing these procedures increases the clinician's ability to visualize the pulpal floor and read the road map to the canal orifices detailed in the subtle color changes and patterns of calcification left by the receding pulp. This is extremely difficult or impossible to do through a "mouse hole" endodontic access.

Removal of the Coronal Pulp

Removal of the coronal pulp so that the canals may be located is necessary in cases with vital pulp. One advantage of removing the coronal pulp is that the radicular fragments may hemorrhage slightly, aiding in location of the canal orifices. This is especially useful in maxillary molar cases for locating the second mesiobuccal (MB$_2$) canal.

Facilitation of Instrument Placement

Although contemporary endodontic techniques require fewer instruments, the overall thrust of endodontic cleaning and shaping continues to be the serial placement into the root canal system of variably sized, tapered, or shaped instruments. This serial placement of instruments is greatly facilitated by spending a few extra minutes on the access preparation. Access preparation becomes even more important with the use of rotary NiTi instruments. Placement of these instruments requires considerably more attention to gaining straight-line access.

With the use of traditional stainless steel hand files, the clinician has several advantages in instrument placement over rotary NiTi instruments. First, the stainless steel files may be pre-bent, allowing the clinician to hook the file into difficult-to-access canals. As stated before, a bent NiTi rotary instrument is a discarded NiTi rotary instrument. Second, the stiffness of stainless steel provides the clinician with tactile feedback that can be used to drop the file through the orifice into the canal. The thin, flexible tips of the NiTi files impair the clinician's ability to feel obstacles and obstructions and locate the canal orifice. Further compounding this lack of tactile sensitivity, the NiTi files are used with a handpiece, which greatly decreases the tactile sensation of the sensitive and delicate pads of the fingertips.

Coronal and orifice access should act as a funnel to guide the instruments into the canal. Ideally, the line angles of the access preparation should smoothly guide the instrument into the correct canal. This funnel shape also facilitates the introduction of obturation instruments.

Minimizing of Instrument Flexure

With the greater emphasis on more conservative radicular shapes and the concomitant use of rotary NiTi files, the minimizing of instrument flexure has taken on a new importance. Two obvious reasons for reducing instrument flexure are to combat work hardening and decrease the stresses that the instruments undergo during preparation of the root canal system. This decreases fracture incidence and allows more of the energy applied to the instrument to be used for carving the preparation out of the radicular walls.

Locating Canals

With complete eradication of the radicular contents, obturation of the radicular space, and good coronal seal to prevent ingress of bacteria, endodontic treatment should approach 100% success. However, this does not occur in reality. The second most common error in access, one that is often not noticed until a recall film is taken or the patient complains of persistent symptoms, is missed canals. The greatest teacher of endodontic anatomy is the microscope. Clinicians have learned that all roots (not teeth) with the exception of #6 through #11 may have two or more canals.[2] The MB$_2$ canal of the maxillary first molar is commonly referred to as an "extra" canal, but this is not the case—the fifth and sixth canals are the "extras." Without obtaining adequate access in shape, size, and location, locating the exceedingly complex anatomy present in posterior teeth becomes an exercise in futility.

Many of these canals are hidden under dentin shelves, pulp stones, protrusions, and restorative materials. Successful treatment requires adequate access, knowledge of the radicular anatomy, determination, and the assumption of two canals per root until proven otherwise.

INSTRUMENTS AND ARMAMENTARIUM

The endodontic tray setup should contain an assortment of round and fissure burs, tapered and round diamonds, and (for the adventurous) Mueller burs and ultrasonics. A sharp endodontic explorer is essential. Although they are often helpful in locating canals, hand files are generally not used during the access preparation.

Fissure Burs

In an uncrowned tooth exhibiting a patent canal, initial access is best accomplished by round or fissure carbide burs (Figure 2-1). Fissure burs such as the #558 produce less "chatter" when penetrating intact enamel or dentin

compared with round carbide burs. In contrast, round carbide burs such as the #6 or #8 seem to be more controllable during the removal of carious dentin.

Round Diamond Burs

New round diamond burs in #4 and #6 sizes work predictably and quickly to cut through both porcelain-fused-to-metal (PFM) crowns and the new all-porcelain crowns (Figure 2-2). The clinician should use relatively new diamonds with abundant water and intermittent light pressure to avoid generating excessive heat. If dull diamonds are used, especially without water coolant, the clinician may be tempted to apply excessive pressure to accelerate the cutting process and thereby overheat the crown. This can result in craze lines and fractures, which may chip off during instrumentation (when they are easy to repair) or after treatment completion (when they are not). After removing the porcelain layer of the PFM, the clinician can then use a carbide fissure bur or specially designed metal cutting bur to perforate the metal substructure and underlying foundation.

Tapered Diamonds

Flame-shaped and round-ended tapered crown-preparation style diamonds are excellent for endodontic access (Figure 2-3). They are unequaled for cutting with

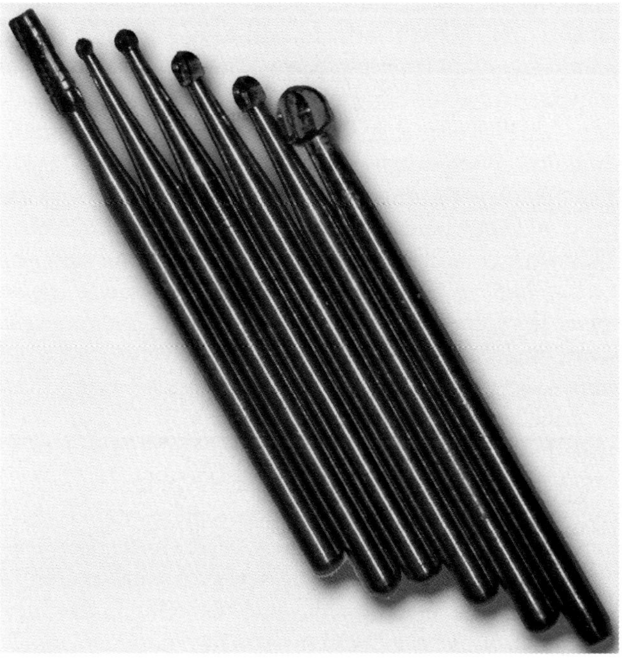

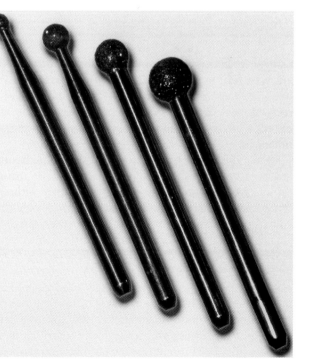

FIGURE 2-1   From *left* to *right,* a #558 surgical length fissure bur followed by #1, #2, #4, #6, and #8 surgical length carbides. These are primarily used for cutting through natural tooth structure.

FIGURE 2-2   From *left* to *right,* round diamonds in sizes #4, #6, #8, and #10. Used with copious water and a very light touch, they can predictably and effortlessly cut through PFM and all-porcelain crowns without fracture.

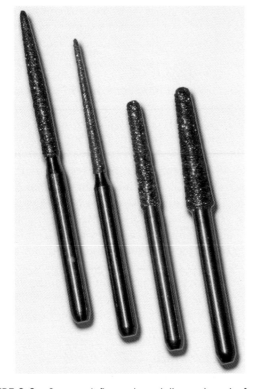

FIGURE 2-3   Coarse grit flame-shaped diamonds and a few sizes of tapered round-ended diamonds can work wonders for refining access outlines and blending canal orifices. These diamonds can safely cut natural and decayed tooth structure, precious and nonprecious crowns, PFM crowns, and all-porcelain crowns.

control, predictability, and ease; this is one reason they are used for the most delicate crown preparations. Perhaps their use should not be restricted to providing restorative treatment. Crown-preparation style diamonds seem to come in more sizes and shapes than any other bur.

After the initial penetration into the pulp chamber has been accomplished, many clinicians advise using a round carbide to finish unroofing the chamber. Although this technique may work in some cases, it is very difficult to perform, especially on a tooth with a small access. The result of this technique is often an overprepared, uneven, gouged wall that catches the tips of files and hampers the placement of files. A much better and safer option is to use an appropriately sized tapered diamond to open and flare the access. The long cutting surface of the diamond can simultaneously open the cavosurface of the access and smooth irregularities in the access walls. The tip removes the last tags and remnants of the chamber roof and blends the dentin from the cavosurface to the canal orifice.

Penetrators and Metal Cutters

Metal cutting burs are highly practical adjuncts for use with full nonprecious castings and nonprecious sub-

structures of PFM crowns (Figure 2-4). The additional expense of using one or two new penetrating burs as opposed to numerous regular carbide fissure burs is offset by the time savings and reduced frustration.

Because of the difficulty in cutting through many restorative materials, especially nonprecious materials, the clinician is often tempted to shortchange the access preparation. Having an arsenal of sharp, new burs specially designed to penetrate these materials helps keep frustration to a minimum.

Surgical Length Burs

Surgical length burs permit displacement of the handpiece away from the incisal or occlusal surface of the tooth, greatly increasing visibility of the cutting tip of the instrument (see Figures 2-1 and 2-4, C). With technical skill, practice, and patience, the clinician can use surgical length burs to gain access in the majority of teeth, including maxillary second molars. Surgical length burs are often useful in teeth that present the greatest problems with access and visibility.

Mueller Burs

Clinicians contemplating tackling difficult or risky cases[3] or those for whom referral is not an option should include Mueller burs in their armamentaria. Mueller burs are long-shaft, carbide-tipped burs used in a low-speed latch handpiece (Figures 2-5 and 2-6). They appear similar to Gates Glidden burs, but have a round carbide tip instead of the noncutting tip of the Gates Glidden bur. The long shaft is useful for working deep in the radicular portion of the tooth. In addition, it displaces the handpiece away from the occlusal surface, allowing the clinician to see the cutting tip in action. An added benefit of Mueller burs that is not well known even in the endodontic community is that unlike ultrasonics that leave a ragged, rough, dusty, debris-filled cut, Mueller burs leave a clean, shiny surface when used on intact dentin. This surface contrasts well with the "white dot" or "white line" connective tissue remnant that was left as the pulp receded. The use of Mueller burs and a microscope makes treating even the most severely calcified teeth less stressful and more predictable.

Mueller burs (Brasseler USA, Savannah, GA) are used after the gross coronal access has been achieved and a reasonable but unsuccessful search for the pulp chamber or canals has been completed. The access preparation is *thoroughly* dried and an appropriately sized Mueller bur is selected. The clinician uses the burs in a brushing motion to search for white dots or white lines representing the calcified canal. While the clinician cuts, the endodontic assistant uses short, light blasts of air to blow out the dentin dust, which is then evacuated by high-volume suction. Water is not used during the process because color differences in the dentin that indicate canal location are more evident in dry dentin. This technique is made even more efficient with the use of a Stropko irrigator on an air-only syringe.

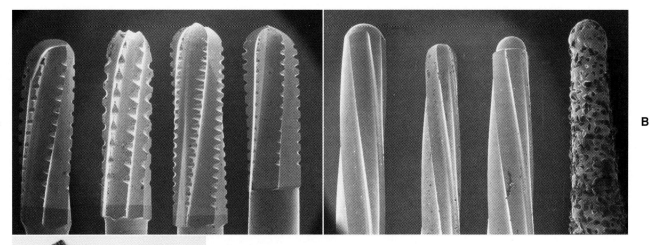

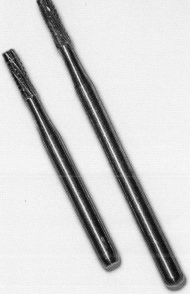

FIGURE 2-4   A, Metal cutting burs are useful for both precious and nonprecious crowns. Pictured from *left* to *right* are the Great White, the Beaver bur, the Transmetal, and the Brassler H34L. They feature a round-ended, crosscut design that minimizes chatter. They can also be used to penetrate the metal substructure of PFM crowns. The conventional-length shank also minimizes handpiece bearing load. **B,** Other burs advocated for endodontic access preparation include the 269GK, the Multipurpose bur, the Endo Z bur, and the Endo access bur. **C,** A surgical length #558 bur compared with a regular #558 bur. The surgical length bur enhances visibility by moving the head of the handpiece away from the tooth. The clinician must exercise care when using extended burs to prevent perforation. (*A* and *B* from Walton RE, Torabinejad M: *Principles and practice of endodontics,* ed 3, Philadelphia, 2002, WB Saunders.)

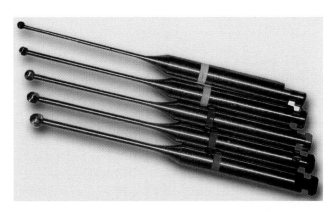

FIGURE 2-5   Mueller burs exhibit a long shank and are used in a slow-speed, latch-type handpiece.

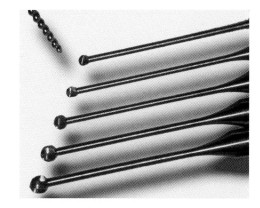

FIGURE 2-6   Mueller burs. The smallest 0.9 mm bur compared with a #70 file.

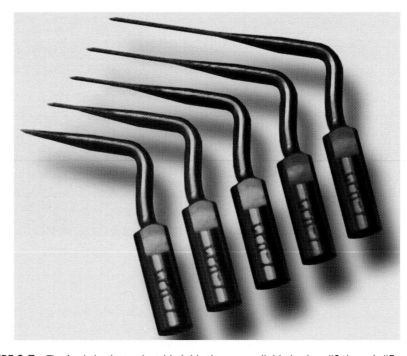

FIGURE 2-7   The Analytic ultrasonic gold nitride tips are available in sizes #2 through #5, and NiTi tips are available in sizes #6 through #8. Pictured *left* to *right* are #2, #3, #6, #7, and #8. Many other configurations are available.

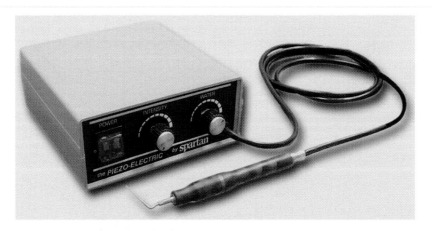

FIGURE 2-8   The Spartan ultrasonic handpiece has been specifically "tuned" to work the CPR tips.

Because these burs are carbide, they do not endure sterilization cycles well and become dull quickly. A few uses are all that can be reasonably expected before they become dull.

Ultrasonics

The CPR tips are available in nitride (gold-yellow) and NiTi (green, blue, and purple) (Figure 2-7). The extremely fine tips coupled with the small handpiece allow unprecedented visibility (Figure 2-8). Ultrasonic tips can be used to remove pulp stones and to cut dentin while locating additional canals.

Canal Orifice Flaring Instruments

An especially important step in preparation for rotary instrumentation is flaring of the canal orifice. As discussed earlier, rotary NiTi instruments cannot be precurved, have very flexible tips, and produce muted tactile sense because of the handpiece. Keeping these limitations in mind, the clinician should spend a few minutes flaring the canal orifices; this technique pays great dividends in increased speed and decreased frustration. Several instruments are available to aid in orifice flaring. These include Gates Glidden drills, GT rotary files (Dentsply Tulsa Dental, Tulsa, OK), and orifice shapers (Figures 2-9 through 2-11).

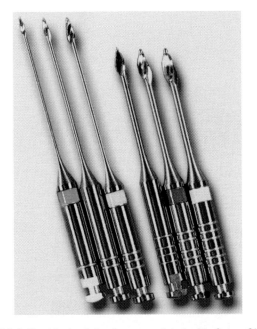

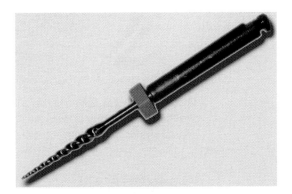

FIGURE 2-9   Much of the fear associated with Gates Glidden burs can be mitigated by using the short versions in sizes #4 to #6. New Gates Glidden drills may tend to be drawn into the canal. They can be run backward until they are slightly dull.

FIGURE 2-10   This GT rotary file has a #35 tip, 1.25 mm maximum flute diameter, and a .12 taper. It can be used at up to 700 RPM for orifice flaring. In patent canal cases, it can be used as a single instrument replacement for the entire set of Gates Glidden burs or orifice shapers.

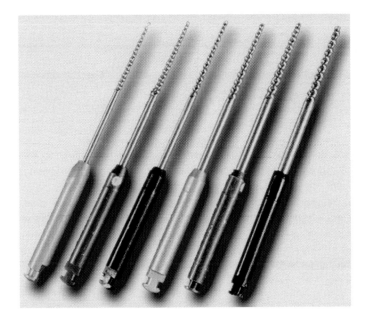

FIGURE 2-11   Orifice shapers are 19 mm long and proceed from a #20/.05 taper to #80/.08. They are used in sequence from left to right to create a funnel within the canal.

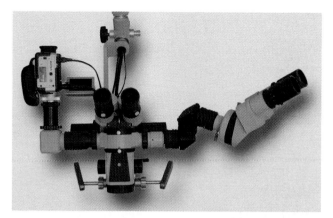

FIGURE 2-12 The operating microscope is an indispensable tool for state-of-the-art endodontic treatment. The specialty practice should not be without a microscope; this instrument is useful in all phases of endodontic treatment from diagnosis to placement of the final restoration.

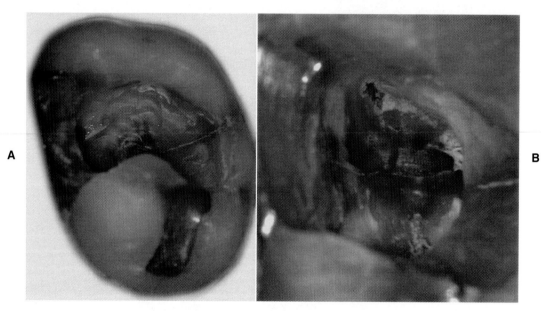

A   B

FIGURE 2-13 **A,** Removal of the amalgam permits inspection of the tooth for fractures. The use of microscopy allows identification of a mesiodistal fracture. The pulp chamber has not been entered. **B,** On entering the pulp chamber, the clinician notes a fracture across the pulpal floor from mesial to distal. Wedging a Glick instrument into the access allows the clinician to visualize the fracture spreading and closing in this hopeless tooth. Although this gross fracture was visible with loupes, the extent of many fractures cannot be seen. Diagnosis and prognostication then become guessing games at best. Note the white dot of the MB$_2$ canal located (in vain) with a Mueller bur above the fracture about halfway between the fracture and the MB canal; this was not visible without the microscope.

VISION, MAGNIFICATION, AND ILLUMINATION

Although ultrasonic and Mueller bur techniques can be used without magnification, they are faster, more predictable, and safer with magnification. The operating microscope is the greatest teacher of endodontic anatomy[4] (Figure 2-12). Previously difficult cases become stress free with microscope use, and previously impossible cases become routine. With the enhanced vision and illumination of the microscope, the clinician operates in an entirely different mode—visually.

To become proficient with the microscope, the clinician should not pull it into service on only the most difficult cases. In fact, without the use of the microscope the clinician may not even be aware of factors increasing

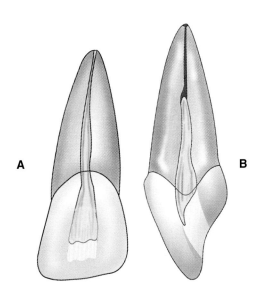

FIGURE 2-14   A, The lingual view shows the incisally repositioned access with the rotary notch. **B,** From the lateral view, the darker wedge-shaped portion of the access shows how incisally this notch may be placed. With the repositioned access, very little cervical dentin needs to be removed.

the difficulty of the case and therefore miss cues only visible with the magnification and illumination the microscope provides (Figure 2-13).

UNCOMPLICATED ACCESS PREPARATIONS

Given the goals and constraints of endodontic access, a distinctive shape is required for each tooth type based on the most common anatomic features of the crown as well as the radicular morphology. Maxillary central and lateral incisors share common coronal and radicular anatomy,[5,6] as do the maxillary premolar and molar tooth groups. The same can be said for the mandibular teeth. Although maxillary and mandibular canine teeth share common coronal and radicular form, the lack of two canals in the maxillary canine as well as less frequent lingual inclination result in a somewhat more constrained access form in the maxillary canine.

Some degree of attrition occurs in the natural adult dentition and dictates some changes in endodontic access design. Because one of the traditional anatomic landmarks (the incisal edge) has been lost, the clinician may be tempted to make the access midway between the "new" incisal edge and the cervical edge. This results in an access that is too cervically positioned.

In light of recent changes in the understanding of canal anatomy, the increased use of rotary NiTi instruments, and the advent of predictable bonding to natural tooth structure with many of new restorative materials, the time may be ripe to reconsider current notions of endodontic access design. Any one of these factors alone might merit rethinking of the access for endodontic treatment, but taken together, they dictate change.

The use of rotary NiTi instruments places even stricter constraints on access design. They are unforgiving of poor access design, irregularities in the access walls, and poor blending of the walls and pulpal floor into the canal orifice.

Maxillary Incisors

In uncomplicated cases, both maxillary central and lateral incisors share a common triangular-shaped access from the lingual surface of the tooth. The classic access design places the access centrally on the lingual surface between the incisal edge and the cervical edge[7] (Figure 2-14). This design is reflective of the poor restorative choices available in the past as well as the limited options for "hiding" the access more cervically. Such a design results in a much larger amount of dentin removal at the lingual cervical edge to gain straight-line access. With improved esthetic bonded composites, the classic access form can be modified by placing it *considerably* more incisally (Figure 2-15). The initial penetration should be approximately in the middle of the lingual surface of the tooth, not just above the cingulum as has been previously described.[8] After locating the canal, the clinician uses a long, tapered diamond to extend the access even further incisally and laterally. An additional modification for use with rotary instrumentation is to slightly notch the middle of the incisal extent of the access (see Figure 2-15). This allows even better straight-line access and greatly decreases the potentially catastrophic cervical flexure of the rotary instruments that can contribute to premature, unexplained fracture.

In anterior teeth the clinician must take care to remove all the coronal tissue and debris from the chamber. Material left in the chamber can cause tooth discoloration. The pulp horns are common locations for residual tissue (Figure 2-16).

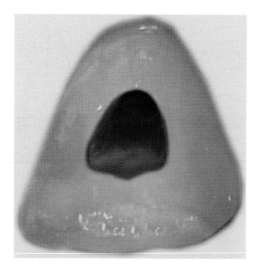

FIGURE 2-15   View of accessed tooth from the incisal and slightly lingual. Note the rotary notch in the middle of the incisal extent of the access. This notch allows more straight-line access for rotary NiTi instruments and greatly helps eliminate cervical flexure that can cause "unexplained" instrument breakage.

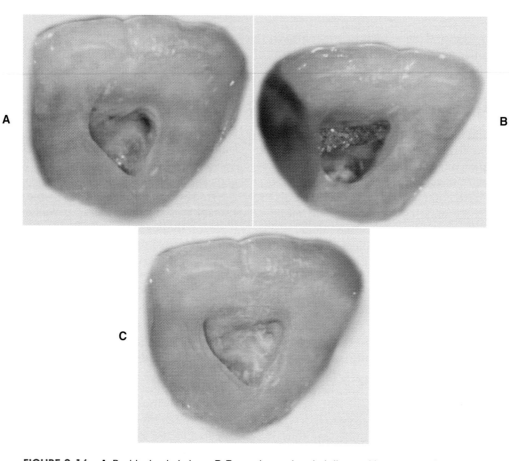

FIGURE 2-16   **A,** Residual pulp in horn. **B,** Tapered, round-ended diamond burs are used to remove debris. The diamond leaves an optimal surface for bonding. **C,** In immature cases with large pulps, the clinician must take care to remove all material in the pulp horns. Often a tapered, round-ended diamond bur can be used to blend the pulp horns into the access form. This blending should be rechecked before the final restoration because any residual pulpal debris, bacteria, sealer, and gutta-percha can contribute to subsequent discoloration.

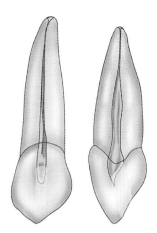

FIGURE 2-17   Access opening for the maxillary canine.

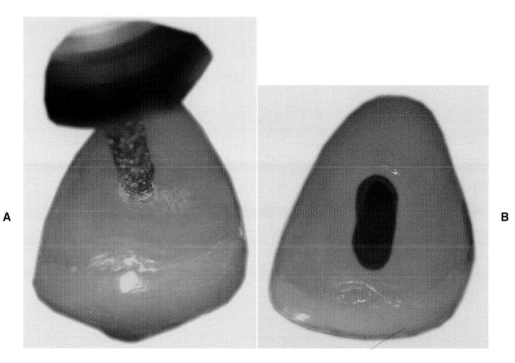

A

B

FIGURE 2-18   A, Initial access penetration occurs in the middle of the incisal-cervical dimension. After locating the canal, the clinician extends the access incisally. Note the facial veneer. **B,** Completed access from the incisal view.

Maxillary Canines

In uncomplicated cases the maxillary canine access is rather broad from buccal to lingual, which reflects the broad buccolingual shape of the root and the canal space (Figures 2-17 and 2-18). In the adult dentition the incisal edge of the maxillary canine has usually undergone significant attrition (Figure 2-19). This alters the normal anatomic landmarks for endodontic access midway between the cervical bulge and the incisal tip (see Figure 2-19). Therefore the endodontic access will be located in a more incisal position than would be the case on a "vir-

gin" tooth. *This modification to access may occur on any tooth but is most common with the maxillary and mandibular anterior teeth.*

Maxillary Premolars

Although not all maxillary premolars have two canals,[8] they should all be approached from the assumption that they have separate buccal and lingual canals (Figure 2-20). This dictates a broad buccolingual access form that is somewhat constrained in the mesiodistal dimension (Figure 2-21). The maxillary premolar access is never round.

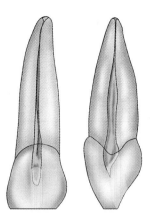

FIGURE 2-19 The effect of attrition. This slightly lingual and incisal view of a tooth shows the access encroaching on the incisal edge.

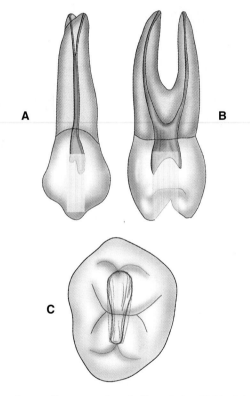

FIGURE 2-20 Access for maxillary premolars. **A,** Buccal view. **B,** Mesial view. **C,** Occlusal view.

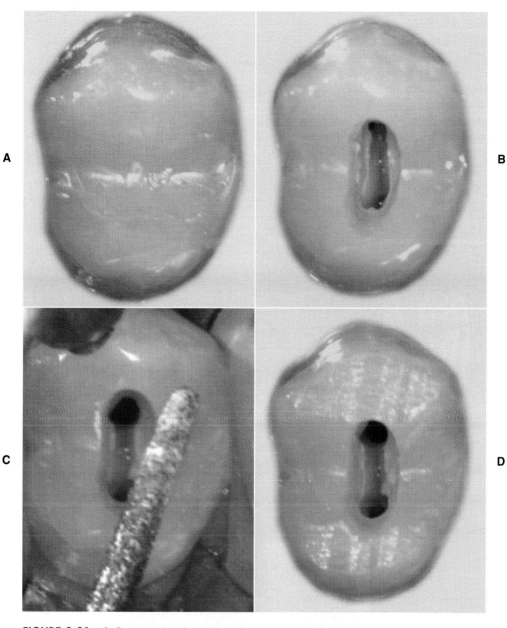

FIGURE 2-21   A, Preoperative view with a distal occlusal (DO) composite. Note the mesial concavity. **B,** Initial access to the pulp chamber is broad buccolingually and narrow mesiodistally. **C,** The cusps are flattened to gain more accurate reference points. **D,** The diamond is used to blend the coronal portion of the access with the cervical portion. This blends the buccal and lingual pulp horns and removes pulp tissue from these areas.

Maxillary Molars

Treatment of maxillary molars is never routine (Figure 2-22). In a recent study of maxillary first and second molars an MB$_2$ canal was found in 96% of the mesiobuccal roots of maxillary first molars and 94% of the maxillary second molars. Approximately 54% were located in the traditional access opening, 31% were found with the use of a bur, and 10% were found with the aid of a microscope. The MB$_2$ canal orifice was found on average 1.82 mm lingual to the main MB canal orifice.[9] In another study of the maxillary first molar using microscopy, the MB$_2$ canal was located in 93% of first molars and 60% of second molars[4] (Figures 2-23 and 2-24). The difficulty in access, high percentage of fourth and even fifth canals, and root curvatures put even the "routine" maxillary molar in a high-risk category.[3] Complicating factors such as limited opening, crowns, changes in tooth angulation, tooth position, and calcification make predictable treatment of these teeth challenging for even the most experienced clinician trained in microscopy, ultrasonics, and rotary instrumentation.

The clinician wishing to treat these high- to extreme-risk cases should perform a 6-month chart review to de-

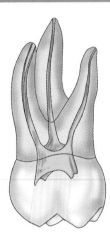

FIGURE 2-22   Buccal view of the access for maxillary molars.

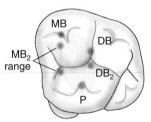

FIGURE 2-23   An occlusal view of the access for maxillary molars.

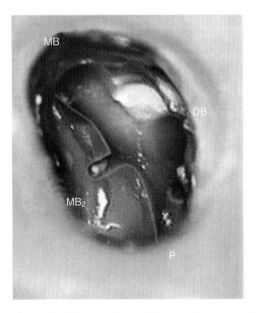

FIGURE 2-24   The location of the MB$_2$ canal is mesial to the line connecting the MB and palatal orifice. In the maxillary first molar the MB$_2$ canal is generally located within the range shown. In the maxillary second molar the location of the MB$_2$ is highly variable and can be located from the MB orifice to the palatal orifice (see Figs. 2-46 and 2-47).

termine the percentage of cases with at least four canals. If the percentage is less than 45% for first molars or less than 35% for second molars, these cases should be carefully screened for referral because the MB_2 canal is being missed and untreated about half of the time.

Guidelines for canal location in the maxillary first molar (Figure 2-25) differ from that in the maxillary second molar. In the maxillary first molar the MB canal is located under the mesial buccal cusp (see Figure 2-25, *D*). The MB_2 canal is located mesial to a line from the MB canal toward the palatal canal (see Figures 2-25, *E*, and 2-26). The DB canal is located distal to the MB canal in the buccal groove area, slightly lingual to the MB canal (see Figure 2-25, *G*). The palatal canal is generally the largest canal and is located under the mesiolingual (ML) cusp (see Figure 2-25, *F*). These general locations remain the same as the pulp calcifies with age (Figure 2-27). Although these general principles apply to the maxillary second molar, the chamber may be narrower, resembling a straight line (see Fig. 2-55).

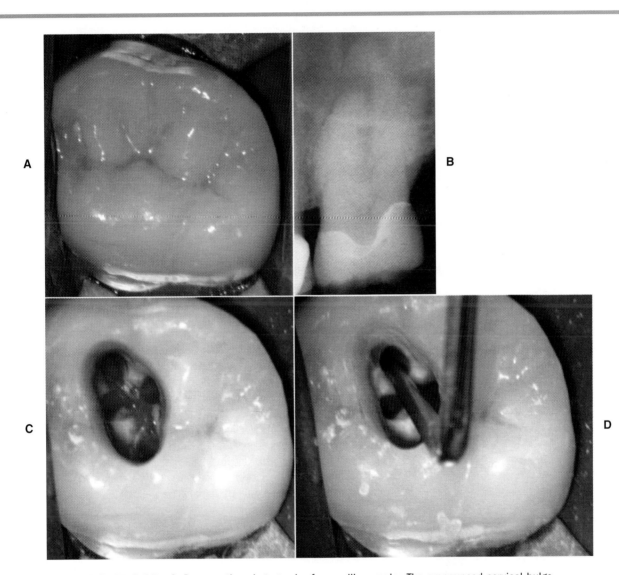

FIGURE 2-25   A, Preoperative photograph of a maxillary molar. The pronounced cervical bulge over the MB is highly suggestive of a large root and two canals. **B,** Preoperative radiograph of this necrotic maxillary first molar. Note the constricted pulp chamber. The angle of entry to the mesial canals is from the distal. **C,** The canals have been prepared to help illustrate their locations and angles. Note that in the following illustrations the access form may need to be extended or modified on the side opposite the canal to clear the rotary instruments and avoid cervical flexure of the instruments. **D,** The angle of entry into the MB canal is markedly from the distal and palatal. The access may need to be extended distally and palatally to allow clean placement of instruments.

Continued

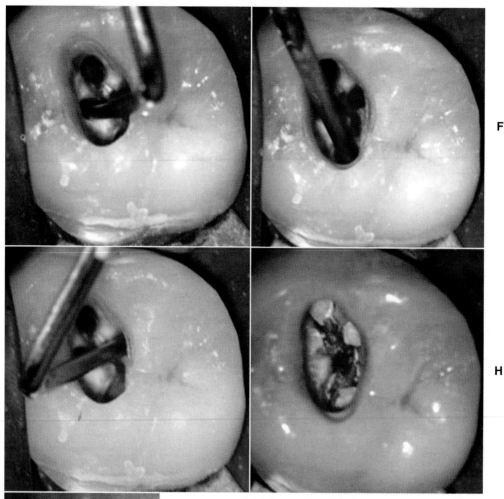

E

F

G

H

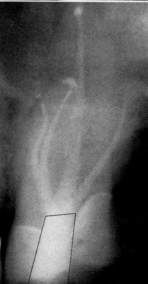

I

FIGURE 2-25, cont'd   **E,** The entrance into the prepared MB$_2$ is from the distal and slightly from the palatal. The access may need to be extended distally to allow clean placement of rotary instruments into the MB$_2$. **F,** The angle of entry into the palatal is from the buccal and mesial. Occasionally the access may need to be extended to the MB to allow clean placement of rotary instruments into the palatal canal. **G,** The angle of entry into the DB canal is from the mesial and palatal. A diamond bur (see Figure 2-26) can be used to relieve the impeding restorative material or tooth structure. **H,** The completed case. Note that the access is not in the center of the tooth. Adequate access to locate, negotiate, prepare, and obturate can be obtained without violating the transverse ridge. Note that the access extends almost to the MB cusp tip. **I,** The HF-etched silanated composite crown repair of the endodontic access is outlined in black. The presence of this type of radicular anatomy is usually unconfirmed until the case is complete. Missing the MB$_2$ canal here would doom the case to failure because of the presence of separate foramina.

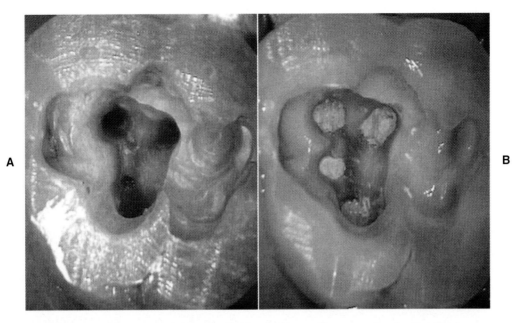

FIGURE 2-26 **A,** On entering the pulp chamber in this maxillary second molar, the clinician can readily locate the MB₂ orifice along a line connecting the MB and palatal orifices. This "false orifice" is a source of frustration for many dentists because although it can be probed, it is often resistant to negotiation. The reason for this is that the MB₂ canal proceeds mesially (horizontally) before making a 90-degree turn down the root. **B,** The prepared and obturated MB₂ canal is considerably more mesial than the original orifice. The red dot to the distal of the obturated MB₂ is the location of the false original orifice. A technique routinely employed is to notch this area with a tapered round-tipped diamond, Mueller bur, or Gates Glidden bur to gain straight line access to the MB₂ canal. This technique is detailed in later figures.

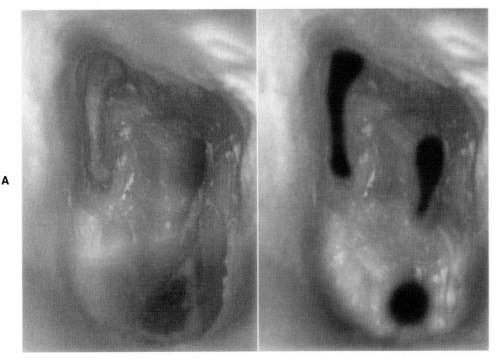

FIGURE 2-27 **A,** Original view of canal shapes in a 9-year-old's maxillary first molar. Note that the very broad MB "canal" is full of debris. **B,** Computer-enhanced view of canal spaces at 9 years.

Continued

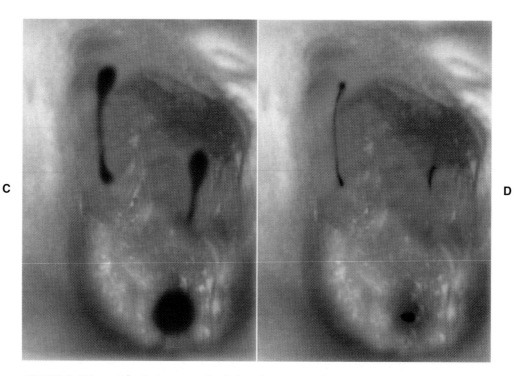

FIGURE 2-27, cont'd C, Computer simulation of typical calcific metamorphosis (calcification) in an adult tooth. **D,** Computer simulation of significant calcific metamorphosis.

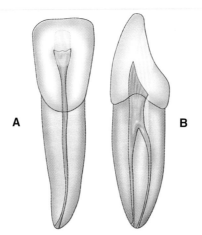

FIGURE 2-28 A, Access for a mandibular incisor as viewed from the lingual. The access is quite high on the lingual surface of the tooth. This gives the clinician a much straighter shot down the canal and minimizes the chance of perforating out the facial surface. **B,** This mesial view shows the access extending nearly to the incisal edge.

Mandibular Incisors

As with the other anterior teeth the traditional access to the mandibular incisor was more cervically placed than necessary because of esthetic constraints. The optimal access for the mandibular central and lateral incisor is actually through the incisal edge, but this is balanced with the desire to maintain an intact incisal edge where possible (Figure 2-28). In the mature adult tooth, attrition has generally caused the access to extend through the incisal edge[10] (Figure 2-29).

Because two canals are present in about 40% of all mandibular incisors,[11] these teeth should be assumed to have two canals until substantial evidence to the contrary is discovered.

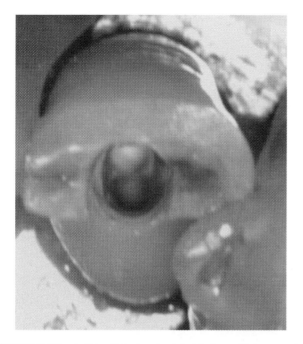

FIGURE 2-29   In this attrited and rotated incisor with two canals, an incisal access greatly facilitated location of the lingual canal.

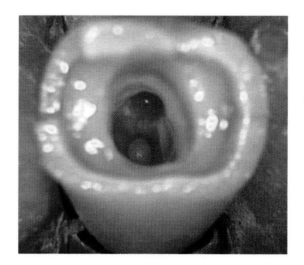

FIGURE 2-30   The typical error in access on a mandibular incisor is to perforate toward the facial (white dot). The clinician had already "located" the canal but bypassed it while continuing to drill down and to the facial. Mandibular incisors are rarely perforated to the lingual.

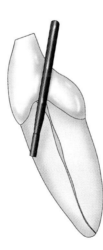

FIGURE 2-31   While searching for a calcified canal, clinicians tend to drill in an apical direction but neglect to take into account the natural angulation of the mandibular incisor, resulting in buccal perforation.

Because of the facial inclination of the tooth, perforation of the facial aspect of the root is a common procedural error in accessing mandibular incisors (Figures 2-30 and 2-31). In cases of rotation or crowding a facial approach to access should be considered.[12]

Mandibular Canines

The mandibular canine has a very broad facial-lingual dimension to its root (Figure 2-32). This root occasion-ally has two canals and therefore requires a broad facial-lingual access. The access opening is ovoid and located on the lingual portion of the crown (see Figures 2-32 and 2-33). As wear occurs, the access may involve the incisal edge (Figure 2-34).

Mandibular Premolars

The broad buccolingual dimension of the mandibular premolar dictates an access form that is about twice as

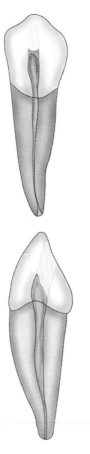

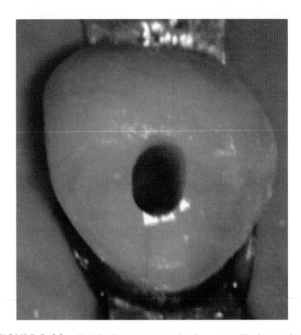

FIGURE 2-32   Access openings for the mandibular canine.

FIGURE 2-33   An ideal access opening in a mandibular canine. Viewed from the incisal surface, the access is slightly to the lingual and can be seen extending to nearly the incisal edge.

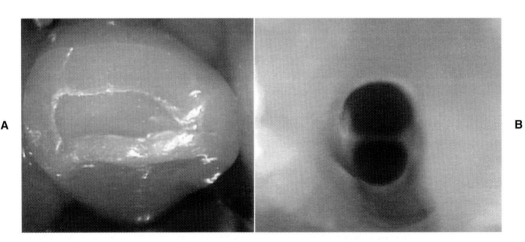

A   **B**

FIGURE 2-34   **A,** Preoperative view of a mandibular canine with incisal attrition. **B,** Occasionally the mandibular canine has two canals. A more incisally and facially positioned access facilitates location of the lingual canal.

broad in the buccolingual dimension than it is mesiodistally (Figures 2-35 through 2-37). Although most mandibular premolars have a single canal, two canals occur about 25% of the time in mandibular first premolars[13]; rarely, three canals are present. When numerous

canals are present, the preoperative radiograph often indicates a "fast break." This appears as a relatively patent canal space in the coronal portion of the tooth that suddenly disappears (Figure 2-38). Locating the two canals requires an appropriate access (Figure 2-39).

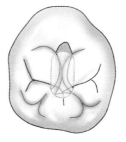

FIGURE 2-35   Viewed from the occlusal, the access is relatively well centered in the buccolingual and mesiodistal dimensions. It is about twice as broad buccolingually as it is mesiodistally.

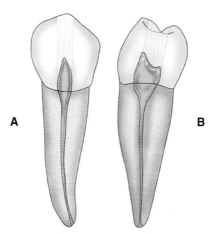

A   B

FIGURE 2-36   A, Viewed from the buccal surface, the access is conservative mesiodistally. **B,** Viewed from the mesial, the crowns of the mandibular premolars have a slightly lingual inclination relative to the root.

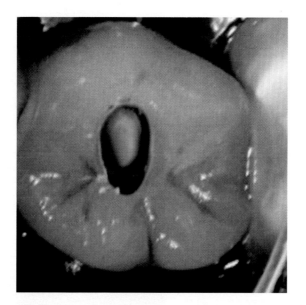

FIGURE 2-37   Occlusal view of access through a PFM crown.

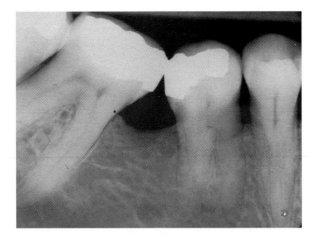

FIGURE 2-38   Radiographic appearance of a fast break in the mandibular right first premolar. The coronal extent of the canal is readily visible but abruptly disappears in the middle of the root, indicating at least two canals. Note that the second premolar has three roots.

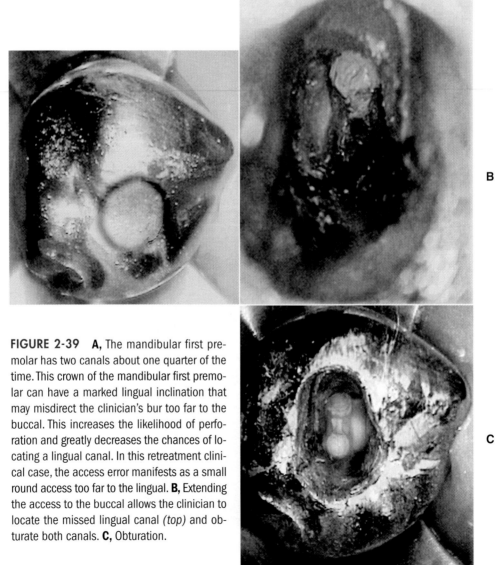

FIGURE 2-39   A, The mandibular first premolar has two canals about one quarter of the time. This crown of the mandibular first premolar can have a marked lingual inclination that may misdirect the clinician's bur too far to the buccal. This increases the likelihood of perforation and greatly decreases the chances of locating a lingual canal. In this retreatment clinical case, the access error manifests as a small round access too far to the lingual. **B,** Extending the access to the buccal allows the clinician to locate the missed lingual canal *(top)* and obturate both canals. **C,** Obturation.

Mandibular Molars

The access to the mandibular molars has been presented by many as triangular in shape. This access shape greatly hinders the clinician's ability to locate the DB canal when one is present and to treat the full buccolingual extent of the broad distal canal when a single distal canal is present. The naturally present slight mesial and lingual inclination of the tooth, coupled with the clinical access to the tooth, dictates an access that is placed more toward the mesial half of the tooth and may extend buc- cally to nearly the MB cusp tip (Figure 2-40). The access may occasionally cross the central pit (Figure 2-41).

In mandibular molars the MB canal lies under the mesiobuccal cusp tip. The ML canal often appears in line with the central groove crossing the mesial marginal ridge. The lingual inclination of the tooth in the arch, coupled with the lingual constriction of the crown, ac- counts for this anatomic relationship (see Figure 2-40, C). The distal canal is generally at the intersection of the buccal, lingual, and central grooves as viewed from the

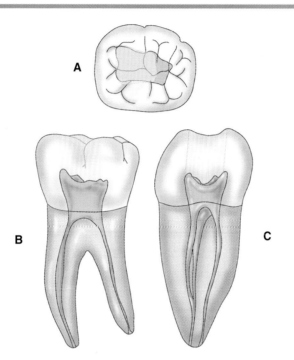

FIGURE 2-40   A, Viewed from the occlusal, the access can be seen to just cross the central pit area and extend to nearly the MB cusp tip. **B,** Viewed from the buccal, the access is slightly mesially inclined. **C,** Viewed from the mesial, the buccal extent of the access can extend to nearly the MB cusp tip.

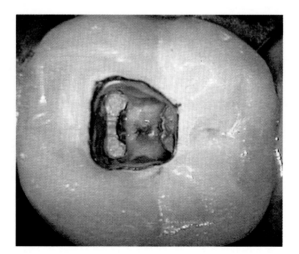

FIGURE 2-41   The ideal access is demonstrated on this mandibular first molar through a PFM crown.

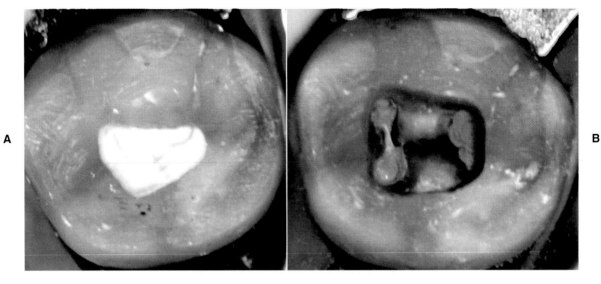

FIGURE 2-42 **A,** The lingually placed triangular form of this access precluded the clinician from locating the MB canal and hindered the ability to instrument the buccal extend of the ovoid distal canal. **B,** Extending the mesial half of the access to the buccal to nearly the MB cusp tip and extending the distal half more buccally allowed the MB canal to be located and greatly facilitated instrumentation.

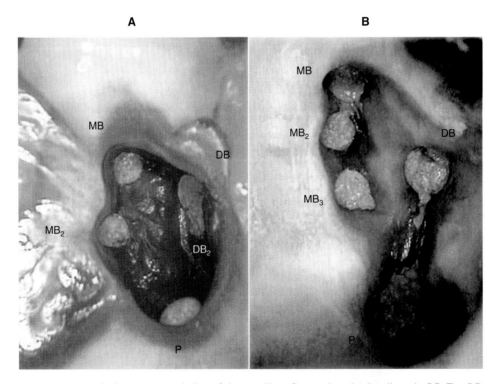

FIGURE 2-43 **A,** A common variation of the maxillary first molar—the bowling pin DB. The DB canal appears similar to an inverted bowling pin. Note the fluting to access the MB_2. The bowling pin appearance can result in two separate canals. **B,** The presence of three MB canals is an additional variation. In this case the MB_2 and MB_3 were confluent, which is not expected given the proximity of the MB_2 to the MB.

occlusal surface. When a DB canal is present, it will be located to the buccal and often slightly mesial to the main distal canal (Figure 2-42). The incidence of four canals is approximately 35%.[14]

In mandibular second molars a C-shaped canal is a morphologic variation.[15] The incidence of this canal morphology is approximately 8% (see Figures 2-54 and 4-3).[16]

CANAL PATTERNS IN MOLARS

With the increased use of the microscope, several additional patterns of canals have been identified. Every clinician has seen unusual radicular anatomy and morphology. Instead of showcasing all of these anatomic anomalies, this section highlights some of the more common variations.

Maxillary First Molars

Although little variation occurs in the root form of the maxillary first molar, several internal patterns can belie the simplicity of the external surface of the tooth. These include variations in the mesiobuccal and distobuccal roots (Figures 2-43 and 2-44).

Maxillary Second Molars

In contrast to the maxillary first molar, the maxillary second molar exhibits a variety of root forms. Any two of the roots can fuse, and occasionally all three of the roots can fuse. Despite these aberrant root forms, the maxillary second molars can have from one to five canals, with four canals being the most common (Figures 2-45 through 2-47).

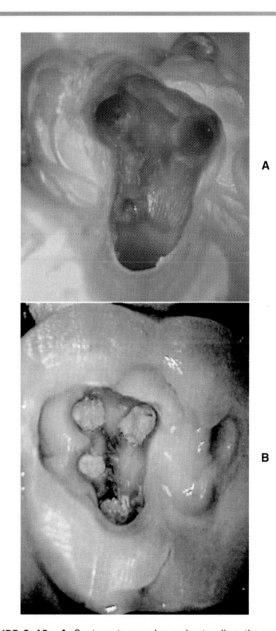

A

B

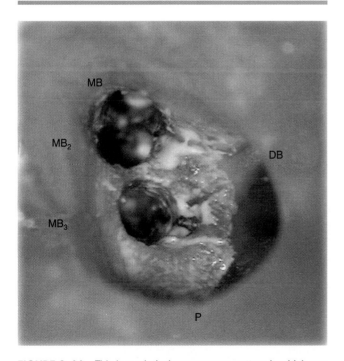

FIGURE 2-44 This is a relatively uncommon pattern in which one coronal orifice gives rise a few millimeters down the canal to an MB and MB$_2$. The case complexity is compounded by the presence of an MB$_3$. The maxillary second molar also can have this pattern of a bifurcation partway down the MB orifice.

FIGURE 2-45 **A,** Contrary to popular understanding, the most common pattern in the maxillary second molar is four canals. In this case the rather large MB$_2$ is visible as a red bleeding point. **B,** The obturated MB$_2$ is just slightly mesial of the line connecting the MB and palatal canals. In the maxillary second molar the location of the MB$_2$ varies greatly, but this case shows a more typical location. Note the fluted access to the mesiobuccal canal.

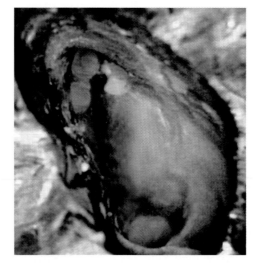

FIGURE 2-46   There is considerable variation in the location of the MB$_2$ in the maxillary second molar. In this case, it is very close to the MB. It is highly variable in the fused root case. It can also be found considerably closer to the palatal canal (see Figure 2-47).

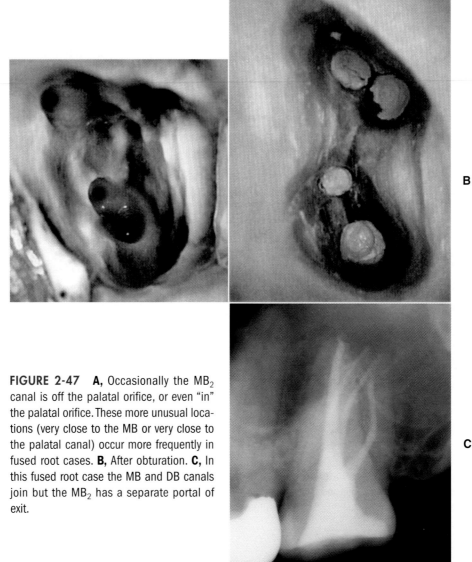

A

B

C

FIGURE 2-47   A, Occasionally the MB$_2$ canal is off the palatal orifice, or even "in" the palatal orifice. These more unusual locations (very close to the MB or very close to the palatal canal) occur more frequently in fused root cases. **B,** After obturation. **C,** In this fused root case the MB and DB canals join but the MB$_2$ has a separate portal of exit.

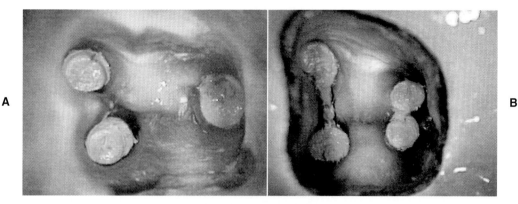

FIGURE 2-48   A, A single round distal canal occurs less commonly than the "figure 8" or oval distal variation. **B,** The most common pattern is two mesial canals with a connecting isthmus and a figure 8–shaped distal canal. The distal canals usually join but can be separate.

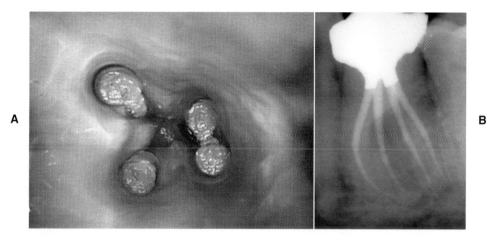

FIGURE 2-49   A, At the orifice level the distal canals appear to be confluent. **B,** The radiograph shows they are not.

Mandibular First Molars

The mandibular first molar traditionally has three or four canals (Figure 2-48), but they are considerably easier to locate than they are in the maxillary first molar. The most commonly missed canal is the DB, probably because the legacy of a triangular access form makes detection of this canal somewhat more difficult. When more than one canal is present in a root the canals can exhibit separate portals of exit (Figure 2-49). Five and six canal variations have been reported in the literature,[15] but taken together they account for a small percentage of the cases (Figures 2-50 and 2-51). As with the maxillary first molar, root fusion is uncommon in the mandibular first molars.

Mandibular Second Molars

As with the maxillary second molars, mandibular second molars have a greatly increased incidence of root form variations. This manifests internally as large variations in the number and locations of the canals (Figures 2-52 through 2-54). Although the initial access form should be somewhat trapezoidal, it may need to be extended to allow more straight-line access for certain canal configurations.

MANAGING COMPLICATIONS

Rarely is the clinician presented with an unrestored, caries-free tooth to treat. The following section illustrates specific clinical techniques and tips to help the clinician manage more complicated cases and avoid procedural mishaps.

Existing Restorative Materials

In cases where the access is surrounded by metallic restorative materials, the restoration should be removed

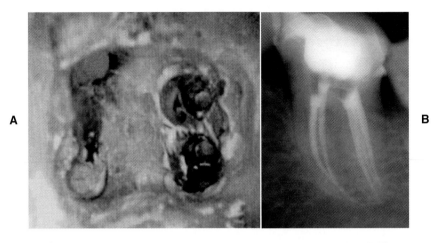

FIGURE 2-50 **A,** The presence of three distal canals is an additional variation. **B,** The postoperative radiograph.

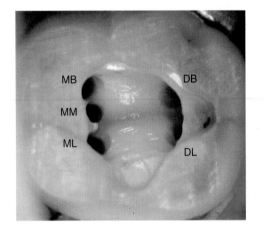

FIGURE 2-51 Three mesial canals occur in a few variations. This pattern is rather evenly spaced. Occasionally the mesial middle (MM) is closer to the ML. The MM can also be closer to the MB.

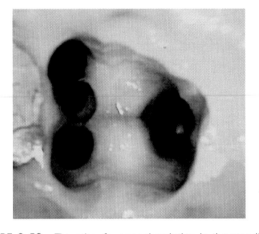

FIGURE 2-52 The other four-canal variation in the mandibular second molar is three mesial canals.

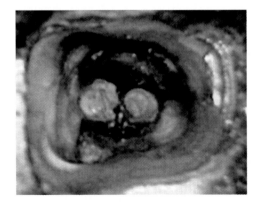

FIGURE 2-53 The fused root variation in the mandibular second molar may have only one mesial and one distal canal. Occasionally only a single canal occurs.

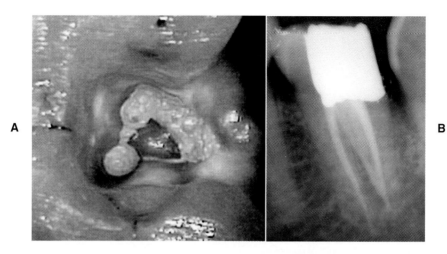

FIGURE 2-54   A, As with the three-rooted mandibular first molar, the C-shaped mandibular second molar occurs more commonly in Asian persons and Native Americans. Typically, the C is open to the lingual, and the ML canal remains somewhat separate. Histologically, this is one large canal that is usually negotiable in three spots: ML, B, and DL. **B,** The postoperative radiograph demonstrates the C configuration.

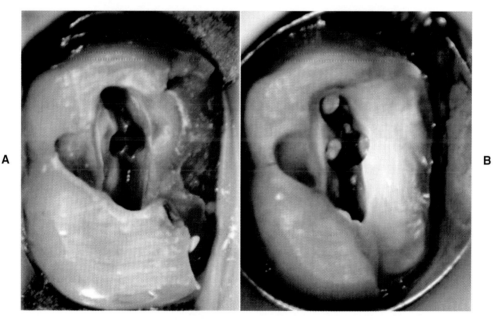

FIGURE 2-55   A, A band of distal caries and unsupported enamel was left to aid in isolation and clamp retention in this maxillary second molar. **B,** Using a caries detector, after obturation the clinician removed decay and placed a band in preparation for a bonded amalgam foundation.

unless it contributes to isolation. If the restorative material contributes to isolation, such as the mesial portion of a mesial occlusal (MO) amalgam, it should be thinned to keep it well away from hand and rotary instruments while the case is treated. After endodontic treatment the clinician removes the material and places a core.

Caries

Although some clinicians advocate removal of all decay before the initiation of endodontic treatment, two reasons exist to leave decay in place during instrumentation. Carious but relatively firm tooth structure may aid in clamp placement and retention and enhance isolation (Figure 2-55).

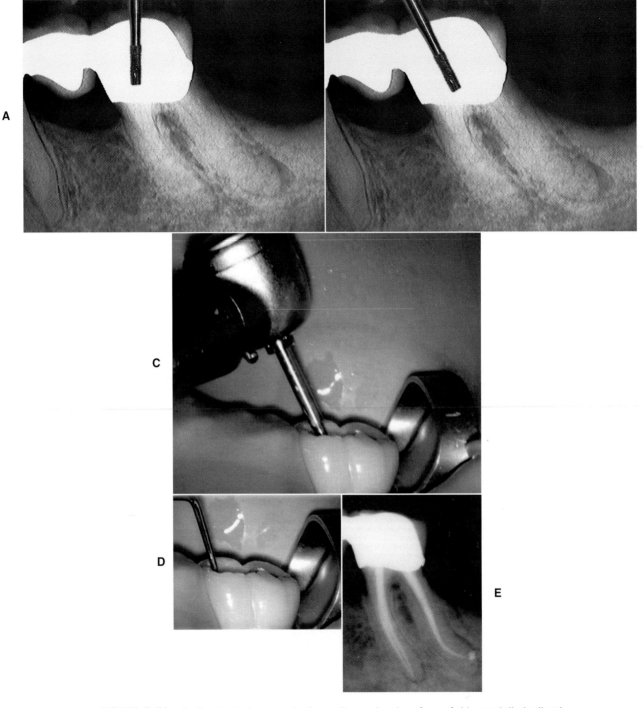

FIGURE 2-56 **A,** Penetrating perpendicular to the occlusal surface of this mesially inclined mandibular second molar bridge abutment will preclude locating the distal canals and could even lead to perforation through the mesial. **B,** Correct angulation relative to the root structure dramatically skews the access to the mesial when viewed from the occlusal. This allows easier location and instrumentation of the canals. **C,** The angle of entry is quite mesial. **D,** The explorer shows the angle of entry into the prepared MB canal. **E,** The postoperative radiograph.

Clearly soft, leathery decay should be removed, especially if it might be abraded or dislodged into the canal. Removal of all caries also aids the clinician in assessing restorability.

Inclined Teeth

Careful inspection of the preoperative radiograph usually indicates an abnormal inclination in the mesiodistal dimension. Mesial inclination is a common finding in molar teeth but can occur in any tooth, especially if an edentulous area is located mesial to the tooth under treatment. Inclinations in the buccolingual plane are considerable less common and can be detected by observing the curve of the arch, the occlusal relationships, and the bony eminences over the roots. Teeth that are routinely inclined include the mandibular incisors, which are usually tilted to the labial, and the mandibular second molars, which are usually tilted to the mesial. The location and occasionally the shape of the endodontic access may need to be modified to take these inclinations into account (Figure 2-56).

Rotated and Malpositioned Teeth

As with inclined teeth, rotated and malposed teeth may require modification to the endodontic access in light of the ultimate goal of straight-line access to the canal spaces. In anterior teeth a buccal access often facilitates treatment and provides the clinician with better visualization for locating the lingual canal in mandibular incisors.[13]

Crowned Teeth

In their efforts to preserve tooth structure, avoid pulpal exposure, and be "conservative," clinicians typically under-prepare teeth receiving crowns. In most cases this does not present a problem, but in more extreme cases of under-reduction and in cases where the restored crown has been shifted relative to the root structure these shifts must be identified and incorporated into the endodontic access. Access through existing crowns may also affect retention by removing the retentive foundation and may influence esthetics if porcelain fracture occurs. Teeth with crowns require careful preclinical assessment and often the use of unique treatment procedures (Figures 2-57 and 2-58).

Calcified and Difficult-To-Locate Canals

Without magnification and illumination, locating canals can be among the most difficult, stressful, and error-prone procedural aspects of endodontics and perhaps of dentistry as a whole. The clinician should carefully and realistically gauge the difficulty in locating canals, the likelihood of a procedural mishap, and the relative importance of the tooth in question (Figure 2-59).

Retreatment

Because most endodontically treated teeth have crowns, retreatment usually occurs through the crown. With use of the microscope, the clinician does not usually need to remove a well-fitting, serviceable crown even when posts are to be removed. Nevertheless, the presence of crowns can and does complicate access (see previous section) and therefore dictates changes in access outline form, especially in retreatment cases.

Access for retreatment should be spacious. The ultimate goal must be kept in mind—if the endodontic component cannot be managed, the tooth may be lost. The clinician does better to risk destroying the crown than fail to achieve the endodontic objective because of too small an access.

Modifications for NiTi Rotary Instruments

Although rotary NiTi instruments do have markedly increased flexibility, the clinician must be attentive in achieving straight-line access. Initially, this may seem counterintuitive. However, the forces placed on these instruments as they rotate around curvatures (especially cervical curvatures) are large. Changes in access design can greatly reduce stress on these instruments and decrease breakage.

Practitioners are often concerned with the difficulty or impossibility of placing rotary NiTi instruments into the access opening of posterior teeth—typically maxillary second molars. As NiTi instruments become the instruments of choice in difficult cases, the difficulty in successfully placing and using these instruments can be traced to inadequate access. Clinicians should therefore keep in mind that even in the specialty practice, only in very rare cases can the access form not be modified to facilitate rotary instruments (Figures 2-60 through 2-62).

Limited Opening

In patients with limited opening, clinicians may be tempted to skimp on the access because fitting the head of the handpiece into the interocclusal space is so difficult. In these cases the clinician needs to redouble the effort to gain adequate access. Limited opening coupled with poor endodontic access is a setup for a difficult, frustrating, less than satisfying case. Typically, in patients with limited opening, the endodontic access should actually be larger and more mesial to facilitate instrument placement. The clinician should be acutely aware of the location and angulation of the bur head because perforations and missed canals are considerably more likely in these cases.

Author's Statement on Manipulation of Digital Images

The radiographs and images used in this chapter are almost all digital in origin. The radiographs are from Trophy RVG and RVGui, with a few scanned radiographs (the suboptimal ones). Color images have been taken with a variety of technologies:

- Hitachi 3CCD microscope-mounted video camera connected to a Trophy video capture board

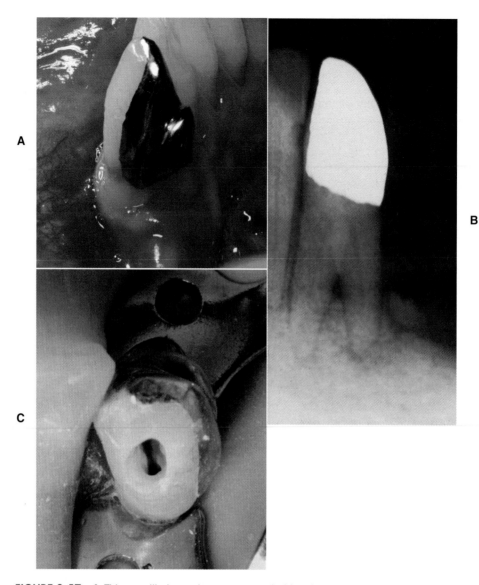

FIGURE 2-57   A, This mandibular canine was restored with a three-quarter crown to provide a rest for a removable partial denture. After restoration the pulp became necrotic. Access opening through the existing restoration may compromise retention and the rest configuration. **B,** A preoperative radiograph reveals two separate roots. **C,** Access from the buccal approach enhances access to the lingual canal and preserves the integrity of the existing restoration.

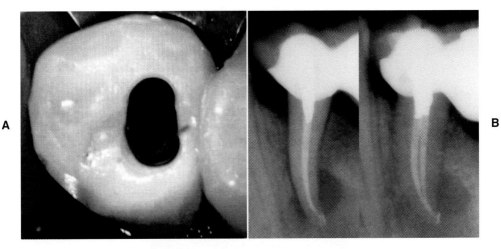

FIGURE 2-58   A, This mandibular premolar was positioned distally before fabrication of a fixed partial denture. As a result the contact was overextended to the mesial by the laboratory to close the contact. In this occlusal view the access is distally placed relative to the occlusal surface. **B,** This final radiograph with a combination amalgam/composite repair reveals that even though the access was quite distal, it was still slightly mesial of true straight-line access.

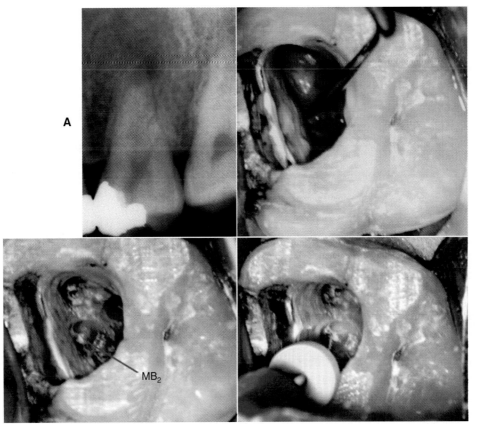

FIGURE 2-59   A, The preoperative view of this maxillary first molar is deceptive. The relatively large pulp chamber suggests easy-to-locate, patent canals. Note, however, the bulge into the pulp chamber from the mesial. **B,** The classic mesial bulge. A stick can be felt along this line, but the MB_2 canal cannot be negotiated. Note that the mesial amalgam has been retained for isolation but thinned to about 1 mm so as to not impede instrument placement. **C,** The telltale white dot of the MB_2 orifice can be seen after use of the Mueller bur mesially and very slightly apically. **D,** A #10 file can be seen to be somewhat sprung toward the distal, conforming the angle of entry.

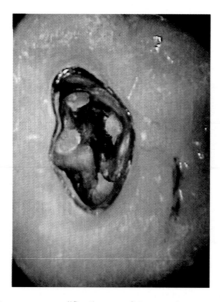

FIGURE 2-60 The most common modification, useful even when rotary NiTi instruments are not used, is to create a notch in the access that enhances visibility and straight-line access to the MB$_2$ canal. In most cases, creating this notch also provides a cleaner path of insertion for the DB canal.

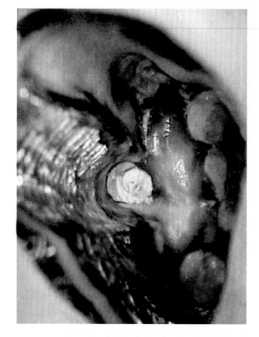

FIGURE 2-61 The amalgam buildup under the crown on this maxillary first molar exhibiting five canals encroached on access to the MB$_2$ canal. The area was fluted aggressively to eliminate the possibility of the rotary NiTi instruments abrading the amalgam during instrumentation and consequently creating amalgam scraps and prematurely dulling the instruments. Note the dentin apical to the amalgam.

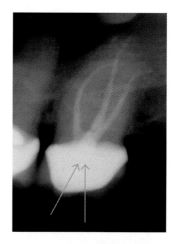

FIGURE 2-62 In this patient with limited opening, the entire access outline was shifted to the mesial. The *arrows* represent the views to the canals perpendicular to the occlusal surface and from the mesial, as the clinician would see when clinically treating the tooth. Note that the arrows are the same length, but the angled arrow requires less interocclusal space.

- Sony DCR-PC 100 DV microscope-mounted camera using the MemoryStick and imported to the Trophy software
- Sony DCR-PC 100 DV microscope-mounted camera using the S-Video output connected to a Trophy video capture board
- Nikon Coolpix 950 microscope-mounted camera using compact flash card and imported to the Trophy software
- DMD Telicam Elite connected to a Trophy video capture board

Images have been globally adjusted and spot adjusted for brightness, contrast, and color balance. Images have also been rotated, flipped, and cropped and converted from the RGB colorspace used in CRTs to the CMYK palette used in printing. These adjustments were made to highlight the relevant anatomic features; correct for the differences among cameras, light sources, and capture mechanisms; and overcome the limitations of technology when working down in deep, dark holes.

References

1. Walton R: Access preparation and length determination. In Walton RE, Torabinejad M, editors: *Principles and practice of endodontics*, Philadelphia, 2002, WB Saunders.
2. Green D: Double canals in single roots, *J Oral Surg* 35:689, 1973.
3. American Association of Endodontists: *Endodontic case difficulty assessment form*, Chicago, American Association of Endodontists.
4. Stropko JJ: Canal morphology of maxillary molars: clinical observations of canal configurations, *J Endodon* 25(6):446, 1999.
5. Vertucci FJ: Root canal anatomy of human permanent teeth, *Oral Surg Oral Med Oral Pathol Oral Radiol Endod* 58:589, 1984.
6. Kasahara E et al: Root canal system of the maxillary central incisor, *J Endodon* 16(4):158, 1990.
7. Burns RC, Herbranson EJ: Tooth morphology and cavity preparation. In Cohen S, Burns RC, editors: *Pathways of the pulp*, ed 8, St Louis, 2002, Mosby.
8. Carns EJ, Skidmore AE: Configuration and deviation of root canals of maxillary first premolars, *J Oral Surg* 36:880, 1973.
9. Kulild JC, Peters DD: Incidence and configuration of canal systems in the mesiobuccal root of maxillary first and second molars, *J Endodon* 16(7):311, 1990.
10. Mauger MJ et al: Ideal endodontic access in mandibular incisors, *J Endodon* 25(3):206, 1999.
11. Benjamin KA, Dowson J: Incidence of two canals in human mandibular incisor teeth, *J Oral Surg* 38:122, 1974.
12. Clements RE, Gilboe DB: Labial endodontic access opening for mandibular incisors: endodontic and restorative considerations, *J Can Dent Assoc* 57:587, 1991.
13. Baisden MK, Kulild JC, Weller RN: Root canal configuration of the mandibular first premolar, *J Endodon* 18(10):505, 1992.
14. Hartwell G, Bellizzi R: Clinical investigation of in vivo endodontically treated mandibular and maxillary molars, *J Endodon* 8(12):555, 1982.
15. Melton DC, Krell KV, Fuller MW: Anatomical and histological features of C-shaped canals in mandibular second molars, *J Endodon* 17(8):384, 1991.
16. Weine FS: The C-shaped mandibular second molar: incidence and other considerations. Members of the Arizona Endodontic Association, *J Endodon* 24(5):372, 1998.

LENGTH DETERMINATION

DAVID J. HOLTZMANN

Cleaning and shaping of the root canal system are among the most important phases of endodontic treatment because they ease pain and eliminate debris and bacterial pathogens. The most challenging step in cleaning and shaping is determining working length, which is defined as the distance from a coronal reference point to the point at which canal preparation and obturation should terminate.[7] After establishing the working length, the clinician can eliminate many etiologies of endodontic pathosis and prepare the root canal system for obturation.

If a proper working length cannot be determined, the canal cannot be cleaned properly, shaped, or obturated. If instruments and obturating materials are not kept within the canal space, unnecessary inflammation can occur.[1] More importantly, when endodontic filling is either too long or too short, the prognosis is decreased.[2-6]

CORONAL REFERENCE POINT

Before calculating working length, the clinician should remove all caries, unsupported cusps, and restorations from the tooth being treated. If occlusal reduction is required for patient comfort or to prevent continued propagation of cracks, it should be completed before the working length is determined. This ensures the reference point to be used will remain unchanged.

The most common method of marking the instruments used for cleaning and shaping is with manufactured silicone "stops." Several devices have been developed to assist in dispensing these stops (Figure 3-1) and setting them on individual files at predetermined lengths (Figure 3-2). The stop should be placed perpendicular to the file to ensure an exact measurement.[8] Alternatively,

the clinician can make rubber stops from rubber bands, using a rubber dam punch set at the largest setting. One benefit of this method is that it produces smaller, more rigid stops, which improve visualization when several instruments are in the canals simultaneously during radiographic working length determination. As an alternative to rubber stops, some files are manufactured with hash marks etched at various levels on the file shank. Endometric probes are etched at millimeter increments and can be identified on radiographs.[9]

The coronal reference point from which the working length is measured should be an exact point to which the file stopper can touch. It should be repeatable and recorded for future reference. If the working length instrument and stop are merely "eyeballed" several millimeters from a particular reference point, the exact position cannot be repeated if the patient or the operator's view is slightly altered because of repositioning or if a second appointment is needed to complete the case. Intracoronal reference points should not be used to prevent movement of the stopper during measurement.[10] The reference is ideally recorded after straight line access in most cases because the stopper may change position in relation to a particular cusp.

The reference point can either be the cusp tip of the canal being measured or the same cusp tip for all canals. If the file is deflected away from a particular cusp tip, the cavosurface margin of that particular cusp may also be used. If no particular definable point can be located, a ledge can be made in the tooth structure that can act as a reference point. When treating a tooth that is longer than the longest set of files available, the clinician may need to find the reference in this fashion. Alternatively, if a crown restoration is planned, the cusp tip can be reduced before length calculation.

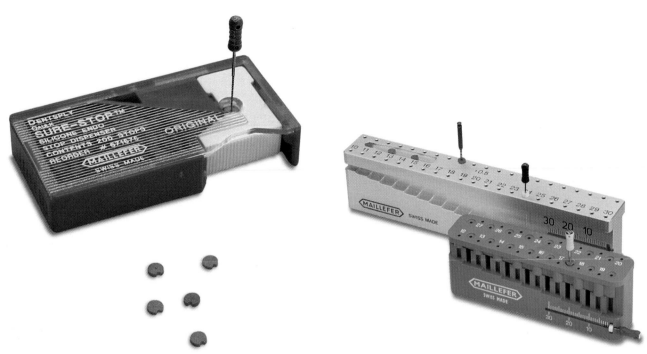

FIGURE 3-1   Sure-Stop silicone endodontic stop dispenser. (Courtesy Dentsply Maillefer, Tulsa, OK.)

FIGURE 3-2   Endo-M-Bloc and File-mate stop setting and measuring devices. (Courtesy Dentsply Maillefer, Tulsa, OK.)

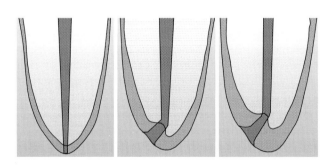

FIGURE 3-3   Chronological cementum deposition with subsequent deviation of the apical foramen. (Redrawn from Kuttler Y: Microscopic investigation of root apexes, *J Am Dent Assoc* 50:544, 1955.)

APICAL REFERENCE POINT

Where should endodontic treatment terminate? In 1916 the theory was advanced that pulp tissue extends through the apical foramen.[11] Later, Grove contradicted this and stated that the tissue in the foramen is periodontal tissue, not pulp tissue, and is important for cementum formation via periodontal ligament cells after pulp tissue removal.[12] Grove later discussed the importance of always filling the root canal to the dentinocemental junction (DCJ), which is "a definable point in all cases."[13,14] This was based on a few histologic sections taken from extracted immature teeth.

Coolidge also evaluated several histologic sections of root ends and described the DCJ as an imaginary line. He stated that the removal of pulp tissue near the apical foramen is required for success, not pulp removal at the DCJ or any other definable point.[15] Grove was also challenged by several other authors who reported that the DCJ is rarely a definable point in teeth. After examining more precise histologic data, they found that not only is the DCJ rarely located near apical constriction, but also that it occasionally is found on the external root surface because of root resorption and anatomic variation.[16,17]

The first extensive investigation of root apex anatomy was performed by Kuttler in 1955.[18] He evaluated 268 teeth (primarily from cadavers) from which 402 root ends were split through the apical foramen and

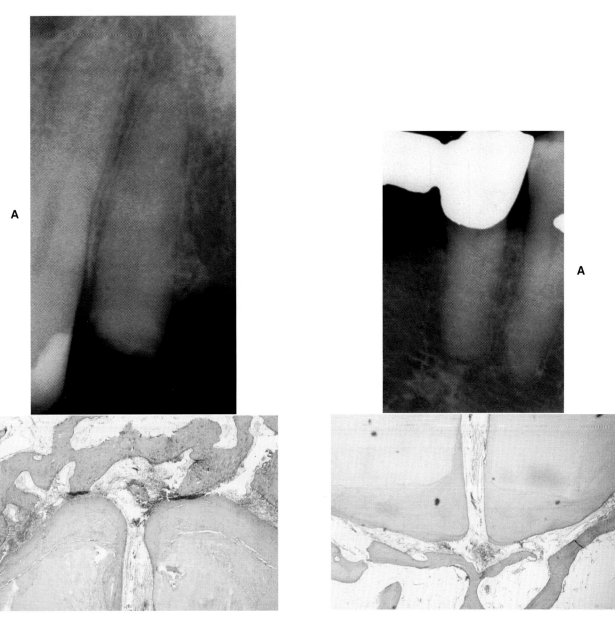

FIGURE 3-4   Radiograph **(A)** and histologic section **(B)** of ideal apical constriction on tooth #7.

FIGURE 3-5   Radiograph **(A)** and histologic section **(B)** of tooth #29 with a slight apical constriction.

examined. He reported several findings, including deviation of the center of the foramen further from the apical vertex with age and subsequent cementum deposition (Figure 3-3). The minor diameter was usually found in dentin. Kuttler concluded that the root canal should be filled as far as 0.5 mm from the foramen because the average distance from the minor diameter to the foramen is roughly 0.6 mm. Only 40% to 47% of apices had two DCJs at the same level on the sections.

Burch confirmed Kuttler's results by finding the average deviation of the apical foramen from the anatomic apex to be 0.59 mm in 877 teeth. He found that 40% of these deviated in a buccal or lingual direction, making

radiographic detection difficult.[19] Others have reported average distances as large as 0.8 mm, 0.99 mm, 0.9 mm, and 0.86 mm.[20-23] Different tooth types have variable anatomic configurations. The average distance between the major foramen and the apex of anterior teeth has been reported to be 0.26 mm, with 31% opening directly at the apex. For molars the average distance is 0.44 mm, with 39% opening directly at the apex.[24,25]

The variability in apical canal anatomy makes working length determination extremely challenging. Canal variations range from an ideal apical constriction (Figure 3-4), to slight apical constriction (Figure 3-5), to no constriction at all (Figure 3-6). Frequently canals can

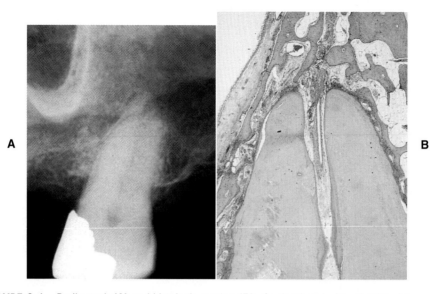

FIGURE 3-6   Radiograph **(A)** and histologic section **(B)** of palatal root of tooth #15 with no apical constriction.

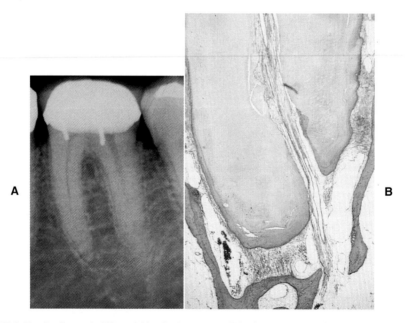

FIGURE 3-7   Radiograph **(A)** and histologic section **(B)** of mesial root of tooth #19 with apical foramen well short of radiographic apex.

terminate several millimeters from the radiographic apex (Figures 3-7 and 3-8). This variability in apical canal anatomy has been reported by Dummer, who examined 270 extracted teeth and categorized the apical anatomy into five types of constrictions[26] (Figure 3-9):

1. Typical single constriction
2. Tapering constriction with the narrowest portion near the actual apex

3. Several constrictions
4. Constriction followed by a narrow, parallel canal
5. Complete blockage of the apical canal by secondary dentin

Besides causing cementum deposition, resorptive processes can also affect the relationships of the apical anatomy and decisions regarding endodontic treatment termination (Figures 3-10 and 3-11). Malueg examined

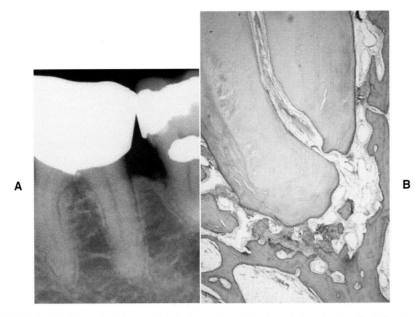

FIGURE 3-8   Radiograph **(A)** and histologic section **(B)** of mesial root of tooth #19 with apical foramen well short of radiographic apex.

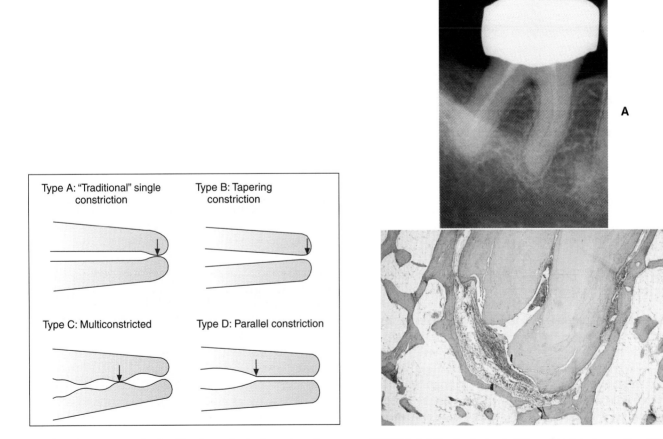

Type A: "Traditional" single constriction

Type B: Tapering constriction

Type C: Multiconstricted

Type D: Parallel constriction

FIGURE 3-9   Dummer's classifications of apical canal anatomy. (Redrawn from Dummer PMH, McGinn JH, Rees DG: The position and topography of the apical canal constriction and apical foramen, *Int Endod J* 17:192, 1984.)

FIGURE 3-10   Radiograph **(A)** and histologic section **(B)** of mesial root of tooth #31 with inflammatory root resorption.

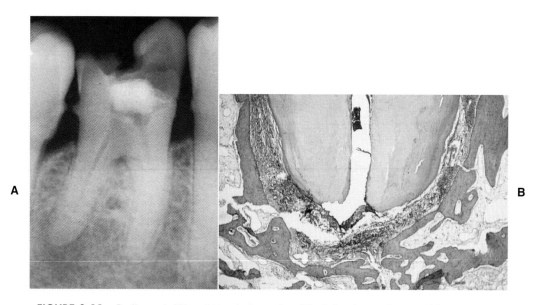

FIGURE 3-11 Radiograph **(A)** and histologic section **(B)** of distal root of tooth #30 with inflammatory root resorption.

49 root ends in 40 teeth with scanning electron microscopy and described the amount of apical resorption occurring with preextraction pulpal and periapical diagnosis.[27] Out of 25 roots with necrotic pulps, 18 demonstrated funneling (root resorption extending into the internal surface of the foramen), a number significantly higher than that observed in vital pulps. Therefore "the status of the pulp and periapical tissues should be considered when determining the length for preparation or obturation."[27] Traumatic tooth injury also can cause root resorption. Approximately 20% to 40% of the root structure must be demineralized before buccal or lingual root resorption can be detected radiographically.[28] Some researchers suggest calculating the working length 1 mm short of the radiographic apex with normal apical anatomy, 1.5 mm short with bone but no root resorption, and 2 mm short with bone and root resorption.[29]

METHODS OF DETERMINING WORKING LENGTH

Methods for determining working length include using average root lengths from anatomic studies, preoperative radiographs, tactile detection, or the "eye twitch" response. Other common methods include bleeding on a paper point and using working length radiographs made with a variety of different film types or digital sensors, electronic apex locators, or any combination of the above.

Ideally, the clinician should measure working length after attaining straight line access to the apical third of the root canal system. The length may change slightly after working length determination because of the elimination of the coronal deflection of the working length.[30,8] This is especially true in the mesial canals of molars, where much of the total curvature of the canal is eliminated after the cervical bulge is removed. Moreover, attaining straight line access and preflaring the canal space greatly improves tactile detection of the apical constriction.[31]

Radiography

Since Wilhelm Roentgen's discovery of the x-ray in 1895, continued efforts have been made to reduce the amount of ionizing radiation exposure to the patient while improving or maintaining image quality. Otto Walkhoff's production of the first dental radiograph required 25 minutes of exposure time.[32] Current methods to reduce radiation exposure include using the paralleling technique instead of the bisecting angle technique and employing rectangular long cone techniques, faster radiographic film, digital radiographic techniques, and electronic apex locators to assist in endodontic treatment.[33] Rectangular collimation can decrease the radiation exposure by 40% compared with a 6 cm round beam, E-speed film can decrease exposure by 40% over D-speed film, and constant potential x-ray units can decrease exposure by 40% compared with conventional alternating current units.[34]

As steps are made to reduce patient radiation exposure, the quality of working length determination must not be sacrificed.[35] When radiographs are used to determine working length, the quality of the image is important for accurate interpretation. Paralleling techniques have been demonstrated as superior to bisecting angle radiographic techniques in interpretation of length determination and reproduction of apical anatomy.[36-38] As the angle increases away from parallel, the quality of the image decreases.[37] This occurs because as the angle is increased, the tissue that the x-rays must pass through includes a greater percentage of bone mass and root anatomy becomes less discernible. To limit some of these problems, the "modified paralleling" technique has been suggested by Walton; in this technique the central beam is oriented perpendicular to the radiographic film, but not to the tooth.[29]

Several choices are available regarding radiographic film and processing. No significant difference has been demonstrated in the diagnostic quality of E-Plus radiographic film compared with D-speed film.[39-43] For this reason, E-Plus film should be used to reduce radiation exposure to the patient. Rapid processing chemicals are also used in endodontics to expedite the development of film for treatment radiographs. When tested, these rapid techniques provided similar diagnostic quality to normally processed radiographs for working length determination.[42]

Parallel working length radiographs can be difficult to attain because of misorientation, shallow palatal vault, and tori. Products such as the "Endo-Ray II" (Figure 3-12) (Dentsply Rinn, Elgin, IL) may help produce more predictable results. This alignment device assists in making a parallel working length radiograph without removing the rubber dam clamp or files from the tooth. Dental students using hemostats produced acceptable radiographs in 66% of maxillary and 75% of mandibular teeth on patients undergoing endodontic treatment. When the Endo-Ray II was used, acceptable radiographs were made in 87% of maxillary and 85% of mandibular teeth.[44]

Because increased vertical angulation is often necessary when making maxillary radiographs, zygomatic arch interference becomes a significant problem in interpreting apical anatomy and determining working length. Approximately 42% of maxillary second molars and 20% of first molars exhibit this interference.[45]

An understanding of the buccal object rule (BOR) is essential to endodontic treatment. The main concept of the rule is that as the vertical or horizontal angulation of the x-ray source or tube head changes, the object buccal or closest to the tube head moves to the opposite side of the radiograph compared with the lingual object. For example, if a working length radiograph is of a maxillary first premolar with no horizontal angulation (buccal and lingual roots are superimposed) and too little vertical angulation (apex is not captured on radiograph), a new working length radiograph is necessary. To separate the buccal and lingual roots to visualize the individual working length file's relationship to the apical root structure, the clinician should place the tube head from a 20 degree mesial angulation. This captures the buccal root on the opposite or distal side of the radiograph and the lingual root on the mesial side of the radiograph. To cap-

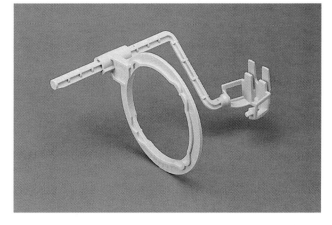

FIGURE 3-12   Endo-Ray II film holder. (Courtesy Dentsply Rinn, Elgin, IL.)

ture the entire apical portion of the roots, the vertical angulation of the tube head should be increased from a positive, or superior, position. This is demonstrated on the radiograph as the buccal root appearing more inferior, or coronal, to the lingual root (the opposite direction of the tube head angulation) and the lingual root appearing toward the superior, or top, of the film. This rule can also be applied to locating root resorptive processes in relation to a tooth, identifying anatomic landmarks and pathosis, locating a canal in relation to a radiopaque marker such as a bur in the access, or locating the position of additional roots.[46] Additionally, to increase visualization of apical anatomy, this rule can be used to "move" anatomic landmarks such as the zygomatic process or impacted teeth.[47] It also helps identify the angle at which a particular radiograph was made even if the information was not recorded. For example, the palatal root of a maxillary molar curves to the distal side and is located toward the distobuccal root rather than between the two buccal roots when the angle of the radiograph is from the mesial side. Extensive information on the BOR has been reported by Richards.[48] Other names for the BOR include the SLOB (*Same Lingual, Opposite Buccal*) rule, the BOMM (*Buccal Object Moves Most*) rule, Clark's rule, and Walton's projection.[49] Walton suggests an easy method to simplify this concept. Place two or three fingers in front of your eyes to represent the roots of a particular tooth. As you move your head to the "mesial," or for demonstration purposes to the right, while keeping your fingers in the same position, you will notice that the "buccal" object, or the finger closest to your face, will move to the "distal" or left. This is exactly the way a structure would be projected on the radiographic film and can be applied to vertical angulation in a similar fashion.[29]

Although the individual canals can usually be deciphered by applying the BOR and knowing the angle at

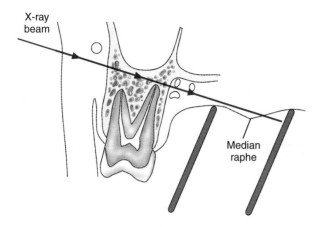

FIGURE 3-13   Film placement for maxillary working length radiographs. (Redrawn from Walton RW, Torabinejad M: *Principles and practice of endodontics,* ed 3, Philadelphia, 2002, WB Saunders.)

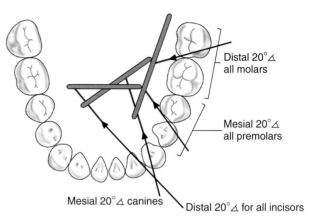

FIGURE 3-14   Film placement for mandibular working length radiographs. (Redrawn from Walton RW, Torabinejad M: *Principles and practice of endodontics,* ed 3, Philadelphia, 2002, WB Saunders.)

which the radiograph was made, misinterpretation is still possible. This can be reduced by using different file types (e.g., Hedstrom, K-file) or different file sizes (e.g., 15, 25, 35) in adjacent canals.[35]

Preoperative periapical radiographs have been used to calculate the working length for endodontic treatment.[36] Because a magnification of about 5.4% is employed in the paralleling technique, 1 to 2 mm must be subtracted from the measurement on the preoperative radiograph.[50] Pantographic radiographs have not been advocated for calculating the estimated working length because of the gross magnification of 13% to 28% that is employed.[51] "Radiographic incrementation" is the process of using a millimeter grid stamped on the film or a copper grid to measure working length. Using these measurements alone can produce unfavorable results.[52,36] Rather than using this method alone to measure working length, which was commonly done in the early years of endodontic treatment, this measurement can be used as an "estimated working length" that can then be confirmed by placing an endodontic instrument into the canal and taking a second radiograph. The "corrected working length" can then be calculated by adding or subtracting the distance between the instrument tip and the desired apical termination of the root. This technique was first introduced by John Ingle.[53] When measuring the distance from the file tip to the adjusted stop with a metric ruler, it is important to straighten any curvatures present in the working length file to prevent misinterpretation.

When rubber dams are in place, working length radiographs can be challenging. The rubber dam frame should be left in place to maintain isolation, but one corner of the dam can be released to facilitate placement of the film. For this reason, plastic rubber dam frames should be used in endodontic treatment.

Angled working length radiographs help separate overlapping canals, especially in mandibular teeth and maxillary premolars. Walton outlined the ideal orientation and angles for working length radiographs in maxillary and mandibular teeth (Figures 3-13 through 3-15). Maxillary anterior teeth only contain single canals, and maxillary molars require straight-on radiographs. The palatal canal is centered between the mesiobuccal and distobuccal roots in maxillary molars. When a second mesiobuccal canal (MB$_2$) is suspected, a mesial radiograph is often required to identify it. However, as the horizontal angulation increases, the clarity of the radicular anatomy decreases. A 20 degree mesial shift is sufficient to separate the canals while limiting distortion. When making maxillary radiographs, the operator places the film parallel to the tooth and perpendicular to the central ray and as far apical as possible. Generally the radiograph is placed at the junction of the hard and soft palate for maxillary anterior teeth and on the opposite side of the palate for maxillary posterior teeth (see Figure 3-13). Mandibular radiography also has some challenges. The radiographic film is placed as close to the tooth and as parallel to the tooth as possible to limit distortion. Generally this can be achieved by placing the film deep in the vestibule. If the patient closes the mouth slightly, the film generally can be placed more apically as the mylohyoid muscle relaxes.[29]

New Technology

Advances in electronics and computers are generating many treatment adjuncts in endodontics and specifically in working length determination. Careful analysis and use of these devices is crucial to provide improved patient care now and in the future. Bender stated on his ninetieth birthday celebration, "The clinical practice of yesterday's endodontics becomes the heresy of today and today's en-

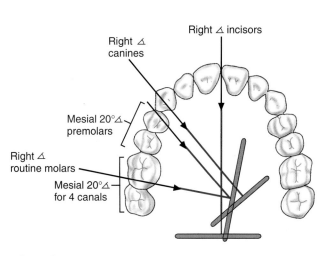

Right △ incisors

Right △
canines

Mesial 20°△
premolars

Right △
routine molars

Mesial 20°△
for 4 canals

FIGURE 3-15   Orientation of film on opposite side of palate when making maxillary posterior working length radiograph. (Redrawn from Walton RW, Torabinejad M: *Principles and practice of endodontics,* ed 3, Philadelphia, 2002, WB Saunders.)

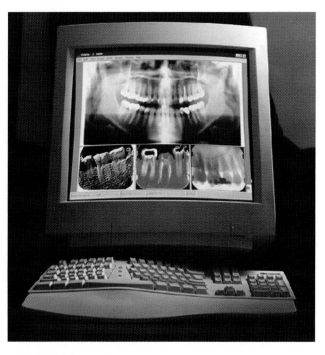

FIGURE 3-16   Gendex GX-S CCD-based digital radiography system. (Courtesy Dentsply Gendex, Des Plaines, IL.)

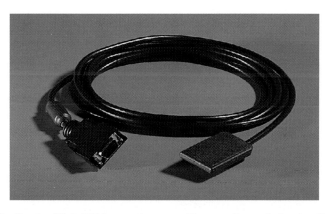

FIGURE 3-17   Gendex GX-S CCD intraoral sensor. (Courtesy Dentsply Gendex, Des Plaines, IL.)

dodontic practice becomes the heresy of tomorrow. So don't be so rigid in your techniques or beliefs."[29a]

DIGITAL RADIOGRAPHY.   For the past 100 years, film-based radiography has been the dominant imaging technique used in dentistry. Although commonplace in medicine for many years, charged coupled device (CCD) sensor-based digital radiography was first introduced to dentistry by Trophy (Trophy Radiologie, Vincennes, France) with the RadioVisioGraphy (RVG) system in 1987. Since that time, other digital systems have entered the market. These include Sens-A-Ray (Regam Medical

Systems AB, Sundsvall, Sweden), Gendex GX-S (Dentsply Gendex, Des Plaines, IL) (Figure 3-16), Flash Dent (Villa Sistem Medicale srd, Buccinasco, Italy), Schick CDR (Schick Technologies, New York, NY), and several others. Modifications of the original systems include larger sensor sizes comparable to size #2 film, thinner and more manageable intraoral sensors (Figure 3-17), and integration with intraoral cameras and patient management database software (Figure 3-18).

Since the introduction of dental digital radiography by Trophy in 1987, its use in endodontics has increased because of the ability to produce instantaneous images dur-

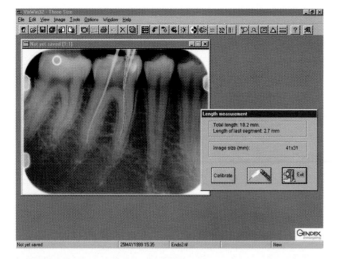

FIGURE 3-18 Gendex DenOptix software demonstrating working length estimation. (Courtesy Dentsply Gendex, Des Plaines, IL.)

ing working length determination. This technology uses a CCD chip inside an intraoral sensor that produces an immediate digital image on the monitor after exposure to about 50% or less of the radiation exposure required by E-speed film. This image can be stored, enhanced, or placed in the patient record. If the apical anatomy cannot be visualized, another image can be made by readjusting the position indicating device (PID) or the intraoral sensor. CCD-based digital radiography systems such as the Trophy RVG, Seamens Sidexis, Regam Sens-A-Ray, and Visualix Vixa all have been demonstrated to be similar in working length determination to D- and E-speed film.[54-62]

Although first described in the medical literature in 1983 by Sonoda et al, storage phosphor–based digital radiography was introduced by Fuji (Fuji Inc., Tokyo, Japan) in 1981. More recently, Soredex (Orion Corp. Ltd., Helsinki, Finland) has introduced an intraoral computed radiography system called the Digora. This system also uses the Fuji sensor and was first described in 1994 by Kashima.[63] It uses a flat imaging plate containing phosphor granules that fluoresce when exposed to ionizing radiation. About 50% of the latent energy remains stored in the imaging plate, similar to an intensifying screen, until the image is read by the scanner. After exposure, the imaging plate is disinfected, removed from its sealed plastic cover, and placed into a laser reader that produces a digital image within 30 seconds. The image can then be viewed on the monitor, enhanced, or stored in the patient record. These systems are similar in cost to intraoral CCD-based sensor systems. Although the image is not immediately viewed on the monitor after exposure, its benefits include a sensor that is similar in thickness and flexibility to a #2 size conventional film (Figure 3-19).

The largest Digora sensor is similar in size and thickness to a #2 dental film. The sensor dimension is 35 ×

45 × 1.6 mm. The imaging area is 30 × 40 mm and 416 × 560 pixels. Each pixel is 70 × 70 μm. The resolution has been reported as more than six line pairs per millimeter. The uncompressed image file size is 234 kilobytes.[64]

Working length determination using storage phosphor radiography has also been demonstrated to be similar to that using D- and E-Plus speed film.[62,65,66] Brettle demonstrated that Digora images of similar quality to Kodak Ektaspeed (E-speed) film were acquired with exposure times 80% less than those of film.[67]

Gendex has introduced a storage phosphor system called DenOptix (Dentsply Gendex, DesPlaines, IL) (Figure 3-20). This new technology uses the same processing equipment to read numerous sizes of storage phosphor–based film (Figure 3-21).

Other emerging digital technologies using the CCD-based sensor are being explored. One example is Panoramic Corporation's latest innovation called RTLX (Panoramic Corporation, Fort Wayne, IN). This is a preliminary product that boasts full-motion digital radiography with minimal radiation dosage. This system allows radiographic imaging during treatment procedures similar to those used in interventional radiography. Although the technology is exciting, protective barrier techniques must be further explored because of the constant radiation exposure to patients and health care providers from the fluoroscope. A similar technology was reported in the literature in 1983; it was called the DXT-100.[68]

ELECTRONIC APEX LOCATORS. Radiographs are often misinterpreted because of the difficulty of discerning radicular anatomy and pathosis from normal structures.[69,70] Electronic apex locators are used for working length determination as an adjunct to radiography. They should be used when the apical portion of the canal system is obstructed by impacted teeth, tori, the malar process, the zygomatic arch, excessive bone density, overlapping roots, shallow palatal vaults, or even normal medullary and cortical bone patterns. In these cases they can provide information that radiography cannot. They may also be used in the treatment of pregnant patients to reduce radiation exposure, in children who may not tolerate taking radiographs, and in disabled or heavily sedated patients. If a patient does not tolerate radiograph placement because of the gag reflex, electronic apex locators can be a valuable tool. Sewerin evaluated full mouth radiographic series taken on 478 patients and found that 13% exhibited a significant gag reflex and 1.3% were unable to tolerate completion of the radiographic examination.[71] Patients with disabilities or debilitating disorders such as Parkinson's disease may not be able to hold the film in place. Children also may have difficulty with this task. Because as many as 40% of deviations of canal foramen from the apical center are in

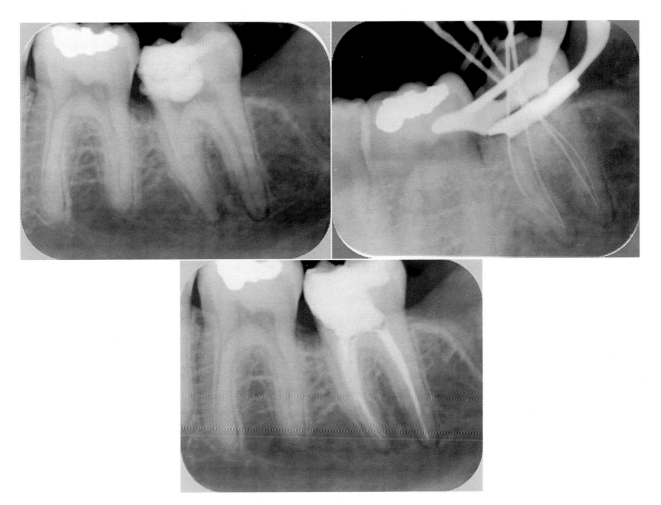

FIGURE 3-19   Endodontic case treated with Soredex Digora digital radiography system.

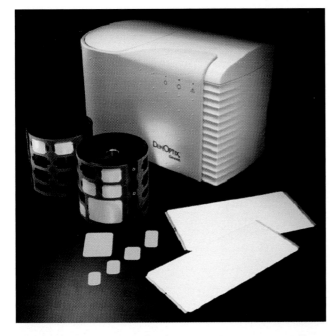

FIGURE 3-20   Gendex DenOptix storage phosphor system. (Courtesy Dentsply Gendex, Des Plaines, IL.)

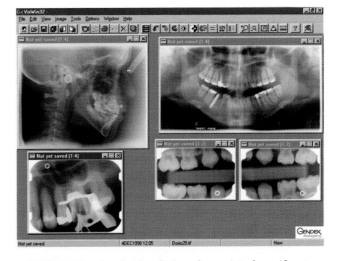

FIGURE 3-21   Gendex DenOptix software interface. (Courtesy Dentsply Gendex, Des Plaines, IL.)

the buccal or lingual plane and apical canal curvature is in the buccal or lingual plane, electronic apex locators can provide good information where unknown curves may otherwise go undetected with radiographic film.[72,73] Electronic devices such as electronic apex locators should not be used on patients who have cardiac pacemakers. The "demand" type pacemakers (the most commonly used today) that stimulate the heart only when necessary are most affected by electronic equipment.[74,75]

In 1942, Suzuki found in experiments on dogs that the electrical resistance between an instrument in the canal and the mucous membrane is a consistent value. These principles were not examined further until Sunada performed a series of experiments on patients and found that the electrical resistance in the canal at the apex, mucosa, and periodontal ligament was 39 to 41 mA with very little variance when measured with an ohmmeter.[76] He then demonstrated that when a reading of 40 mA was attained, the apex was consistently located. Huang found the same constant resistance in vitro.[77] Therefore he claims it is a physical and not a biologic phenomenon. Inuoe developed a sonic readout system using a transistor equalizer-amplifier that converts the feedback to sound.

One of the most widely used apex locators in the 1970s and 1980s was the Sono-Explorer (Union Broach, New York, NY). An article was published reporting the accuracy of the Sono-Explorer to be only 48% compared with a digital-tactile sense accuracy of 64%.[78] A flurry of letters was published in later issues of the *Journal of the American Dental Association* condemning this article by practitioners who felt they used their instruments with a great deal of success. Since that time, more sound clinical testing has been performed and apex locators continue to evolve and improve.

Because of the problems caused by the interaction of electronic apex locators with moisture and endodontic irrigants in the canals, devices were developed to operate in moist conditions. The Endocator (Hygienic Corporation, Akron, OH) was the first to do this, using a Teflon-coated probe instead of files for working length determination. This insulated the measuring device from canal irrigants and tissue, but the instruments were not always fine enough to pass through the apical constriction. Also, the Teflon coating tended to break away from the probes with time, altering the accuracy of the device.

Most recently, third-generation electronic apex locators have entered the market. They can operate in a wet environment, even one containing sodium hypochlorite, and appear to be much more accurate compared with previous devices. They use two different frequencies and average the change as the apex is reached to provide a much smoother reading in different conditions. The first of this generation was the Osada Endex, or Apit as it is called outside the United States (Osada Electrical Co., Tokyo, Japan). This apex locator must be used in a moist environment and is calibrated by being reset with the file a few millimeters into the canal before a measurement is taken of each canal. The apical terminus is reported with a constant tone as well as a meter that reflects the position in the canal. The J. Morita Root ZX (Figure 3-22)

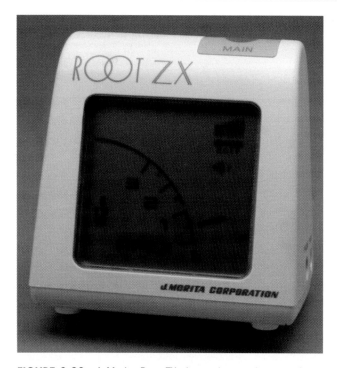

FIGURE 3-22 J. Morita Root ZX electronic apex locator. (Courtesy J. Morita Co., Kyoto, Japan.)

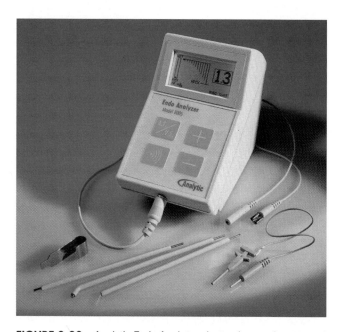

FIGURE 3-23 Analytic Endo Analyzer electronic apex locator and electronic pulp tester. (Courtesy Analytic Endodontics, Orange, CA.)

(J. Morita Co., Kyoto, Japan) can be used in either a wet or dry environment, including blood, sodium hypochlorite, and saline. It uses a tone as well as a digital readout. The Root ZX has been demonstrated in the literature to be the most accurate apex locator on the market. The Analytic Apex Finder (Analytic Endodontics, Orange, CA) uses three different frequencies with a digital readout, but no studies have been reported yet to demonstrate its performance. Analytic also produces the Endo Analyzer (Figure 3-23), which acts as an electronic apex locator as well as an electric pulp tester.

The working length measured to clean, shape, and obturate a canal space may not always be measured to the apical constriction. In cases of root perforation, the point of exit of the canal to the periodontal ligament space is a crucial measurement. If the perforation occurs on the buccal or lingual or furcal surface of the tooth, it may be difficult to detect. Apex locators can be reliable instruments to detect perforations and the length to the area where the perforation exits the tooth structure.[79-82] An electronic apex locator can also be placed on a post to confirm that the post is perforated or on a pin to detect whether it has been placed into the pulp space.[83]

When electronic apex locators are compared for accuracy in the literature, scientific methods used include simulated acrylic canals, animal, cadaver, and human studies (Table 3-1). A defined acceptable range of accuracy among working length determinations is plus or

TABLE 3-1

Literature Regarding Electronic Apex Locators

FIRST AUTHOR	YEAR	EAL 1	EAL 2	TRUTH	STUDY TYPE	0.5 MM 1	0.5 MM 2	N (CANALS)	TOOTH TYPE
Sunada	1962	37 μA	40 μA				100%	27	
Arora	1995	Endex	RCM Mark II	Direct	Patient–Extract	64%	34%	61	
Felippe	1994	Endex		Direct	Extract–Mount	97%		350	All
Fouad	1993	Endex	Exact-A-Pex	Direct	Extract–Mount	Endex best			
Frank	1993	Endex	Rad	Rad	Only patient	90%		185	All
Lauper	1996	Endex	Odontometer	Direct	Patient–Extract	93%	73%	22	
Ounsi	1998	Endex	Rad	Direct	Extract–Mount	85%	97%	33	
Pratten	1996	Endex	D-speed	Direct	Cadavers	0.26 mm	0.58 mm	27	All
Keller	1991	Endocator	Film	Direct	Patient–Extract	52%	80%	99	All
McDonald	1990	Endocator	Film	Direct	Patient–Extract	93%		59	All
Pallares	1994	Endocator	Odontometer	Direct	Patient–Extract	90%	85%	34	Molars
Ricard	1991	Evident Mark II		Direct	Patient–Extract	87%		37	All
Czerw	1994	Exact-A-Pex	Foramatron 4	Direct	Extract–Mount	100%	100%	45	Anterior
Fouad	1989	Exact-A-Pex	Neosono-D	Direct	Extract–Mount	95%	100%	20	All
Becker	1980	Forameter	Film	Direct	Pig mandible	24%	44%	41	Pig premolars first
Foramen	1986	Homemade	Commercial	Rad	Only patient	93%	93%	15	
Suchde	1977	Homemade Ant	Posterior teeth	Rad	Only patient	83%	88%	51/25	
Berman	1984	Neosono-D	Open apex	Direct	Patient–Extract	Average 0.49	Average 3.25	24	
Rivera	1993	Neosono-D	Without recap	Direct	Extract–Mount			15	Anterior
Stein	1990	Neosono-D		Direct	Extract–Mount	66% short		47	All
Stein	1991	Neosono-D	Film	Direct	Patient–Extract	58% short	0.24-2.39	47	All
Czerw	1995	Root ZX	Apex Finder	Direct	Extract–Mount	100%	83%	30	Anterior
Dunlap	1998	Root ZX		Direct	Patient–Extract	82%		35	All
Dunlap	1998	Root ZX		Direct	Patient–Extract	82%		34	
Katz	1996	Root ZX	Ingle's	Direct	Extract–Mount	100%		20	First molars

Continued

TABLE 3-1

Literature Regarding Electronic Apex Locators—cont'd

FIRST AUTHOR	YEAR	EAL 1	EAL 2	TRUTH	STUDY TYPE	0.5 MM 1	0.5 MM 2	N (CANALS)	TOOTH TYPE
Pagavino	1998	Root ZX		Direct	Patient–Extract	100%		15	
Shabahang	1996	Root ZX		Direct	Patient–Extract	96%		26	
Vajrabhaya	1997	Root ZX		Direct	Patient–Extract	100%		19	Single root
Kaufman	1989	SE Mark II	Ingle's	Rad	Only patient	87%	87%	75	All
Hembrough	1993	SE Mark III	Rad	Direct	Patient–Extract	73%	89%	52	Maxillary molars
Inoue	1985	SE Mark III		Rad	Only patient	58%		310	
Trope	1985	SE Mark III		Rad	Only patient	91%		127	All
Wu	1992	Se Mark III		Direct	Patient–Extract	78%		20	Single root
Blank	1975	Sono Explorer	Endometer	Direct	Patient–Extract	89% (0.2)	85% (0.2)	91	
Busch	1976	Sono Explorer		Rad	Only patient	93%			All
Fouad	1990	Sono Explorer	Apex Finder	Direct	Patient–Extract	75%	67%	20	Single root
Inoue	1973	Sono Explorer		Rad	Only patient	74%	92%	201	
Kaufman	1979	Sono Explorer	Ingle's	Rad	Only patient	48%		106	All
O'Neill	1974	Sono Explorer		Direct	Patient–Extract	100%		53	All
Seidberg	1975	Sono Explorer	Digital-Tactile	Rad	Only patient	48%	64%	50	

minus 0.5 mm from the apical constriction. Researchers averaged the accuracy of 12 studies assessing the Sono-Explorer, a second-generation apex locator, and found that 76% of the measurements fall within this range.[78,84-94] A third-generation electronic apex locator, the Endex, has been shown to be 86% accurate according to the average of five studies.[95-99] Researchers averaging the accuracy of another third-generation apex locator, the Root ZX, in seven studies found it to be 94% accurate.[100-105] The most clinically relevant data can be gathered from blinded studies where working length is determined with any test method, cementation of the file in position, extraction of the tooth, and direct measurement of the file tip from the apical constriction. When only these types of studies are used to compare apex locators, the Sono-Explorer is found to be 83% accurate (five studies), the Endex is 79% accurate (two studies), and the Root ZX is 92% accurate (five studies). The percent accuracy of these three commonly used electronic apex locators is summarized in Table 3-2.

Recently, apex locators have been married to other endodontic instruments. The Tri Auto ZX (J. Morita Co., Kyoto, Japan) (Figure 3-24) is a rechargeable electric handpiece that rotates nickel titanium files at 240 to 280 rpm and has the electronic components of an apex locator built in. When the file reaches the preset working length (e.g., 1.0 or 1.5 mm short of the apical constriction as read by the electronic apex locator), the file automatically reverses direction and backs out of the canal. This auto-reverse mechanism also begins when excessive torque is sensed by the handpiece to avoid possible instrument separation.[106] When tested on extracted teeth, the canals were instrumented to 0.1 mm short of the electronically measured length when set at 1.0 mm; however, the apical constriction was commonly overprepared.[107] An ultrasonic device called the Solfy ZX (J. Morita Co., Kyoto, Japan) has also been introduced. It combines an ultrasonic handpiece with electronic apex locator technology. This instrument also can be set to stop vibrating when a preset length is detected by the electronic apex locator. It has been demonstrated that when the auto-stop function is set at 2, the chance of over-enlarging the apical constriction is lessened compared with a setting of 1.[108]

When using electronic apex locators to determine working length, the clinician should keep in mind that metallic restorations may interfere with the reading of the device if the working length file comes into contact

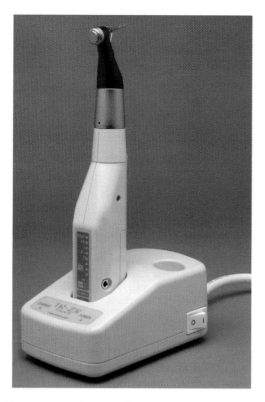

FIGURE 3-24   J. Morita Tri Auto ZX. (Courtesy J. Morita Co., Kyoto, Japan.)

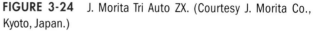

TABLE 3-2

Summary of Literature on Three Apex Locators

APEX LOCATOR	ALL STUDIES COMBINED		PATIENT TREATMENT, THEN EXTRACTION	
	NUMBER	ACCURACY	NUMBER	ACCURACY
Sono-Explorer	12	76%	5	83%
Endex	5	86%	2	79%
Root ZX	7	94%	5	92%

with the restoration or fluid that is in contact with the restoration. This problem can be avoided by initially drying the coronal canal space and chamber before measurement or by using a silicone-containing material within the canal spaces, such as Gly-Oxide (Marion Laboratories, Inc., Kansas City, MO).

The most important thing to do when determining working length is to use as many of the techniques as possible during the course of treatment. First the clinician should secure a stable coronal reference point(s). The next step is to estimate working length from the historical average lengths and the preoperative radiograph and keep this estimate in mind throughout treatment. Finally, the clinician should use rational thought in combining tactile sense, radiography, and electronic devices to arrive at the desired apical terminus of the endodontic preparation.

References

1. Seltzer S, Soltanoff W, Smith J: Periapical tissue reactions of root canal instrumentation beyond the apex, *Oral Surg Oral Med Oral Pathol Oral Radiol Endod* 36:725, 1973.
2. Strindberg L: The dependence of pulp therapy on certain factors: an analytic study based on radiographic and clinical follow-up examinations, *Acta Odontol Scand* 14:1, 1956.
3. Grahnén H, Hansson L: The prognosis of pulp and root canal therapy, *Odontol Rev* 12:146, 1961.
4. Seltzer S, Bender I, Turkenkopf S: Factors affecting successful repair after RCT, *J Am Dent Assoc* 67:651, 1963.
5. Swartz DB, Skidmore AE, Griffin JA, Jr: Twenty years of endodontic success and failure, *J Endod* 9:198, 1983.
6. Sjögren U: Factors affecting the long-term results of endodontic treatment, *J Endod* 16:498, 1990.
7. American Association of Endodontists: *Contemporary terminology for endodontics,* ed 6, Chicago, 1998, American Association of Endodontists.
8. Gutmann JL, Leonard JE: Problem solving in endodontic working length determination, *Compend Cont Ed Dent* 16:288, 1995.

9. Dummer PMH, Lewis JM: An evaluation of the endometric probe in root canal length estimation, *Int Endod J* 20:25, 1987.

10. Schilder H: Cleaning and shaping the root canal, *Dent Clin North Am* 18:269, 1974.

11. Grove CJ: The biology of multi-canaliculated roots, *Dent Cosmos* 58:728, 1916.

12. Grove CJ: Nature's method of making perfect root fillings following pulp removal, with a brief consideration of the development of secondary cementum, *Dent Cosmos* 63:968, 1921.

13. Grove CJ: Why root canals should be filled to the dentinocemental junction, *J Am Dent Assoc* 17:293, 1930.

14. Grove CJ: The value of the dentinocemental junction in pulp canal surgery, *J Dent Res* 11:466, 1931.

15. Coolidge ED: Anatomy of the root apex in relation to treatment problems, *J Am Dent Assoc* 16:1456, 1929.

16. Orban B: Why root canals should be filled to the dentinocemental junction, *J Am Dent Assoc* 17:1086, 1930.

17. Skillen WG: Why root canals should be filled to the dentinocemental junction, *J Am Dent Assoc* 17:2082, 1930.

18. Kuttler Y: Microscopic investigation of root apexes, *J Am Dent Assoc* 50:544, 1955.

19. Burch JG, Hulen S: The relationship of the apical foramen to the anatomic apex of the tooth root, *Oral Surg Oral Med Oral Pathol Oral Radiol Endod* 34:262, 1972.

20. Tamse A et al: Morphologic and radiographic study of the apical foramen in distal roots of mandibular molars, Part II: the distance between the foramen and the root end, *Int Endod J* 21:211, 1988.

21. Blaskovic-Subat V, Maricic B, Sutalo J: Asymmetry of the root canal foramen, *Int Endod J* 25:158, 1992.

22. Mizutani T, Ohno N, Nakamura H: Anatomic study of the root apex in the maxillary anterior teeth, *J Endod* 18:344, 1992.

23. Pagan JC, Santa CA, Alvarez JA: Working length in root canal fillings, *NY State Dent J* 59:41, 1993.

24. Green D: A stereomicroscopic study of the root apices of 400 maxillary and mandibular anterior teeth, *Oral Surg Oral Med Oral Pathol Oral Radiol Endod* 9:1224, 1956.

25. Green D: Stereomicroscopic study of 700 root apices of maxillary and mandibular posterior teeth, *Oral Surg Oral Med Oral Pathol Oral Radiol Endod* 13:728, 1960.

26. Dummer PMH, McGinn JH, Rees DG: The position and topography of the apical canal constriction and apical foramen, *Int Endod J* 17:192, 1984.

27. Malueg LA, Wilcox LR, Johnson WT: Examination of external apical root resorption with scanning electron microscopy, *Oral Surg Oral Med Oral Pathol Oral Radiol Endod* 82:89, 1996.

28. Andreasen JO: Luxation of permanent teeth due to trauma: a clinical and radiographic follow-up study of 189 injured teeth, *Scand J Dent Res* 78:273, 1970.

29. Walton RW, Torabinejad M: *Principles and practice of endodontics,* ed 3, Philadelphia, 2002, WB Saunders.

29a. Bender IB: The past, present, and future of endodontics, Delivered at the IB Bender conference, *The biologic basis and clinical practice of endodontics,* on the occasion of his ninetieth birthday celebration.

30. Caldwell JL: Change in working length following instrumentation of molar canals, *Oral Surg Oral Med Oral Pathol Oral Radiol Endod* 41:114, 1976.

31. Stabholz A, Rotstein I, Torabinejad M: Effect of preflaring on tactile detection of the apical constriction, *J Endod* 21:92, 1995.

32. Rezai RF, Salamat K: In commemoration of endodontic patriarch Friedrich Otto Walkhoff (April 23, 1860-June 8, 1934), *J Endod* 11:45, 1985.

33. Lecomber AR, Faulkner K: Organ absorbed doses in intraoral dental radiography, *Br J Radiol* 66:1035, 1993.

34. Hirschmann PN: Dose limitation in dental radiography, *Dent Update* 20:257, 1993.

35. Nixon PP, Robinson PB: Endodontic radiography, *Dent Update* 24:165, 1997.

36. Abdul Razak AA, Abdul Razak I: Accuracy of tooth length measurements from periapical radiographs, *Dent J Malays* 8:27, 1985.

37. Forsberg J: Radiographic reproduction of endodontic "working length" comparing the paralleling and the bisecting-angle techniques, *Oral Surg Oral Med Oral Pathol Oral Radiol Endod* 64:353, 1987.

38. Forsberg J: Estimation of the root filling length with the paralleling and bisecting-angle techniques performed by undergraduate students, *Int Endod J* 20:282, 1987.

39. Girsch WJ, Matteson SR, McKee MN: An evaluation of Kodak Ektaspeed periapical film for use in endodontics, *J Endod* 9:282, 1983.

40. Donnelly JC, Hartwell GR, Johnson WB: Clinical evaluation of Ektaspeed X-ray film for use in endodontics, *J Endod* 11:90, 1985.

41. Powell-Cullingford AW, Pitt Ford TR: The use of E-speed film for root canal length determination, *Int Endod J* 26:268, 1993.

42. Rushton VE et al: An in vitro comparison of 10 radiographic methods for working length estimation, *Int Endod J* 28:149, 1995.

43. Brown R, Hadley JN, Chambers DW: An evaluation of Ektaspeed Plus film versus Ultraspeed film for endodontic working length determination, *J Endod* 24:54, 1998.

44. Gound TC, DuBois L, Biggs SG: Factors that affect the rate of retakes for endodontic treatment radiography, *Oral Surg Oral Med Oral Pathol Oral Radiol Endod* 77:514, 1994.

45. Tamse A, Kaffe I, Fishel D: Zygomatic interference with correct radiographic diagnosis in maxillary molar endodontics, *Oral Surg Oral Med Oral Pathol Oral Radiol Endod* 50:563, 1980.

46. Khabbaz MG, Serefoglou MH: The application of the buccal object rule for the determination of calcified root canals, *Int Endod J* 29:284, 1996.

47. Goerig AC, Neaverth EJ: A simplified look at the buccal object rule in endodontics, *J Endod* 13:570, 1987.

48. Richards AG: The buccal object rule, *Dent Radiogr Photogr* 53:37, 1980.

49. Chenail B, Aurelio JA, Gerstein H: A model for teaching the buccal object moves most rule, *J Endod* 9:452, 1983.

50. VandeVorde HE, Bjorndahl AM: Estimating endodontic "working length" with paralleling radiographs, *Oral Surg Oral Med Oral Pathol Oral Radiol Endod* 27:106, 1969.

51. Thanyakarn C et al: Measurements of tooth length in panoramic radiographs. 1: the use of indicators, *Dentomaxillofac Radiol* 21:26, 1992.

52. Everett FG, Fixott HC: Use of an incorporated grid in the diagnosis of oral roentgenograms, *Oral Surg Oral Med Oral Pathol Oral Radiol Endod* 16:1061, 1963.

53. Ingle JI: Endodontic instruments and instrumentation, *Dent Clin North Am* p 805, Nov 1957.

54. Ong EY, Pitt Ford TR: Comparison of radiovisiography with radiographic film in root length determination, *Int Endod J* 28:25, 1995.

55. Leddy BJ et al: Interpretation of endodontic file lengths using radiovisiography, *J Endod* 20:542, 1994.

56. Versteeg KH et al: Estimating distances on direct digital images and conventional radiographs, *J Am Dent Assoc* 128:439, 1997.

57. Shearer AC, Horner K, Wilson NH: Radiovisiography for length estimation in root canal treatment: an in-vitro comparison with conventional radiography, *Int Endod J* 24:233, 1991.

58. Hedrick RT et al: Radiographic determination of canal length: direct digital radiography versus conventional radiography, *J Endod* 20:320, 1994.

59. Garlock JA et al: Measurement algorithm accuracy of the RVG-PCi in vertical and diagonal assessments at various beam energies, *J Endod* 22:646, 1996.

60. Sanderink GC et al: Image quality of direct digital intraoral x-ray sensors in assessing root canal length, *Oral Surg Oral Med Oral Pathol Oral Radiol Endod* 78:125, 1994.

61. Garcia AA et al: Evaluation of digital radiography to estimate working length, *J Endod* 23:363, 1997.

62. Velders XL, Sanderink GC, van der Stelt PF: Dose reduction of two digital sensor systems measuring file lengths, *Oral Surg Oral Med Oral Pathol Oral Radiol Endod* 81:607, 1996.

63. Kashima I et al: Intraoral computed radiography using the Fuji computed radiography imaging plate. Correlation between image quality and reading condition, *Oral Surg Oral Med Oral Pathol Oral Radiol Endod* 78:239, 1994.

64. Digora: *Installation, setup, and user's guide,* Helsinki, Finland, 1995, Orion Corporation Soredex.

65. Cederberg RA et al: Endodontic working length assessment. Comparison of storage phosphor digital imaging and radiographic film, *Oral Surg Oral Med Oral Pathol Oral Radiol Endod* 85:325, 1998.

66. Borg E, Grondahl HG: Endodontic measurements in digital radiography acquired by a photostimulable storage phosphor system, *Endod Dent Traumatol* 12:20, 1996.

67. Brettle DS et al: The imaging performance of a storage phosphor system for dental radiography, *Br J Radiol* 69:256, 1996.

68. Higashi T et al: New intraoral x-ray fluorographic imaging for dentistry, *Oral Surg Oral Med Oral Pathol Oral Radiol Endod* 55:628, 1983.

69. Goldman M, Pearson AH, Darzenta N: Endodontic success—who's reading the radiograph?, *Oral Surg Oral Med Oral Pathol Oral Radiol Endod* 33:432, 1972.

70. Zakariasen KL, Scott DA, Jensen JR: Endodontic recall radiographs: how reliable is our interpretation of endodontic success or failure and what factors affect our reliability?, *Oral Surg Oral Med Oral Pathol Oral Radiol Endod* 57:343, 1984.

71. Sewerin I: Gagging in dental radiography, *Oral Surg Oral Med Oral Pathol Oral Radiol Endod* 58:725, 1984.

72. Burch JG, Hulen S: The relationship of the apical foramen to the anatomic apex of the tooth root, *Oral Surg Oral Med Oral Pathol Oral Radiol Endod* 34:262, 1972.

73. Palmer MJ, Weine FS, Healey HJ: Position of the apical foramen in relation to endodontic therapy, *J Can Dent Assoc* 8:305, 1971.

74. Beach CW, Bramwell JD, Hutter JW: Use of an electronic apex locator on a cardiac pacemaker patient, *J Endod* 22:182, 1996.

75. Woolley LH, Woodworth J, Dobbs JL: A preliminary evaluation of the effects of electric pulp testers on dogs with artificial pacemakers, *J Am Dent Assoc* 89:1099, 1974.

76. Sunada I: New method for measuring the length of the root canal, *J Dent Res* 41:375, 1962.

77. Huang L: An experimental study of the principle of electronic root canal measurement, *J Endod* 13:60, 1987.

78. Seidberg BH et al: Clinical investigation of measuring working lengths of root canals with an electronic device with digital-tactile sense, *J Am Dent Assoc* 90:379, 1975.

79. Kaufman AY et al: Reliability of different electronic apex locators to detect root perforations in vitro, *Int Endod J* 30:403, 1997.

80. Fuss Z, Assooline LS, Kaufman AY: Determination of location of root perforations by electronic apex locators, *Oral Surg Oral Med Oral Pathol Oral Radiol Endod* 82:324, 1996.

81. Kaufman AY, Keila S: Conservative treatment of root perforations using apex locator and thermatic compactor—case study of a new method, *J Endod* 15:267, 1989.

82. Nahmias Y, Aurelio JA, Gerstein H: Expanded use of the electronic canal length measuring devices, *J Endod* 9:347, 1983.

83. Knibbs PJ, Foreman PC, Smart ER: The use of an analog type apex locator to assess the position of dentine pins, *Clin Prev Dent* 11:22, 1989.

84. Kaufman AY, Keila S: Conservative treatment of root perforations using apex locator and thermatic compactor—case study of a new method, *J Endod* 15:267, 1989.

85. Hembrough JH et al: Accuracy of an electronic apex locator: a clinical evaluation in maxillary molars, *J Endod* 19:242, 1993.

86. Inoue N, Skinner DH: A simple and accurate way of measuring root canal length, *J Endod* 11:421, 1985.

87. Trope M, Rabie G, Tronstad L: Accuracy of an electronic apex locator under controlled clinical conditions, *Endod Dent Traumatol* 1:142, 1985.

88. Wu YN et al: Variables affecting electronic root canal measurement, *Int Endod J* 25:88, 1992.

89. Blank LW, Tenca JI, Pelleu GB, Jr: Reliability of electronic measuring devices in endodontic therapy, *J Endod* 1:141, 1975.

90. Busch LR et al: Determination of the accuracy of the Sono-Explorer for establishing endodontic measurement control, *J Endod* 2:295, 1976.

91. Fouad AF et al: Clinical evaluation of five electronic root canal length measuring instruments, *J Endod* 16:446, 1990.

92. Inoue N: An audiometric method for determining the length of root canals, *J Can Dent Assoc* 9:630, 1973.

93. Kaufman AY, Heling B, Sechaiek M: What apex does the Sono-Explorer really read?, *Quintessence Int* 12:63, 1979.

94. O'Neill LJ: A clinical evaluation of electronic root canal measurement, *Oral Surg Oral Med Oral Pathol Oral Radiol Endod* 38:469, 1974.

95. Felippe MCS, Soares IJ: In vitro evaluation of an audiometric device in locating the apical foramen in teeth, *Endod Dent Traumatol* 10:220, 1994.

96. Arora RK, Gulabivala K: An in vivo evaluation of the Endex and RCM Mark II electronic apex locators in root canals with different contents, *Oral Surg Oral Med Oral Pathol Oral Radiol Endod* 79:497, 1995.

97. Frank AL, Torabinejad M: An in vivo evaluation of Endex electronic apex locator, *J Endod* 19:177, 1993.

98. Lauper R, Lutz F, Barbakow F: An in vivo comparison of gradient and absolute impedance electronic apex locators, *J Endod* 22:260, 1996.

99. Ounsi HF, Haddad G: In vitro evaluation of the reliability of the Endex electronic apex locator, *J Endod* 24:120, 1998.

100. Czerw RJ et al: In vitro evaluation of the accuracy of several electronic apex locators, *J Endod* 21:572, 1995.

101. Dunlap CA et al: An in vivo evaluation of an electronic apex locator that uses the ratio method in vital and necrotic canals, *J Endod* 24:48, 1998.

102. Katz A, Mass E, Kaufman AY: Electronic apex locator: a useful tool for root canal treatment in the primary dentition, *ASDC J Dent Child* 63:414, 1996.

103. Pagavino G, Pace R, Baccetti T: A SEM study of in vivo accuracy of the Root ZX electronic apex locator, *J Endod* 24:438, 1998.

104. Shabahang S, Goon WW, Gluskin AH: An in vivo evaluation of Root ZX electronic apex locator, *J Endod* 22:616, 1996.

105. Vajrabhaya L, Tepmongkol P: Accuracy of apex locator, *Endod Dent Traumatol* 13:180, 1997.

106. Kobayashi C, Yoshioka T, Suda H: A new engine-driven canal preparation system with electronic canal measuring capability, *J Endod* 23:751, 1997.

107. Campbell D et al: Apical extent of rotary canal instrumentation with an apex-locating handpiece in vitro, *Oral Surg Oral Med Oral Pathol Oral Radiol Endod* 85:319, 1998.

108. Kobayashi C, Yoshioka T, Suda H: A new ultrasonic canal preparation system with electronic monitoring of file tip position, *J Endod* 22:489, 1996.

4

CANAL PREPARATION

KEITH V. KRELL

lthough complete débridement of all tissue and debris from the root canal system is the goal of root canal treatment, it is still an "impossible dream" given the current instruments, irrigants, and instrumentation techniques. The task of manipulating endodontic instruments along the length and circumference of a noncircular irregular space while maintaining the original canal shape and position within the root is difficult. The process of developing a cylindrical taper is complicated even more if the root and canal exhibit curvature.

The complexity of the preparation process can be demonstrated by looking at the cross-section of a "simple" mandibular central incisor. The canal(s) usually exhibit a ribbon shape when viewed in cross-section, and frequently have both a buccal and lingual canal that join at the apex.[1] The confluence of the two canals has an area that instruments cannot effectively clean, resulting in debris accumulation (Figures 4-1 and 4-2). In some instances, the initial canal diameter of these teeth may be less than the smallest instruments manufactured (less than 0.06 mm). Trying to débride these small canals without radically altering the existing canal morphology is a meticulous task.

With the more complex anatomy seen in a C-shaped mandibular second molar (Figure 4-3), the challenge of complete débridement becomes even more formidable because of irregularities such as fins and cul-de-sacs within the root canal system. These are areas that the instruments used for cleaning and shaping cannot reach.

Faced with complex canal morphology and current instrument technology, the crusade for the "holy grail" of complete débridement remains elusive. Although general guidelines exist for root canal preparation, each case presents unique characteristics requiring the clinician to vary the armamentarium and technique to clean and shape the root canal space without procedural errors. A variety of instrumentation techniques are discussed in this chapter as they relate to cleaning and shaping procedures.

CLEANING AND SHAPING

Traditional discussions of canal preparation have recognized cleaning and shaping as two distinct processes. Schilder used the terms *cleaning* to refer to the débridement of the root canal space and *shaping* as the step to prepare the canal for obturation.[2] During treatment a clear demarcation does not exist between these two concepts. All clinically accepted endodontic instruments and instrumentation techniques attempt to perform both processes concurrently.

Débridement of the root canal space includes removal of vital and necrotic tissue, bacteria, bacterial byproducts, and dentinal debris created during the cleaning and shaping process. Irrigation and disinfection are integral parts of débridement.

The principles of shaping are as follows[2]:

1. Develop a continuously tapering funnel from the apex to the coronal orifice.
2. Maintain the original shape of the canal.
3. Maintain the apical foramen in its original position.
4. Keep the apical opening as small as possible.

The principles related to shaping are universal and hold true for all obturation techniques, although some techniques may necessitate larger canal preparations to facilitate placement of the root canal filling.

Irrigants and Irrigation

All of the instrumentation techniques rely on the use of irrigants to help flush debris from the canal. The ideal

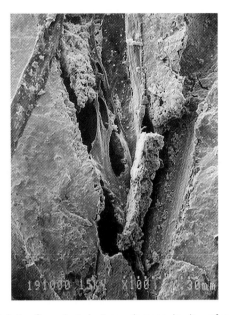

FIGURE 4-1 Scanning electron microscopic view of an unprepared type II canal in a mandibular incisor.

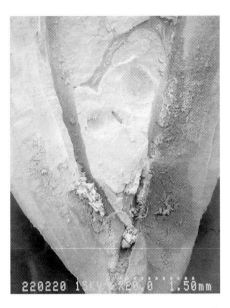

FIGURE 4-2 Scanning electron microscopic view of a prepared type II canal in a mandibular incisor. Note the areas of debris and uncleaned canal space.

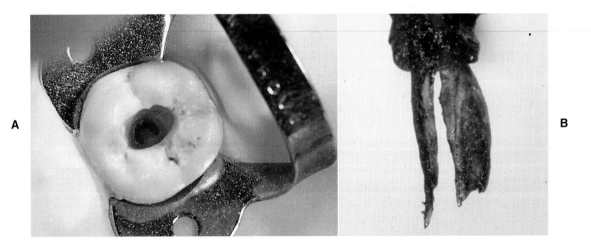

FIGURE 4-3 **A,** C-shaped morphology in this mandibular second molar complicates instrumentation. **B,** Resin cast of a C-shaped canal from a mandibular second molar.

irrigant should be nontoxic, capable of dissolving both vital and necrotic pulp tissue, kill bacteria, lubricate, and remove the smear layer.[3-10] At least one study has found that the smear layer seems to inhibit bacterial growth.[11] Presently, no single irrigant possesses all of these traits.

The most common intracanal irrigant used is sodium hypochlorite. Other irrigants that have been studied alone or in combination with sodium hypochlorite include 3% hydrogen peroxide, ethylenediaminetetraacetic acid (EDTA), citric acid, and lactic acid.[10,12-20]

Sodium hypochlorite has been shown to be an effective antimicrobial agent when placed in contact with bacteria.[21-23] However, bacteria are never totally eliminated because a sufficient volume of irrigant does not reach all aspects of the canal space or dentinal tubules.

To facilitate penetration of the canal system, the use of 27- or 28-gauge irrigating needles with a Luer-Lok syringe is suggested. As the apical preparation approaches a size 45 file, the ability of the solution to reach the apical extent of the canal through a 27-gauge needle improves.[24] One study comparing closed-tip needles with a side portal with other irrigation techniques found these syringe tips were the most effective in removing dye from plastic artificial canals.[25]

Sonic and ultrasonically activated devices are capable of delivering larger volumes of irrigant in smaller canals, but they require special equipment and instruments.[26,27] Few of these current vibrating devices are capable of delivering sodium hypochlorite because of its corrosive action on aluminum components.

Lubricating pastes are often employed in canal preparation with sodium hypochlorite. In addition to facilitating placement of the file, these pastes also entrap debris. Dentin chips are held in suspension and are less likely to be packed in the apical portion of the canal.

Instruments

Over the second half of the twentieth century, advances in endodontic instruments and techniques allowed millions of previously condemned teeth to be saved. The early pioneers in endodontics recognized the significance of complete débridement and disinfection of the canal space in ensuring eventual endodontic success. However, their initial selection of endodontic files and reamers from various manufacturers was limited. In a cooperative effort, both the American Dental Association (ADA) Council on Dental Materials and the American Dental Manufacturers worked together to develop instrument standardization and ADA specification No. 28.[28]

In the early 1970s, most accepted instrumentation techniques emphasized hand débridement with minimal use of handpiece-driven instruments except for orifice enlargement. Specification No. 28 was developed for hand-operated K-type files and reamers and was first published in 1976. This specification established tip diameter, taper (increase of diameter for each millimeter of length), torsional limits, and other physical attributes for files. Specification No. 58 was developed for Hedstrom files and was published in 1982.[29] Revised standards for specifications No. 28 and No. 58 were published in 1989.[30]

Presently, no approved standards are available for rotary instruments, but the American National Standard/ADA Council on Scientific Affairs has proposed Specification No. 95 for root canal enlargers.[31] This document is based largely on published reports from a Marquette University group that examined the torsional, bending, and metallurgical properties of all stainless steel engine– and carbon steel engine–driven endodontic enlargers.[32-36] No recognized standards are available for nickel-titanium instruments; however, the manufacturers must meet the United States Food and Drug Administration's (FDA's) Good Manufacturing Practice Regulations before introducing a new device.

The following discussion of canal preparation techniques assumes that all files or reamers are hand operated unless otherwise stated. Instrumentation techniques that require specific instruments are identified at the time of their discussion.

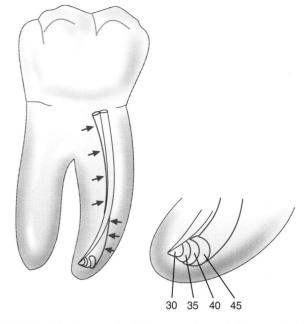

30 35 40 45

FIGURE 4-4 The standardized preparation technique resulted in procedural errors when used in a curved canal. Dentin was removed from the inner wall of the canal coronal to the curve and from the outer wall of the canal apical to the curve. This resulted in an "hourglass" preparation. In the apical portion the canal was transported, or "zipped," when larger, less flexible instruments were used at the correct working length.

Canal Preparation Techniques

From a historical perspective, clinical techniques tend to build on previously successful techniques. Therefore the various canal preparation techniques will be introduced in chronologic order, beginning with hand débridement techniques using stainless steel instruments. A few assumptions are made here to facilitate understanding of the differences among the techniques. These assumptions may not apply in actual clinical cases. The primary goal of all these techniques is to shape the canals to the apical constriction of the canal space, regardless of the radiographic appearance of the actual tooth. The guidelines for shaping outlined by Schilder are followed in this discussion.[2]

Before initiating any treatment, the clinician should evaluate each case and determine the degree of difficulty. As the complexity increases, the ability to clean and shape decreases, and the potential for procedural errors increases. Procedural errors include loss of working length, transportation of the apex (or zipping), apical perforation, lateral stripping, and instrument breakage (Figure 4-4). The following criteria are suggested for evaluation of cases before treatment:

Root length—Longer roots are generally more difficult to treat.
Root width—Narrow, curved roots are at risk for apical and lateral stripping perforations.

Canal size—Small canals are more difficult to prepare and may not exhibit any natural taper.

Canal curvature—Difficulty increases as curves progress from gentle to sharp dilacerations.

Calcifications—Calcification makes location and negotiation more difficult.

Resorptions—Resorptions present potential problems for negotiation, cleaning, shaping, and obturation.

Restorations—Restorations may change the orientation of the tooth in the dental arch, block canals, and restrict vision.

Previous treatment—Teeth exhibiting previous root canal treatment are more difficult to manage for a variety of reasons. Normal anatomic landmarks may have been removed, procedural errors may be present, and debris in the root canal system may be difficult to remove.

STANDARD TECHNIQUE.   John Ingle was a member of the first committee to propose standardization of endodontic instruments and introduced the classic "standardized preparation."[37] Standardized files were used sequentially to produce a canal preparation that had the same size and shape (taper) as the last standardized instrument used. The canal could then be obturated with a filling material that was also the same size and shape. Essentially, the canal was made to fit the filling material. At this same time, obturation with silver points having the same shape as the files was an accepted and popular obturation technique.

The technique was easy to perform in straight canals of mature teeth exhibiting natural taper but posed problems in small, curved canals. As the instruments got larger, the ability to finesse the stiff instruments to different lengths decreased because of the restoring force of the metal. This often resulted in ledging, apical transportation, and apical perforation, or "zipping" (see Figure 4-4).[38-40]

STEP-BACK TECHNIQUE.   The realization that curved canals may require less aggressive instrumentation resulted in the introduction of the step-back preparation technique.[41] Several comparative débridement studies have been performed that demonstrate the superiority of the step-back preparation over the standard technique.[42] The step-back technique emphasizes keeping the apical preparation small, in its original position, and producing a gradual taper. The working length is established and then the first file to bind is set as the master apical file (MAF). Subsequent larger files are introduced at 1-mm or shorter increments (Figure 4-5). After each step back, the canal is irrigated and the MAF replaced to the established working length to remove any loosened debris. The step-back "telescoped" preparation produces a canal with greater taper compared with the standard technique and results in more dentin removal and cleaner canal walls.[43,44]

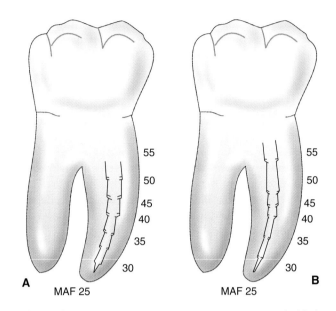

FIGURE 4-5   A, To reduce procedural errors encountered with the standardized preparation technique, the step-back technique was developed. After the working length and MAF were established, successive instruments were shortened by 1-mm increments and used to develop a more tapered preparation. **B,** Canal bed enlargement permits the development of a tapered preparation using a more flexible process. After working length determination and establishment of the MAF, successive instruments are introduced to the initial point of binding and then rotated one half turn. No attempt is made to force the instrument to the working length or artificial predetermined length.

As an alternative to the step-back preparation, Schilder advocated canal bed enlargement.[2] After determining the length determination and establishing the largest MAF, the clinician places the next larger instrument into the canal to the point of initial contact and rotates it one half turn. Force is not applied to the instrument in an apical direction and no effort is made to advance the instrument to the working length. The canal is then irrigated and the process repeated with increasingly larger instruments (see Figure 4-5). The technique allows the body of the canal to be prepared without the procedural errors inherent in the standardized preparation technique. In addition, the technique permits the natural morphology of the canal to influence the preparation, in contrast to the more ridged incremental step-back technique. After completion of the tapering process, Schilder advocates the use of Gates Glidden drills in the canal orifice to remove coronal obstructions.

Weine emphasized pre-curving files to minimize canal alteration. However, pre-curving does not guarantee total canal symmetry and alterations occur despite the best efforts of the clinician.[45-47]

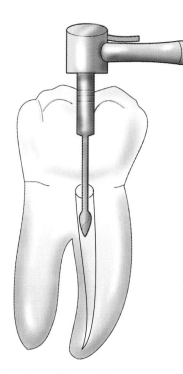

FIGURE 4-6   Gates Glidden drills are used in the coronal portion of the canal for orifice enlargement and straight line access. Before using the Gates Glidden drills, the clinician should evaluate the sizes of the canal and root as they relate to the diameter of the instrument.

FIGURE 4-7   Straight line access is facilitated by removing overhanging ledges of dentin before using the Gates Glidden drills. This can be accomplished by either slow- or high-speed instrumentation.

Later variations of the original step-back technique incorporated the use of Gates Glidden #2 , #3, and #4 drills to help gain straight line access to the apical third of the canal (Figure 4-6).[44,48,49] This facilitated the placing of a tapered instrument into the canal; previously, progress toward the apex was impeded when the diameter of the tapered file exceeded the diameter of the cylindrical canal. Before using Gates Glidden drills, the clinician facilitates access to the canal orifice by removing overlying dentinal structure (Figure 4-7).

Coronal enlargement before apical preparation provides straighter access to the apical region; eliminates interferences and canal irregularities in the coronal two thirds of the root; permits deeper placement of instruments that otherwise might not go to length; removes the bulk of tissue, debris, and microorganisms; and allows deeper penetration of irrigating solutions. One disadvantage of coronal enlargement and the use of Gates Glidden drills is the excessive removal of tooth structure. A comparison of the size of the Gates Glidden drills to standardized files is presented in Box 4-1. The routine use of #5 and #6 Gates Glidden instruments results in excessive removal of tooth structure and increases the incidence of stripping perforations in the furcation area.

The Gates Glidden drills are used after a size 25 MAF can be introduced to the corrected working length.

BOX 4-1

Comparison of Gates Glidden Drills with Standardized Files

GATES GLIDDEN DRILL	INSTRUMENT SIZE IN MILLIMETERS
#1	0.50
#2	0.70
#3	0.90
#4	1.10
#5	1.30
#6	1.50

After lubricating the chamber with an irrigant, a #2 bur is placed into the canal orifice and run at medium speed with a light force. The deepest penetration of the canal occurs with the #2 Gates Glidden. Next, the #3 Gates Glidden is used at a shorter length and directed to the perimeter of the canal (Figure 4-8). Finally, a #4 Gates Glidden is used to the depth of the head of the bur to finalize the straight line access. This step helps establish the space for the hand files to reach the apical third without interference.

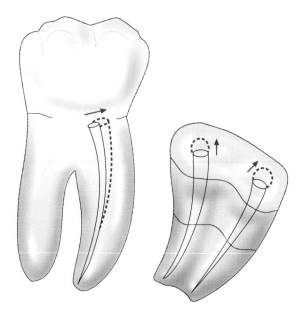

FIGURE 4-8 Although the #1 and #2 Gates Glidden drills are used to remove dentin uniformly from the canal walls, the #3 to #6 drills have the strength to permit lateral movement and selective removal of tooth structure away from the furcation or danger zone. Directing the Gates Glidden drill toward the line angles in molars enhances straight line access and reduces the risk of stripping perforations.

STEP-DOWN TECHNIQUE.   A variation on the timing of the use of the Gates Glidden drills was presented by Goerig.[50] He advocated using a #4 round bur to establish coronal access, followed by Hedstrom files size 15, 20, and 25 in the coronal two thirds of the estimated canal length. Only a filing or rasping motion is used and apical patency is maintained with a size #10 K-file. Patency should be checked as necessary. A #2 Gates Glidden drill is then used 14 to 16 mm in the canal, a #3 Gates Glidden is inserted 11 to 13 mm into the canal, and a #4 Gates Glidden is used as needed by the canal size. This procedure allows straight line access to the apical one third before active instrumentation takes place, thereby eliminating many of the interferences usually encountered.

Several studies have supported this general technique with respect to reducing procedural accidents such as stripping perforations and apical transportation. Greater apical enlargement without apical transportation can be achieved if coronal obstructions are eliminated.[51,52] One group of authors demonstrated significant improvement in tactility with files following coronal pre-flaring.[53] In a direct comparison between pre-flaring before the establishment of working length and flaring after working length establishment, Morgan and Montgomery found that the "crown-down pressureless" technique resulted in a rounder canal shape

significantly more often than when the step-back flaring technique was used.[54]

PASSIVE STEP-BACK TECHNIQUE.   The passive step-back technique developed by Torabinejad uses a combination of hand and rotary instruments to develop a flared preparation.[55] This technique provides gradual enlargement of the root in an apical to coronal direction without the application of force and reduces the risk of procedural accidents caused by transportation. It is a modification of the canal bed enlargement advocated by Schilder, in which shaping consisted of placing instruments larger than the MAF to a point of first binding and then using a reaming action to enlarge the coronal portion of the canal. This permits the morphology (shape) of the canal to influence the preparation and differs from the arbitrary step-back procedures of millimeter increments.[2]

The passive step-back technique involves establishing a corrected working length using a #15 file. The #15 file is inserted to the corrected working length with light pressure and then rotated one eighth to one quarter turn. Additional K-type files between #20 and #40 are then inserted passively as far as they will go and rotated one eighth to one quarter turn with light pressure. Gates Glidden drills (#2 to #4) are then used coronally, and apical preparation is accomplished. Narrow, curved canals should not be enlarged beyond a #25 or #30 file. The apical portion of the canal is prepared by placing sequentially larger files passively in the canal and rotating them one eighth to one quarter turn. Advantages to the passive step-back technique include knowledge of canal morphology, removal of debris and minor canal obstructions, and a gradual passive enlargement of the canal in an apical to coronal direction. With this process the canal morphology influences the preparation shape.

The passive step-back technique has also been advocated for use with ultrasonic instruments after the working length is established. Copious irrigation with sodium hypochlorite is suggested. A #15 endosonic file is passively placed in the canal, driven ultrasonically for 30 seconds, and worked circumferentially. Hand instruments are then introduced into the canal. This alternating use of ultrasonic and hand instruments is performed in a stepwise fashion until a mildly flared canal is achieved. A #2 Gates Glidden drill is then inserted until it binds, withdrawn 1 to 1.5 mm, and activated with an up-and-down motion. A #3 Gates Glidden drill is used after irrigation with 2.5% sodium hypochlorite. Working length is then reestablished, and the apical preparation is completed.

BALANCED FORCE TECHNIQUE.   The balanced force technique was developed and introduced by Roane.[56] This technique employs a unique instrument tip design and method of cutting dentin. One principle of the balanced

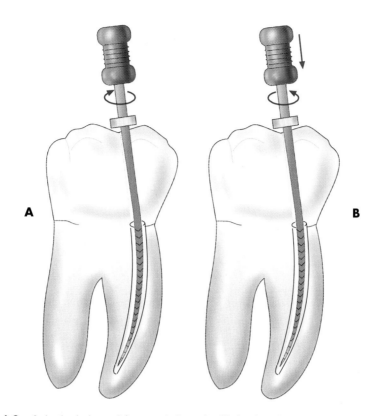

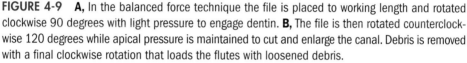

FIGURE 4-9 **A,** In the balanced force technique the file is placed to working length and rotated clockwise 90 degrees with light pressure to engage dentin. **B,** The file is then rotated counterclockwise 120 degrees while apical pressure is maintained to cut and enlarge the canal. Debris is removed with a final clockwise rotation that loads the flutes with loosened debris.

force technique is the recognition that traditional K-type files have pyramidal tips with cutting angles that can be quite aggressive with clockwise rotation. Roane modified traditional K-type files to reduce the transitional angle at the tip, producing a parabolic shape that alters the ability of the instrument to respond to distortion in a concentrated area. Forces are distributed over the file flutes and are not concentrated at the tip. The subsequent Flex-R (Union Broach, York, PA) file has a unique "safe" tip design with a guiding land area behind the tip that allows the file to follow canal curvature without binding in the outside wall of the curved canal. In addition, Roane advocated the use of a triangular cross-sectional instrument because the decreased mass of the instrument and its deeper cutting flutes improve flexibility and decrease the restoring force of the instrument when placed in a curved canal.

Before instrumentation, #1 to #6 Gates Glidden drills are used for straight line access. In balanced force instrumentation, the files cut in both clockwise and counterclockwise rotation. Instruments rotated in a clockwise direction tend to move apically as the instrument engages the dentinal wall, pulling the instrument into the canal. Instruments rotated in a counterclockwise direc-

tion tend to move coronally or out of the canal. Rotation of the instrument 120 degrees ensures that each blade reaches the beginning position of the initial blade and enlarges the entire canal.

In the balanced force technique the file is placed to working length and rotated clockwise 90 degrees with light pressure to engage the dentin (Figure 4-9). The file is then rotated counterclockwise 120 degrees while apical pressure is maintained to cut and enlarge the canal. Further counterclockwise rotation ensures enlargement of the full diameter of the canal. A final clockwise rotation then loads the flutes of the file with loosened debris, and the file is withdrawn. An advantage to the technique is the ability to manipulate the files at any point in the canal without ledging or blockage.

In small, curved canals, one study using extracted teeth demonstrated that the apical canal preparation up to a size 40 MAF remained centered in the original canal space in 80% of the cases.[57] Another study found less debris extrusion with the balanced force technique compared with step-back filing and endosonic filing.[58]

Overall, the technique has been shown to reduce canal transpiration compared with other techniques.[59-61] However, one shortcoming of the technique is that the use of #5 and #6 Gates Glidden drills results in a higher incidence of stripping perforations. Also, no clinical studies have demonstrated superior success rates over other techniques.[62]

NICKEL-TITANIUM INSTRUMENTS.   In 1988, researchers at Marquette University published a study examining endodontic files that had been fabricated from nitinol orthodontic wire for use as hand instruments.[63] Nickel–titanium (nitinol) alloy possesses a modulus of elasticity that is one fourth to one fifth that of stainless steel and has a wide range of elastic deformation, resulting in greater flexibility. An advantage of this increased flexibility is that the file follows the canal curvature with less deformation of the curvature during enlargement.[64] Better instrument centering in the apical preparation has been reported for both engine-driven and hand-manipulated nickel-titanium instruments.[65,66] A disadvantage of increased flexibility is the inability to pre-curve the file for introduction into canals of posterior teeth when the size of the interocclusal opening is decreased. Because of its greater elasticity, the cutting efficiency of nickel–titanium files may be reduced with clinical use compared with stainless steel.[67-69] Therefore, to take advantage of the properties of nickel–titanium files, engine–driven instruments have been developed. The present nickel–titanium instruments incorporate a U-shaped groove with a flat land area. When the instrument is rotated, the flutes plane the canal wall while the land area keeps the instrument centered, especially in fine, curved canals.[70-73]

As might be expected, instrumentation techniques with the newer nickel-titanium files have been evolutionary as well as revolutionary. After the initial introduction of nickel-titanium files, step-back preparations using hand files and engine-driven files were common. Dentsply, Tulsa Dental (Tulsa, OK) has always advocated the use of a "crown down" technique with their Profile brand instruments. However, changes in instrument design over the past several years have resulted in at least three different sets of instruments (Profile, Quantec, and Lightspeed) and subsequent instrumentation techniques (see Chapter 5).

EVALUATION OF CANAL PREPARATION TECHNIQUES

Several techniques have been advocated for the evaluation of root canal débridement and enlargement. Plastic blocks with uniform, preformed curves have been used by many researchers to evaluate the appearance of the canal before and after the instrumentation technique.[26,27,42,74] This methodology provides some answers to general questions of instrument action or irrigation patterns, but does not address concerns regarding the starting point for teeth with cross-sections and curves that are far more complex than the circular artificial

canal. In addition, these studies do not provide information regarding the cleaning phase of treatment.

Some researchers have performed histologic evaluations of remaining debris or pulp tissue while relying on estimates for dentinal walls that were planed.[44,75,76] The limitations of these studies lie in the fact that no method exists to "pre-test" for existing debris and therefore all results are post-test estimates. These histologic studies are extremely time-consuming and can also have artifacts from processing errors. They do not lend themselves to evaluation of the complete length of the canal.

An attempt at a "pre-test, post-test" model was developed by Bramante et al.[77] The model consisted of teeth that were mounted in dental stone or acrylic that could then be sectioned and reassembled in a jig.[77-79] This allows photographs or micrographs of the canal to be made before instrumentation. Post-instrumentation evaluation can then compare several of the aforementioned criteria with the differences found between the two photographs or micrographs. Limitations include tooth loss resulting from sectioning, a lack of precision in the instruments used to compare before and after instrumentation, and an inability to observe the entire length of the canal.

Recently a technique has been developed that eliminates many of the shortcomings of the previous studies. A three-dimensional, nondestructive technique for detailing root canal geometry by means of high-resolution tomography has been developed.[80] A micro-computed tomography scanner (microCT, cubic resolution of 34 microns) is used to record the precise canal anatomy before and after instrumentation. A three-dimensional analysis of root canal geometry by high-resolution computed tomography is then performed. The first report of this technique studied hand instrumentation with K-flex files, Lightspeed rotary instruments, Profile .04 taper rotary instruments, and GT rotary files. They found no differences in volume removed, canal straightening, and the amount of untreated area among the techniques. Significantly, they reported that all the techniques left more than a third of the canal surface uninstrumented.[81] This advance in the technology of canal preparation evaluation leads to only one conclusion—all instrumentation techniques fail to débride 100% of the canal space.

CLINICAL SIGNIFICANCE

Canal preparation is only one phase of endodontic treatment. Although current instruments and techniques vary, straight line access, step-back instrumentation, and apical preparation are three common concepts (Figure 4-10). Major differences in technique involve the order in which each step is accomplished and the instruments used. Although clinicians may use a specific process routinely, each case is unique and astute clinicians modify their techniques when necessary to achieve success.

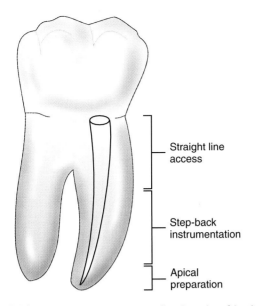

Straight line access

Step-back instrumentation

Apical preparation

FIGURE 4-10   Canal preparation can be thought of in three phases: 1) straight line access, 2) step-back instrumentation, and 3) apical preparation. Although the instruments used and order of these three steps may vary, the end result should be a tapered canal in its original position with a small apical opening.

The clinical success that occurs in endodontic practice far exceeds 66%, which is the theoretical predicted success if débridement is the only criterion for predicting success. The importance of adequately sealing the canal after débridement and then sealing the coronal space are integral parts of the process and undoubtedly contribute to the reported success rates in practice.[82-86]

References

1. Leuck M: Root canal morphology of human mandibular incisors and canines. In Bjorndal A, Skidmore AE, editors: *Anatomy and morphology of human teeth*, ed 2, Iowa City, IA, 1987, University of Iowa Press.
2. Schilder H: Cleaning and shaping the root canal, *Dent Clin North Am* 18(2):269, 1974.
3. Rosenfeld EF, James GA, Burch BS: Vital pulp tissue response to sodium hypochlorite, *J Endod* 4(5):140, 1978.
4. The SD: The solvent action of sodium hypochlorite on fixed and unfixed necrotic tissue, *Oral Surg Oral Med Oral Pathol Oral Radiol Endod* 47:558, 1979.
5. Baumgartner JC, Cuenin PR: Efficacy of several concentrations of sodium hypochlorite for root canal irrigation, *J Endod* 18(12):605, 1992.
6. Svec TA, Harrison JW: Chemomechanical removal of pulpal and dentinal debris with sodium hypochlorite and hydrogen peroxide vs normal saline solution, *J Endod* 3(2):49, 1977.
7. Foley DB et al: Effectiveness of selected irrigants in the elimination of *Bacteroides melaninogenicus* from the root canal system: an in vitro study, *J Endod* 9(6):236, 1983.
8. McComb D, Smith DC: A preliminary electron microscopic study of root canals after endodontic procedures, *J Endod* 1:238, 1975.
9. McComb D, Smith DC, Beagrie GS: The results of in vivo endodontic chemomechanical instrumentation—a scanning electron microscopic study, *J Br Endod Soc* 9(1):11, 1976.
10. Goldman LB et al: The efficacy of several irrigating solutions for endodontics: a scanning electron microscopic study, *Oral Surg Oral Med Oral Pathol Oral Radiol Endod* 52(2):197, 1981.
11. Drake DR et al: Bacterial retention in canal walls in vitro: effect of smear layer, *J Endod* 20(2):78, 1994.
12. Trepagnier CM, Madden RM, Lazzari EP: Quantitative study of sodium hypochlorite as an in vitro endodontic irrigant, *J Endod* 3(5):194, 1977.
13. Cecic PA, Peters DD, Grower MF: The comparative efficiency of final endodontic cleansing procedures in removing a radioactive albumin from root canal systems, *Oral Surg Oral Med Oral Pathol Oral Radiol Endod* 58(3):336, 1984.
14. Baumgartner JC, Mader CL: A scanning electron microscopic evaluation of four root canal irrigation regimens, *J Endod* 13(4):147, 1987.
15. Svec TA, Harrison JW: The effect of effervescence on débridement of the apical regions of root canals in single-rooted teeth, *J Endod* 7(7):335, 1981.
16. Gambarini G: Shaping and cleaning the root canal system: a scanning electron microscopic evaluation of a new instrumentation and irrigation technique, *J Endod* 25(12):800, 1999.
17. Behrend GD, Cutler CW, Gutmann JL: An in-vitro study of smear layer removal and microbial leakage along root-canal fillings, *Int Endod J* 29(2):99, 1996.
18. Takeda FH et al: A comparative study of the removal of smear layer by three endodontic irrigants and two types of laser, *Int Endod J* 32(1):32, 1999.
19. Yamaguchi M et al: Root canal irrigation with citric acid solution, *J Endod* 22(1):27, 1996.
20. Wayman BE et al: Citric and lactic acids as root canal irrigants in vitro, *J Endod* 5(9):258, 1979.
21. Grahnen H, Krasse B: The effect of instrumentation and flushing of non-vital teeth in endodontic therapy, *Odontol Rev* 14:167, 1963.
22. Bystrom A, Sundqvist G: Bacteriologic evaluation of the efficacy of mechanical root canal instrumentation in endodontic therapy, *Scand J Dent Res* 89(4):321, 1981.
23. Bystrom A, Claesson R, Sundqvist G: The antibacterial effect of camphorated paramonochlorophenol, camphorated phenol and calcium hydroxide in the treatment of infected root canals, *Endod Dent Traumatol* 1(5):170, 1985.
24. Ram Z: Effectiveness of root canal irrigation, *Oral Surg Oral Med Oral Pathol Oral Radiol Endod* 44(2):306, 1977.
25. Kahn FH, Rosenberg PA, Gliksberg J: An in vitro evaluation of the irrigating characteristics of ultrasonic and subsonic handpieces and irrigating needles and probes, *J Endod* 21(5):277, 1995.
26. Krell KV, Johnson RJ, Madison S: Irrigation patterns during ultrasonic canal instrumentation. Part I. K-type files, *J Endod* 14(2):65, 1988.
27. Krell KV, Johnson RJ: Irrigation patterns of ultrasonic endodontic files. Part II. Diamond-coated files, *J Endod* 14(11):535, 1988.
28. American Dental Association, Council on Dental Materials: New American Dental Association specification no. 28 for endodontic files and reamers, *J Am Dent Assoc* 93:813, 1976.
29. American Dental Association, Council on Dental Materials: ANSI/ADA specification no. 58 for root canal files, type H (Hedstrom), *J Am Dent Assoc* 104:88, 1982.
30. American Dental Association, Council on Dental Materials, Instruments and Equipment: Revised ANSI/ADA specifications no. 28 for root canal files and reamers, type K, and no. 58 for root canal files, type H (Hedstrom), *J Am Dent Assoc* 118:239, 1989.
31. American National Standard/American Dental Association, Council on Standards: *Proposed specification no. 95 for root canal enlargers*, Chicago, 2000, American Dental Association.

32. Luebke NH, Brantley WA: Physical dimensions and torsional properties of rotary endodontic instruments. 1. Gates Glidden drills, *J Endod* 16(9):438, 1990.

33. Luebke NH, Brantley WA: Torsional and metallurgical properties of rotary endodontic instruments. 2. Stainless steel Gates Glidden drills, *J Endod* 17(7):319, 1991.

34. Luebke NH et al: Physical dimensions, torsional performance, and metallurgical properties of rotary endodontic instruments. 3. Peeso drills, *J Endod* 18(1):13, 1992.

35. Luebke NH et al: Physical dimensions, torsional performance, bending properties, and metallurgical characteristics of rotary endodontic instruments. VI. Canal Master drills, *J Endod* 21(5):259, 1995.

36. Brantley WA et al: Performance of engine-driven rotary endodontic instruments with a superimposed bending deflection: V. Gates Glidden and Peeso drills, *J Endod* 20(5):241, 1994.

37. Ingle JI: A standardized endodontic technique using newly designed instruments and filling materials, *Oral Surg Oral Med Oral Pathol Oral Radiol Endod* 14:83, 1961.

38. Haga CS: Microscopic measurements of root canal preparations following instrumentation, *J Br Endod Soc* 2(3):41, 1969.

39. Jungmann CL, Uchin RA, Bucher JF: Effect of instrumentation on the shape of the root canal, *J Endod* 1:66, 1975.

40. Schneider SW: A comparison of canal preparations in straight and curved root canals, *Oral Surg Oral Med Oral Pathol Oral Radiol Endod* 32(2):271, 1971.

41. Clem WH: Endodontics: the adolescent patient, *Dent Clin North Am* 13(2):482, 1969.

42. Weine FS, Kelly RF, Lio PJ: The effect of preparation procedures on original canal shape and on apical foramen shape, *J Endod* 1(8):255, 1975.

43. Coffae KP, Brilliant JD: The effect of serial preparation versus nonserial preparation on tissue removal in the root canals of extracted mandibular human molars, *J Endod* 1(6):211, 1975.

44. Walton RE: Histologic evaluation of different methods of enlarging the pulp space, *J Endod* 2:304, 1976.

45. Weine FS et al: Pre-curved files and incremental instrumentation for root canal enlargement, *J Can Dent Assoc* 36(4):155, 1970.

46. Weine FS, Kelly RF, Bray KE: Effect of preparation with endodontic handpieces on original canal shape, *J Endod* 2(10):298, 1976.

47. Johnson WT: Instrumentation of the fine curved canals found in the mesial roots of maxillary and mandibular molars, *Quintessence Int* 17(5):309, 1986.

48. Weine F: *Endodontic therapy*, ed 5, St Louis, 1996, Mosby.

49. Mullaney TP: Instrumentation of finely curved canals, *Dent Clin North Am* 23(4):575, 1979.

50. Goerig AC, Michelich RJ, Schultz HH: Instrumentation of root canals in molars using the step-down technique, *J Endod* 8(12):550, 1982.

51. Abou-Rass M, Frank AL, Glick DH: The anticurvature filing method to prepare the curved root canal, *J Am Dent Assoc* 101(5):792, 1980.

52. Leeb J: Canal orifice enlargement as related to biomechanical preparation, *J Endod* 9(11):463, 1983.

53. Stabholz A, Rotstein I, Torabinejad M: Effect of preflaring on tactile detection of the apical constriction, *J Endod* 21(2):92, 1995.

54. Morgan LF, Montgomery S: An evaluation of the crown-down pressureless technique, *J Endod* 10(10):491, 1984.

55. Torabinejad M: Passive step-back technique. A sequential use of ultrasonic and hand instruments, *Oral Surg Oral Med Oral Pathol Oral Radiol Endod* 77(4):402, 1994.

56. Roane JB, Sabala CL, Duncanson, MG, Jr: The "balanced force" concept for instrumentation of curved canals, *J Endod* 11(5):203, 1985.

57. Southard DW, Oswald RJ, Natkin E: Instrumentation of curved molar root canals with the Roane technique, *J Endod* 13(10):479, 1987.

58. McKendry DJ: Comparison of balanced forces, endosonic, and step-back filing instrumentation techniques: quantification of extruded apical debris, *J Endod* 16(1):24, 1990.

59. Sabala CL, Roane JB, Southard LZ: Instrumentation of curved canals using a modified tipped instrument: a comparison study, *J Endod* 14(2):59, 1988.

60. Sepic AO et al: A comparison of Flex-R files and K-type files for enlargement of severely curved molar root canals, *J Endod* 15(6):240, 1989.

61. Backman CA, Oswald RJ, Pitts DL: A radiographic comparison of two root canal instrumentation techniques, *J Endod* 18(1):19, 1992.

62. Zuolo ML, Walton RE, Imura N: Histologic evaluation of three endodontic instrument/preparation techniques, *Endod Dent Traumatol* 8(3):125, 1992.

63. Walia HM, Brantley WA, Gerstein H: An initial investigation of the bending and torsional properties of Nitinol root canal files, *J Endod* 14(7):346, 1988.

64. Zmener O, Balbachan L: Effectiveness of nickel-titanium files for preparing curved root canals, *Endod Dent Traumatol* 11(3):121, 1995.

65. Glossen CR et al: A comparison of root canal preparations using Ni-Ti hand, Ni-Ti engine-driven, and K-Flex endodontic instruments, *J Endod* 21(3):146, 1995.

66. Esposito PT, Cunningham CJ: A comparison of canal preparation with nickel-titanium and stainless steel instruments, *J Endod* 21(4):173, 1995.

67. Camps JJ, Pertot WJ: Machining efficiency of nickel-titanium K-type files in a linear motion, *Int Endod J* 28(6):279, 1995.

68. Schafer E, Tepel J: Cutting efficiency of Hedstrom S and U files made of various alloys in filing motion, *Int Endod J* 29(5):302, 1996.

69. Schafer E, Lau R: Comparison of cutting efficiency and instrumentation of curved canals with nickel-titanium and stainless-steel instruments, *J Endod* 25(6):427, 1999.

70. Harlan AL, Nicholls JI, Steiner JC: A comparison of curved canal instrumentation using nickel-titanium or stainless steel files with the balanced-force technique, *J Endod* 22(8):410, 1996.

71. Coleman CL, Svec TA: Analysis of Ni-Ti versus stainless steel instrumentation in resin simulated canals, *J Endod* 23(4):232, 1997.

72. Short JA, Morgan LA, Baumgartner JC: A comparison of canal centering ability of four instrumentation techniques, *J Endod* 23(8):503, 1997.

73. Carvalho LA, Bonetti I, Borges MA: A comparison of molar root canal preparation using stainless-steel and nickel-titanium instruments, *J Endod* 25(12):807, 1999.

74. Wildey WL, Senia ES: A new root canal instrument and instrumentation technique: a preliminary report, *Oral Surg Oral Med Oral Pathol Oral Radiol Endod* 67(2):198, 1989.

75. Hill RL, del Rio CE: A histological comparison of the canal wall planing ability of two new endodontic files, *J Endod* 9(12):517, 1983.

76. Reynolds MA et al: An in vitro histological comparison of the step-back, sonic, and ultrasonic instrumentation techniques in small, curved root canals, *J Endod* 13(7):307, 1987.

77. Bramante CM, Berbert A, Borges RP: A methodology for evaluation of root canal instrumentation, *J Endod* 13(5):243, 1987.

78. Calhoun G, Montgomery S: The effects of four instrumentation techniques on root canal shape, *J Endod* 14(6):273, 1988.

79. Leseberg DA, Montgomery S: The effects of Canal Master, Flex-R, and K-Flex instrumentation on root canal configuration, *J Endod* 17(2):59, 1991.

80. Peters OA et al: Three-dimensional analysis of root canal geometry by high-resolution computed tomography, *J Dent Res* 79(6):1405, 2000.

81. Schöenberger K, Laib A, Peters O: Four NiTi canal preparation techniques evaluated by micro computed tomography, *Oral Res Poster Res Abstr* p 1, March 2000.

82. Sivers JE, Johnson WT: Restoration of endodontically treated teeth, *Dent Clin North Am* 36(3):631, 1992.

83. Orstavik D: Time-course and risk analyses of the development and healing of chronic apical periodontitis in man, *Int Endod J* 29(3):150, 1996.

84. Sjögren U et al: Influence of infection at the time of root filling on the outcome of endodontic treatment of teeth with apical periodontitis [published erratum appears in *Int Endod J* 31(2):148, 1998], *Int Endod J* 30(5):297, 1997.

85. Sundqvist G et al: Microbiologic analysis of teeth with failed endodontic treatment and the outcome of conservative re-treatment, *Oral Surg Oral Med Oral Pathol Oral Radiol Endod* 85(1):86, 1998.

86. Zmener O, Banegas G: Clinical experience of root canal filling by ultrasonic condensation of gutta-percha, *Endod Dent Traumatol* 15(2):57, 1999.

5

ROTARY CANAL PREPARATION

TY E. ERICKSON *and* WILLIAM T. JOHNSON

NICKEL-TITANIUM FILES

Traditional cleaning and shaping techniques employing hand instruments have a variety of steps, depend on the clinician's skill, and are often complex. Each canal is unique and requires adaptation of varied techniques for successful cleaning and shaping. Recent advances, including the use of nickel-titanium in instrument manufacture and the introduction of high-torque rotary handpieces, have made canal preparation less arduous and more standardized. Rotary instrumentation with nickel-titanium files results in a more uniform preparation with regard to taper and can enhance obturation by providing resistance.

The concept of rotary canal preparation is not new. Early systems employing traditional stainless steel instruments were found to produce procedural errors.[1] The introduction of instruments made of nickel-titanium has permitted the development of rotary instrumentation because nickel-titanium is two to three times more flexible than stainless steel and considerably more resistant to clockwise torsional stress.[2] Nickel-titanium instruments are as successful as stainless steel instruments in removing dentin and are more durable than stainless steel instruments.[3] The instruments do not corrode in the presence of sodium hypochlorite and are not affected by sterilization procedures.[4-8]

The main advantage to nickel-titanium instruments is that they permit canal preparation with less transportation and ledging.[9-17] Nickel-titanium rotary instruments also enhance the ability of the operator to shape the canal uniformly. The cleaning ability of nickel-titanium instruments is comparable to that of other instrumentation techniques. Moreover, sodium hypochlorite can be used as an adjunct to enhance the cleaning ability of these instruments.[18-21] Additional advantages of rotary instrumentation include reduced operator fatigue and improved efficiency.

Regardless of the system employed, rotary nickel-titanium instrumentation is not indicated for all cases. Rotary instruments should not be used in cases where calcifications, ledges, severe curvatures, canals with a type II configuration, and S-shaped canals are present.

When employing nickel-titanium instruments, the operator must clean the files frequently to prevent the buildup of debris and use a lubricant to reduce friction. Instruments should not be extended beyond the apical foramen in curved canals because their tips will no longer have circumferential dentin to guide them.

Nickel-titanium instruments are in the austenite phase at rest. When deformed under stress they convert to the martensite phase.[22] While they are in this phase the instruments are more prone to permanent deformation and fracture. Fracture can occur with no visible defects in the instruments, making visual inspection an unreliable method of instrument evaluation.[23] For this reason the instruments' life spans are limited and they should generally be discarded after five clinical cases.[24] In difficult cases the instruments should be used only once. When visible evidence of damage is evident the instrument must be discarded immediately.

Fracture can occur from torsional or flexural fatigue.[25] Torsional fatigue occurs when a portion of the instrument locks in the canal and the shaft continues to rotate. This frequently occurs with small files that bind at the tip. Large files are more likely to tolerate greater forces. Flexural fracture is related to work hardening the instrument, which causes metal fatigue. Fracture occurs as the instrument rotates in a curved canal until it reaches a maximal point of flexure. Larger instruments are more likely to fail in this manner. Evidence suggests that instruments are less prone to fracture when the rotational speed is decreased.[26,27]

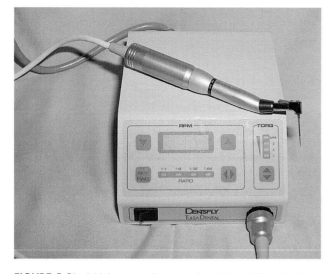

FIGURE 5-1   A high-torque, low-rpm electric handpiece designed for nickel-titanium rotary instrumentation.

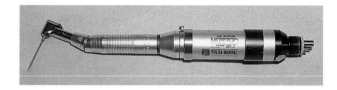

FIGURE 5-2   A high-torque, low-rpm air-driven handpiece designed for nickel-titanium rotary instrumentation.

To facilitate rotary instrumentation, high-torque low-RPM handpieces have been developed. Electric (Figure 5-1) and air-driven handpieces (Figure 5-2) are available and perform equally well in regard to file distortion and breakage, with the speed of operation being the most significant factor in these failures.[28] The type of handpiece used does not appear to be as important as the force applied and the operational speed. Some electric handpieces can sense instrument stress and reverse when their limits are exceeded. Quiet operation is an additional advantage of electric handpieces.

The sequential insertion of files with a standardized .02 taper ensures that each file inserted into the canal has maximal contact with the canal walls throughout the working length of the instrument. This contact induces frictional resistance on rotation. The principle of sequential insertion applies to rotary canal preparation techniques. However, nickel-titanium instruments can separate if they are stressed during rotation. As the surface area of contact between the file and the canal wall increases, so too does the frictional resistance and the force required to rotate the file, thereby increasing the potential for fracture. A variety of tapered nickel-titanium instruments used in a crown-down method reduces the contact area and therefore the frictional resistance and stress. In addition, the flute design of the instruments aids in removal of debris and the decreased cutting length of the files reduces stress.

Nickel-titanium instruments fail at a lesser torque compared with stainless steel instruments of the same size.[29] This means nickel-titanium fails under lighter pressure. Although stainless steel files often give a visual clue that stress has occurred, nickel-titanium files fail without warning. Inspection of the files should be performed with magnification.[28]

Most rotary systems employ a crown-down approach. With this technique the canal is cleaned and shaped as the coronal structure is removed. The crown-down technique provides space for succeeding instruments to pass unobstructed to the unprepared apical portion of the root. As coronal space is created, interferences are removed. Therefore when the radicular portion of the canal is prepared, the instruments tend to center in the canal and remove dentin uniformly. This reduces procedural errors such as ledging, zipping, and apical perforation. An additional advantage to the crown-down approach is that it causes less extrusion of debris through the apex.[30,31] Evidence suggests that clinicians should exercise care when using .04 tapered instruments because file contact with dentin is concentrated at the tip.[32]

PROFILE INSTRUMENTS

The nickel-titanium files manufactured by Dentsply/Tulsa Dental (Tulsa, OK) exhibit a cross-sectional configuration consisting of three radial lands. These keep the instruments centered in the canal and plane or scrape the canal walls during use.[33] U-shaped flutes that remove debris separate the radial lands. A non-cutting pilot tip provides guidance to the instruments.

Profile 29 Series

The Profile 29 series of instruments has a progressive 29% increase in diameter size at D_0. The first eight files replace the 11 files necessary with the traditional size 0.10 through 0.60 files. The instruments are better spaced, with more instruments in smaller sizes (where procedural errors occur) and fewer large instruments. The transition between sizes is enhanced by a more gradual increase in diameter. The clinician should keep in

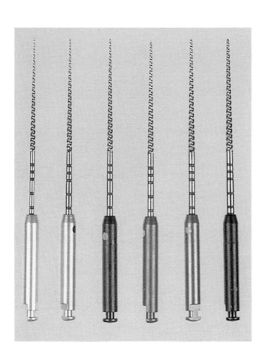

FIGURE 5-3   Profile .04 tapered instruments, sizes 15 to 40.

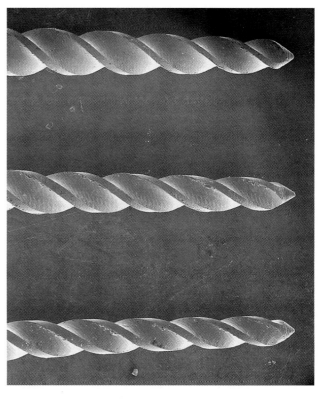

FIGURE 5-4   Scanning electron microscopic view of 25/.02 *(bottom)*, 25/.04 *(middle)*, and 25/.06 *(top)* Profile instruments.

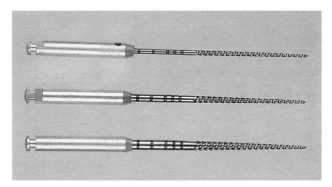

FIGURE 5-5   Profile 15/.02 *(top),* 15/.04 *(middle),* and 15/.06 *(bottom)* instruments. Note the standardized tip diameter and increased taper of the files.

mind that the percent difference in diameter from a traditional size 10 file and a size 15 file is 50%, whereas the difference between a size 55 and a size 60 instrument is only 9%. The first five Profile 29 instruments exhibit narrower diameters at D_0 compared with traditional files.

Profile .02, .04, and .06 Tapered Instruments

The Profile .02, .04, and .06 series of instruments are manufactured to International Standards Organization (ISO) standards with regard to tip diameter (Figure 5-3). The instruments differ only in regard to taper (Figure 5-4). The 25/.02 file has a diameter at D_{16} of 0.57 mm, the 25/.04 instrument has a diameter at D_{16} of 0.89 mm, and the 25/.06 instrument has a diameter of 1.21 mm at D_{16} (Figure 5-5). As the taper of the instruments used increases, the shape of the preparation becomes fuller.[30] The instrument design incorporates radial lands in the flute design (Figure 5-6). In cases of fine, curved canals the .04 (Figure 5-7) and .06 (Figure 5-8) tapered instruments produce excellent clinical results.

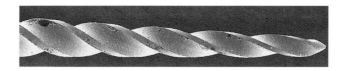

FIGURE 5-6   Scanning electron microscopic view of a Profile 25/.04 instrument with radial lands.

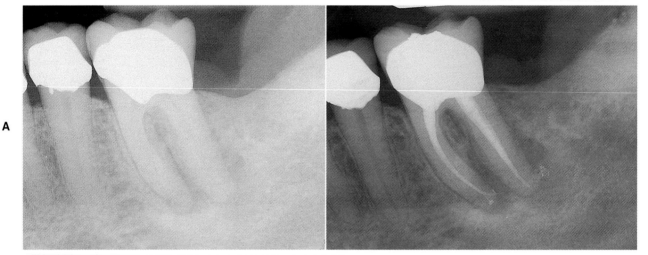

FIGURE 5-7   Preoperative **(A)** and postoperative **(B)** radiographs of a right mandibular first molar prepared with Profile .04 tapered instruments.

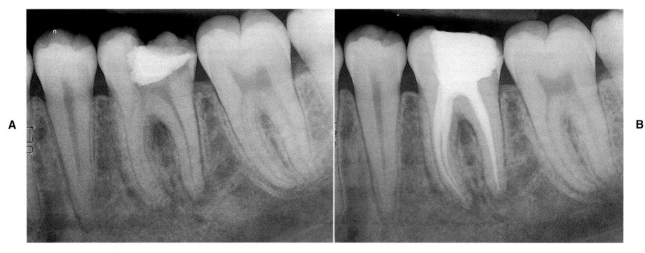

FIGURE 5-8   Preoperative **(A)** and postoperative **(B)** radiographs of a right mandibular first molar prepared with Profile .06 tapered instruments.

Greater Taper Series

The original Profile GT starter kit consists of the standard GT series of instruments, Profile .04 tapered files, and the accessory GT instruments. The standard series is composed of three instruments with 0.06-, 0.08-, and 0.10-mm tapers. The tip diameter of these files remains constant at 0.20 mm. The maximum file diameter is 1.0 mm (Figure 5-9). The instruments exhibit variable taper and variably pitched flutes. The GT files have K-type flute angles at the tip and open, reamer-type flute angles near the shank to preserve strength.[33] This makes the instruments more aggressive and the bulk of metal provides strength. The flute length decreases as the taper increases, and the instruments exhibit radial lands (Figure 5-10). The Profile .04 instruments have files with tip diameters of 0.20, 0.25, 0.30, and 0.35 mm. The accessory GT series has three instruments that are employed when apical diameters exceed 0.3 mm. These instruments can also be used to enlarge the coronal portion of smaller canal systems. The instruments exhibit a common taper of 0.12 mm and the same maximum file diameter of 1.5 mm. The three accessory GT instruments have varied tip diameters of 0.35, 0.50, and 0.70 mm. Typically used in large canals, their increased taper and reduction in flute length on the shaft minimize the area of contact with dentin and subsequent potential for fracture. The GT accessory series tends to produce parallel canal walls coronal to the flutes because of the fixed maximum diameter and short length of the flutes.

A technique advocated by the manufacturer of the Profile GT starter kit (Figure 5-11) involves using the 20/.10 (red), 20/.08 (yellow), and 20/.06 (white) tapers sequentially in a crown-down fashion at 300 rpm. Each instrument is used until resistance is encountered. When the files have reached one half to two thirds of the estimated root length, the clinician can determine the working length. Profile .04 tapers with standardized tip diameters 35/.04 (green), 30/.04 (blue), 25/.04 (red), and 20/.04 (gold) are then employed in a crown-down manner (Figure 5-12). They should be operated at 150 rpm.[27] Clinicians should exercise care when using the .04 tapered instruments because evidence suggests that the area of file contact during use of these instruments is at the tip.[34] For canals with large apical diameters the accessory GT series can be employed.

Recent developments to the original greater taper files include improved flute geometry; the creation of 13-mm instruments for easy introduction in posterior teeth; the development of the 20, 30, and 40 Series ProSystem GT files (each with tapers of 0.04, 0.06, 0.08, and 0.10 mm to facilitate shaping small, medium, and large canals); and modifications to the 35/.12 accessory file that decrease the maximum shank diameter from 1.5 to 1.25 mm so the instrument can be used in the large canals of molars (palatal canals of maxillary molars and distal canals of mandibular molars).[35] In addition, a standardized marking system has been introduced for easy identification of the taper and tip configuration of the instruments. The standard series of GT files was

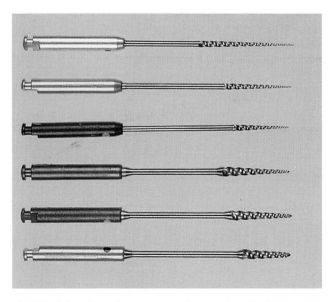

FIGURE 5-9   Files of greater taper. Standard Profile GT files (Silver 20/.06, Gold 20/.08, Red 20/.10) and Profile GT accessory files (Green 35/.12, Brown 50/.12, and Gold 70/.12).

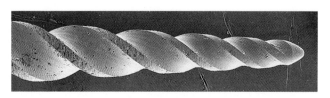

FIGURE 5-10   Scanning electron microscopic view of a Profile GT instrument.

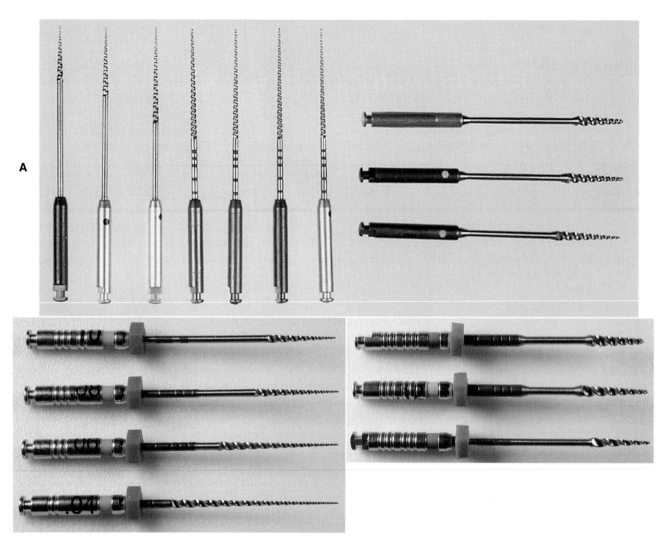

FIGURE 5-11 **A,** Profile GT starter kit. From *left* to *right:* Red 20/.10, Gold, 20/.08, Silver 20/.06, Green 35/.04, Blue 30/.04, Red 25/.04, Gold 20/.04. Profile GT accessory files, from *bottom* to *top:* Green 35/.12, Brown 50/.12, and Gold 70/.12. **B,** The ProSystem 20 series. The instrument tips are 0.20 mm and the instruments have (from *top* to *bottom*) tapers of .10, .08, .06, and .04. Note the color coding for tip diameter and markings for instrument taper. Each ring represents a taper of 0.02 mm. The ProSystem 30 and 40 series instruments are similar, with tip diameters of 0.30 and 0.40 mm, respectively. **C,** The ProSystem GT accessory series consists of instruments with (from *top* to *bottom*) tip diameters of 0.70 mm, 0.50 mm, and 0.35 mm. The taper is 0.12 mm for each instrument, as designated by the six rings.

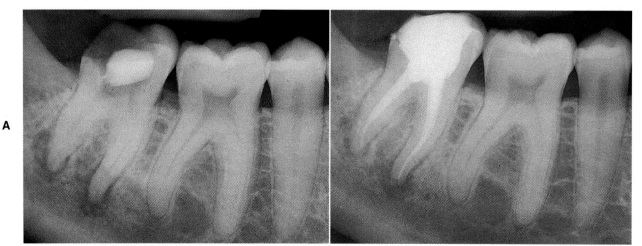

FIGURE 5-12 Preoperative **(A)** and postoperative **(B)** radiographs of a left mandibular second molar prepared with the Profile GT Starter Kit.

TABLE 5-1

General Guidelines for Canal Size by Tooth Group

SMALL CANALS	MEDIUM CANALS	LARGE CANALS
Mandibular incisors Buccal roots of maxillary molars Mesial roots of mandibular molars	Maxillary premolars Mandibular first premolars	Maxillary central incisors Maxillary lateral incisors Maxillary canines Mandibular canines Palatal roots of maxillary molars Distal roots of mandibular molars

modified to include the .04 tapered instrument in addition to the 0.06-, 0.08-, and 0.10-mm tapers.

The crown-down technique with the new ProSystem GT files is designed to provide a uniform predefined shape to the prepared canal while reducing the potential for procedural errors.[35] Because each case is unique, a pretreatment assessment of the final size and shape of the canal is required. The largest file projected for use at the working length, termed the *shaping objective file,* depends on canal anatomy and morphology.[35] This preclinical assessment can be modified during the procedure as more accurate information on canal morphology is obtained.

The primary objective in shaping is to develop a continuous funnel from the orifice to the corrected working length. Establishing adequate taper during the shaping process facilitates obturation and ensures that resistance form is present for obturation. The process begins with an assessment of the canal size and shape. Although general guidelines are presented in Table 5-1, canal size depends on many factors and the clinician should analyze each tooth as projected on a parallel preoperative radiograph. The initial series of instruments can then be selected based on this assessment (Table 5-2).

For cases with small canals, shaping begins with straight-line access to the canal orifice. The canal is then negotiated with standardized 08/.02 and 10/.02 ISO tapered files. If the small files fail to negotiate the canal, the clinician can use a passive step-back procedure to create coronal space for tapered #8 and #10 instruments. The 20/.10 GT file can then be used with light pressure. When the file can progress no further, the 20/.08 GT file is used. This instrument is followed by the GT 20/.06 and then the GT 20/.04. The crown-down process continues until the desired shape has been achieved.

After performing a crown-down preparation with ProSystem GT files, the clinician must evaluate the canal to ensure that adequate taper has been established. This process is termed *apical gauging* and is accomplished by using .02 tapered standardized stainless steel instruments.[35] Because of the coronal taper established by the GT files, the standardized ISO instruments bind only at their tips. The placement of a size #20 standardized ISO

TABLE 5-2

Instrument Tip and Taper Selection for Root Canal Preparation Based on Canal Size and Shape

SMALL CANALS	MEDIUM CANALS	LARGE CANALS
20/.10	30/.10	40/.10
20/.08	30/.08	40/.08
20/.06	30/.06	40/.06
20/.04	30/.04	40/.04

file to the corrected working length and the confirmation of file binding confirm that the apical terminus has a diameter of 0.2 mm. Adequate taper can then be confirmed by placing size #25 and #30 files into the canal to detect binding short of the corrected working length.

When the size #20 file goes beyond the corrected working length or binding fails to occur after shaping with GT files, the apical size of the canal is greater than 0.2 mm. Successively larger instruments are then placed until binding occurs. This assessment of the size of the apical terminus indicates which ProSystem GT series should be used at the corrected working length to establish adequate taper. The 30 series GT files, the 40 series GT files, and the accessory series GT files are useful in these cases. After using additional GT files, the clinician should perform apical gauging and confirmation of taper to ensure the presence of resistance before obturation. For medium and large canals the process of apical gauging is the same, but larger instruments consistent with the increased tip diameter are employed.

Files of greater taper are also manufactured as hand instruments. These are usually used in conjunction with rotary instruments and produce the same standardized shape during root canal preparation.

The use of a combination of GT rotary and hand instruments is an option. Hand files may be used for

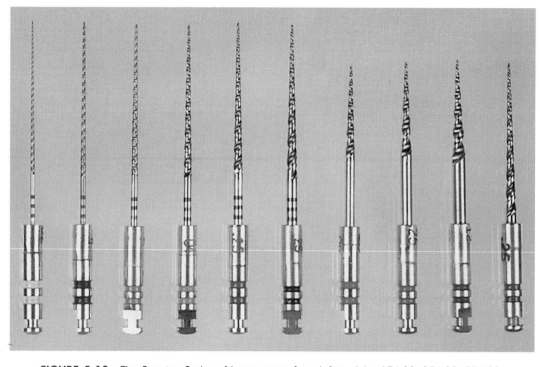

FIGURE 5-13 The Quantec Series of instruments, from *left* to *right:* 15/.02, 25/.02, 25/.03, 25/.04, 25/.05, 25/.06, 25/.08, 25/.10, 25/.12, and 25/.06.

preparation of the apical portion of the canal after coronal use of rotary instruments. Some clinicians employ traditional hand preparation techniques, including the use of Gates Glidden drills, to prepare the radicular space and then use rotary instruments to establish the final shape (taper). The use of GT rotary instruments as a finishing technique enhances the selection of the master cone and facilitates obturation.

ProSystem GT files facilitate obturation with predefined gutta-percha points during warm vertical condensation. Pluggers are available with the System B heat source that are consistent with the taper of the preparation produced by rotary instruments. The uniform taper of the prepared canal and the correlation of the gutta-percha and the plugger to the preparation enhance the hydraulics of warm vertical compaction.

In addition, the ProSystem GT technique combines the use of rotary files with GT obturators. These carrier-based gutta-percha obturators are integrated with the appropriate size rotary files.

Quantec Series

The Quantec series of instruments consists of 10 files made of nickel-titanium (Figure 5-13). The instruments are designed to be used in a high-torque, slow-speed handpiece at 340 RPM. The design of the instruments and the sequence of their use limit the contact surface of the instrument with the canal wall. This is accomplished primarily by the different tapers incorporated into the instruments. The instruments differ from the Profile and Lightspeed instruments (Lightspeed, San Antonio, TX) in that they have a slightly positive rake angle to the cutting flute (Figure 5-14).

The primary Quantec technique employs a three-step process of early orifice enlargement, apical preparation, and merging of the orifice enlargement with apical preparation.[34] An operational speed of 340 RPM is recommended. Orifice enlargement is accomplished with the No. 1 instrument, which has a size 25 tip and exhibits a .06 taper (25/.06). The file is passively advanced in 1-mm increments until pressure is necessary to advance the instrument. Stage two consists of apical preparation. The No. 2 Quantec file with a size 15 tip and conventional .02 taper is used to reach the estimated working length. After establishing the corrected working length, the clinician uses the No. 3 file 20/.02 and the No. 4 file 25/.02 at length. Stage three consists of merging the coronal and apical preparations by flaring the body of the canal. The instruments used in this treatment process all have size 25 tips. The instruments differ in that each file has an increasing taper. The No 5 file has a .03 taper, the No. 6 file has a .04 taper, the No. 7 file has a .05 taper, and the No. 8 file has a .06 taper. Each instrument is used

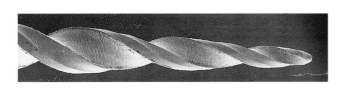

FIGURE 5-14   A scanning electron microscopic view of a Quantec instrument.

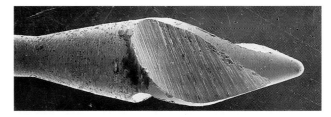

FIGURE 5-15   A scanning electron microscopic view of a Lightspeed instrument. Note the radial lands and non-cutting pilot tip.

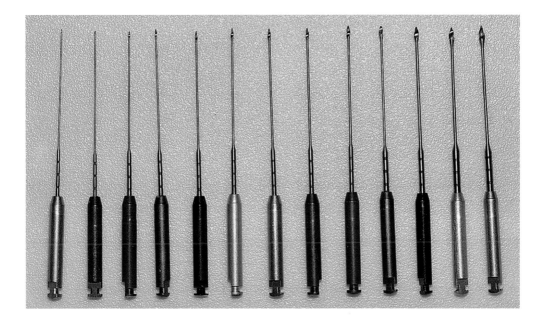

FIGURE 5-16   The Lightspeed series of files.

sequentially to working length. The final two files are used to finish cases when a larger apical preparation is desired. The No. 9 file has a size 40 tip with a conventional .02 taper and is used approximately 1 mm short of working length. The No. 10 instrument has a size 45 instrument tip and a .02 taper. This instrument is used circumferentially to blend irregularities and canal imperfections.

An alternative technique employs a crown-down technique with a sequence of No. 8, No. 7, No. 6, No. 5, No. 4, and No. 3 files. The Quantec Flare (Analytic Endodontics, Sybron Dental Specialties, Orange, CA) series of instruments can be used to facilitate coronal flaring. These instruments have a size 25 tip and tapers of 1.2, 1.0, and .08; they are used sequentially in a crown-down approach.

Advantages to the crown-down technique include reduction of procedural errors, a more uniform preparation and canal shape, coronal removal of debris, reduction of stress on the instruments and operator, and improved efficiency.

Lightspeed

Lightspeed nickel-titanium instruments are similar in appearance to Gates Glidden drills. The U-file design incorporates radial lands, a neutral rake angle, and a non-cutting pilot tip (Figure 5-15). The instruments are manufactured with tip diameters from 20 to 100, with half sizes from 22.5 to 65 (Figure 5-16). The parallel non-cutting shaft provides flexibility and limits the surface area of contact during rotation. The instruments are used at 750 to 2000 RPM, a relatively high speed compared with the Profile and Quantec systems.

The Lightspeed technique requires coronal flaring with Gates Glidden drills, as well as establishment of working length. Apical patency is established with a size 15 file. After this the clinician establishes the size of the canal at working length by placing Lightspeed instruments into the canal, beginning with the size #20 and progressing sequentially through larger sizes, until the first instrument to bind at length is determined. This procedure establishes canal size before preparation and is designated the *first Lightspeed to bind* (FLSB). To speed the process of finding the FLSB, the manufacturer provides guidelines for beginning the process for each tooth group (Table 5-3). Canal preparation begins with the next largest instrument. Rotation of the instrument should be continuous at a recommended speed of 750 to 2000 RPM, with 1300 to 2000 RPM being preferred. The instruments are gently advanced and withdrawn. After encountering resistance the clinician uses a light "pecking" motion to advance the instrument. Instruments should always be in motion and never left in one place. Enlargement of the canal is accomplished by using instruments in sequential order until the master apical rotary (MAR) file is reached. The MAR is defined as the Lightspeed instrument that requires a minimum of 12 "pecks" to reach the working length. After reaching the MAR, the clinician uses the next four instruments in a step-back manner at 1-mm increments. The fifth largest instrument is placed in the canal until it binds and then advanced apically with four light pecks. Recapitulation is accomplished with the MAR. An advantage to the Lightspeed technique is that it preserves tooth structure because the canal does not become extensively tapered. This minimal tapering preserves dentin and tooth strength.

TABLE 5-3

Lightspeed Guidelines for Establishing the First Lightspeed Size to Bind (FLSB) and the Master Apical Rotary (MAR) File

TOOTH TYPE OR GROUP	FLSB	MAR
MAXILLARY		
Maxillary central incisor	45	70
Maxillary lateral incisor	35	60
Maxillary canine	35	60
Maxillary first premolar	35	60
Maxillary second premolar	30	50
Maxillary molars		
Buccal canal	25	40
Palatal canal	30	50
MANDIBULAR		
Mandibular incisor	30	60
Mandibular canine	30	55
Mandibular premolar	30	55
Mandibular first molar		
Mesial canal	25	40
Distal canal	30	50
Mandibular second molar		
Mesial canal	25	45
Distal canal	30	50

References

1. Turek T, Langeland K: A light microscopic study of the efficacy of the telescopic and the Giromatic preparation of root canals, *J Endod* 8:437, 1982.
2. Walia H, Brantley WA, Gerstein H: An initial investigation of bending and torsional properties of nitinol root canal files, *J Endod* 14:346, 1988.
3. Kazemi RB, Stenman E, Spangberg LS: Machining efficiency and wear resistance of nickel-titanium endodontic files, *Oral Surg Oral Med Oral Pathol Oral Radiol Endod* 81:596, 1996.
4. Busslinger A, Sener B, Barbakow F: Effects of sodium hypochlorite on nickel-titanium Lightspeed instruments, *Int Endod J* 31:290, 1998.
5. Stokes OW et al: Corrosion in stainless-steel and nickel-titanium files, *J Endod* 25:17, 1999.
6. Mize SB et al: Effect of sterilization on cyclic fatigue of rotary nickel-titanium endodontic instruments, *J Endod* 24:843, 1998.
7. Canalda-Sahli C, Brau-Aguade E, Sentis-Vilalta J: The effect of sterilization on bending and torsional properties of K-files manufactured with different metallic alloys, *Int Endod J* 31:48, 1998.
8. Hilt R et al: Torsional properties of stainless steel and nickel-titanium files after multiple autoclave sterilization, *J Endod* 26:76, 2000.
9. Zmener O, Balbachan L: Effectiveness of nickel-titanium files for preparing curved root canals, *Endod Dent Traumatol* 11:121, 1995.
10. Royal JR, Donnelly JC: A comparison of maintenance of canal curvature using balanced-force instrumentation with three different file types, *J Endod* 21:300, 1995.
11. Glossen CR et al: A comparison of root canal preparations using Ni-Ti hand, Ni-Ti engine-driven, and K-Flex endodontic instruments, *J Endod* 21:146, 1995.
12. Esposito PT, Cunningham CJ: A comparison of canal preparation with nickel-titanium and stainless steel instruments, *J Endod* 21:173, 1995.
13. Pertot WJ, Camps J, Damiani MG: Transportation of curved canals prepared with Canal Master U, Canal Master U NiTi, and stainless steel K-type files, *Oral Surg Oral Med Oral Pathol Oral Radiol Endod* 79:504, 1995.
14. Shadid DB, Nicholls JI, Steiner JC: A comparison of curved canal transportation with balanced force versus Lightspeed, *J Endod* 24:651, 1998.
15. Short JA, Morgan LA, Baumgartner JC: A comparison of canal centering ability of four instrumentation techniques, *J Endod* 23:503, 1997.
16. Portenier I, Lutz F, Barbakow F: Preparation of the apical part of the root canal by the Lightspeed and step-back techniques, *Int Endod J* 31:103, 1998.
17. Thompson SA, Dummer PM: Shaping ability of Quantec Series 2000 rotary nickel-titanium instruments in simulated root canals: part 1, *Int Endod J* 31:259, 1998.
18. Siqueira JF, Jr, et al: Histological evaluation of the effectiveness of five instrumentation techniques for cleaning the apical third of root canals, *J Endod* 23:499, 1997.
19. Tucker DM, Wenckus CS, Bentkover SK: Canal wall planing by engine-driven nickel-titanium instruments, compared with stainless-steel hand instrumentation, *J Endod* 23:170, 1997.
20. Dalton BC et al: Bacterial reduction with nickel-titanium rotary instrumentation, *J Endod* 24:763, 1998.
21. Shuping GB et al: Reduction of intracanal bacteria using nickel-titanium rotary instrumentation and various medications, *J Endod* 26:751, 2000.
22. Glickman GN, Koch KA: Twenty-first century endodontics, *JADA* 131:39S, 2000.
23. Pruett JP, Clement DJ, Carnes DL: Cyclic fatigue testing of nickel-titanium endodontic instruments, *J Endod* 23:77, 1997.

24. Bonetti Filho I et al: Microscopic evaluation of three endodontic files pre-and postinstrumentation, *J Endod* 24:461, 1998.

25. Boonrat S et al: Defects in rotary nickel-titanium files after clinical use, *J Endod* 26:161, 2000.

26. Deitz DB et al: Effect of rotational speed on the breakage of nickel-titanium rotary files, *J Endod* 26:68, 2000.

27. Gabel WP et al: Effect of rotational speed on nickel-titanium file distortion, *J Endod* 25:752, 2000.

28. Bortnick KL, Steiman HR, Ruskin A: Comparison of nickel-titanium file distortion using electric and air-driven handpieces, *J Endod* 27:57, 2001.

29. Roane JB: Crown-down nickel-titanium and endodontics, *Endod Pract* 2:16, 1999.

30. Hinrichs RE, Walker WA, III, Schindler WG: A comparison of amounts of apically extruded debris using handpiece-driven nickel-titanium instrument systems, *J Endod* 24:102, 1998.

31. Beeson TJ et al: Comparison of debris extruded apically in straight canals: conventional filing versus Profile .04 Taper series 29, *J Endod* 24:18, 1998.

32. Blum JY, Machtou P, Micallef JP: Location of contact areas on rotary Profile instruments in relationship to the forces developed during mechanical preparation on extracted teeth, *Int Endod J* 32:108, 1999.

33. Kanavagh D, Lumley PJ: An in vitro evaluation of canal preparation using Profile .04 and .06 taper series instruments, *Endod Dent Traumatol* 14:16, 1998.

34. Swartz S, McSpadden JT: The Quantec rotary nickel titanium instrumentation system, *Int J Epidemiol* 2:14, 1999.

6

SONICS AND ULTRASONICS IN ENDODONTICS

PHILLIP J. LUMLEY *and* DAMIEN D. WALMSLEY

The concept of using ultrasound in endodontic therapy was suggested in 1957 by Richman,[1] who adapted an ultrasonic scaler for use in apicoectomies. However, its potential was not fully developed until Martin created a commercial system harnessing the properties of ultrasonic energy for the preparation and cleaning of the root canal in 1976.[2] This technique, termed *endosonics,* was readily accepted and continues to be a well-recognized procedure.

The use of ultrasound in endodontics has evolved since its introduction more than a decade ago. Its popularity with regard to root canal preparation, however, has decreased as a result of the development of more efficient techniques. Nevertheless, ultrasonic irrigation remains an extremely effective method of canal débridement after space has been created within the root canal system.

OSCILLATION OF ULTRASONIC FILES

In his early work on endosonics, Martin[2] developed an instrument (Figure 6-1) that was a direct adaptation of the ultrasonic scaler used to clean teeth except that the energy provided an oscillatory action to the file. During operation an irrigant solution (sodium hypochlorite) was passed through a separate channel from a reservoir over the oscillating file. Endosonic instruments initially worked at ultrasonic frequencies of 25 kHz but later developments led to sonic instruments powered by pressurized air. Oscillation of the endodontic file during sonic activation occurred at frequencies of 1 to 6 kHz.

Both ultrasonic and sonic instruments are similar in design in that they consist of a driver onto which an endosonic file is clamped—usually at an angle of 60° to 90° to the long axis of the driver. The oscillatory pattern of the driver determines the nature of movement of the attached file. This transverse oscillation is unique to the ultrasonic instruments.[3,4]

Although the main driver oscillates longitudinally, the file vibrates transversely (Figure 6-2).[3] This sets up a characteristic pattern of nodes (points of minimum oscillation) and antinodes (points of maximum oscillation). The greatest displacement occurs when the working tip of the file is allowed to work without interference. Transverse motion of the file causes filing of the dentine when the instrument is moved vertically within the root canal space (Figure 6-3). Files of different thickness and length oscillate differently and the node/antinode position can vary.[4]

The energy in the transverse oscillation is low, and the file is susceptible to constraint or loading. This in turn produces variability in clinical efficiency. To keep such constraint to a minimum the clinician should keep the file in constant motion when it is activated within the root canal. File constraint is more pronounced in curved canals and when pre-curving is necessary.[5,6] Therefore the clinician should keep the file moving in an up-and-down motion.

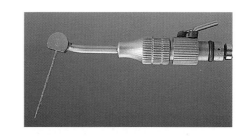

FIGURE 6-1   Close-up of an ultrasonic device, showing the insert head with attached endodontic file.

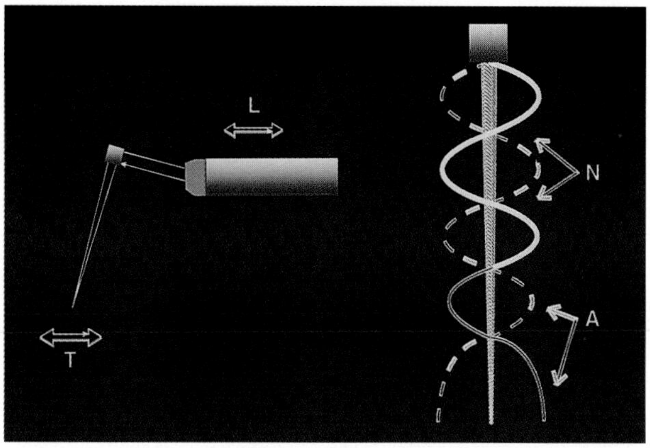

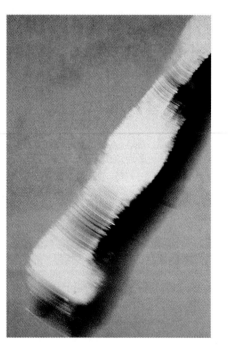

FIGURE 6-2 *Left,* Characteristic ultrasonic movement, showing a longitudinal motion. *Right,* A file set at an angle to the driver has a transverse oscillation with nodes *(N)* and antinodes *(A).*

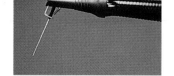

FIGURE 6-4 A sonic handpiece.

FIGURE 6-3 Photomicrograph of an activated K-file (#20).

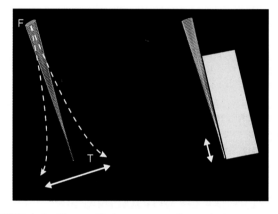

FIGURE 6-5 The oscillation pattern of a sonic instrument. The initial transverse motion in air changes to a vertical action when the file contacts the root canal wall.

Sonic instruments (Figure 6-4) produce an elliptical pattern of transverse oscillation when operated in air, a pattern similar to those powered ultrasonically. However, this large transverse motion is eliminated entirely and replaced by a true longitudinal vibration of the file when the file is activated and loaded in the root canal (Figure 6-5).[4] This longitudinal file motion may offer a superior action within the root canal.

FILE DESIGN

Different file designs are used with sonic and ultrasonic instruments, and different manufacturers have unique designs of files for use with endosonic instruments. The Cavi-Endo (Dentsply, York, Pennsylvania) uses small K-files (#15, #20, #25). Sonic instruments are supplied with two file types: Rispisonic and Shaper (Micro-Mega, Prodonta, Geneva, Switzerland) (Figure 6-6). These files

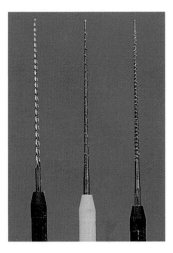

FIGURE 6-6   Files used in sonic instruments. From *left* to *right* are displayed the Heliosonic file (Micro Mega Prodonta, Geneva, Switzerland) (based on a triple file), the characteristic Shaper file, and the Rispisonic file.

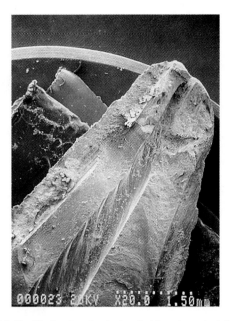

FIGURE 6-7   Photomicrograph showing the characteristic ridging pattern made in the canal by a K-type file. (Courtesy Dr. K.V. Krell, West Des Moines, Iowa.)

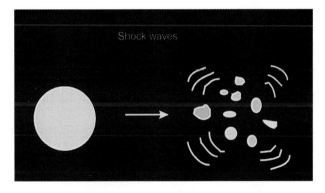

FIGURE 6-8   Cavitational activity.

have spiral blades protruding along their lengths and non-cutting tips. The Rispisonic spirals are closer together than those of the Shaper file. In addition, the Rispisonic file does not follow International Standards Organization (ISO) standards and has a thicker cross-section toward the coronal part of the file.

Although canals prepared with ultrasonics are smooth, the cutting edges of the file produce characteristic markings in a diagonal wave pattern on the canal walls (Figure 6-7). This pattern is caused by the action of the K-file flutes because the distance between the crests produced in the dentine and the cutting edges is similar.[7]

CAVITATION AND ACOUSTIC MICROSTREAMING

During operation of the endosonic file, water or an irrigant such as sodium hypochlorite is passed over the oscillating tip. Cavitation is generated by the movement of the file within the water supply, and is claimed to be one of the primary beneficial effects of the endosonic instrument.[8] Cavitation consists of the growth and subsequent violent collapse of bubbles in fluid (Figure 6-8). This motion results in the development of a shock wave, increased temperature and pressure, and free radical formation in the fluid. Cavitational activity is readily demonstrated within the cooling water supply of the ultrasonic scaler.[9]

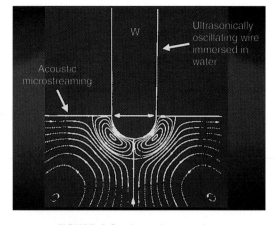

FIGURE 6-9   Acoustic streaming.

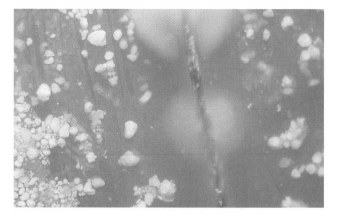

FIGURE 6-10   Acoustic streaming around a sonic file helps clean debris from around the file.

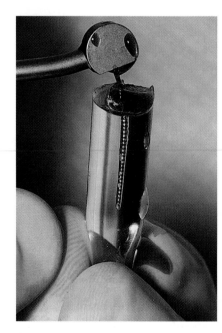

FIGURE 6-11   Streaming within an artificial root canal. Banding occurs where the red dye has been moved in areas of intense streaming. (Courtesy Dr. K.V. Krell, West Des Moines, Iowa.)

Although transient cavitation may theoretically occur during use of an endosonic instrument, sufficiently high sound pressure fields are unlikely to occur around the oscillating file unless it is operated at high displacement amplitudes.[3] The more beneficial biophysical action of the file is likely to result from acoustic microstreaming.

Acoustic streaming is produced around an object oscillating in a liquid. It is characterized by the production of large shear forces that are capable of dislodging or disassociating lumps of material (Figure 6-9). However, the forces of acoustic streaming are not sufficient to break up the bacterial cell wall.

The oscillating file in the endosonic system produces streaming fields along its length, with the great-est shear stresses being generated around points of maximum displacement such as the tip of the file and the antinodes along its length.[3,10] These streaming fields are likely to be responsible for many of the beneficial effects attributed to the use of endosonics and are important in moving the irrigant around the root canal (Figure 6-10). However, the efficiency of such forces depends on the amount of damping and file constraint that occurs when the instrument is working within the canal.[3]

Streaming forces occurring around the file disassociate clumps of bacteria without disruption.[11] The acoustic streaming generated by the file may play a useful role in reducing the number of bacteria in the canal by remov-

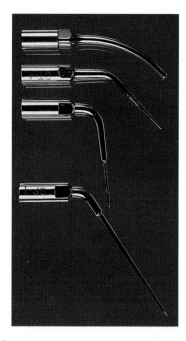

FIGURE 6-12   Analytic (Sybron Dental Specialties, Orange, CA) ultrasonic inserts. These inserts are for prosthetic post vibration; use in the pulp chamber; and use in the suborifice, middle, and apical third regions.

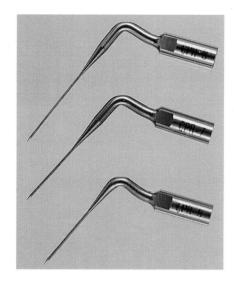

FIGURE 6-13   A selection of ultra-slim titanium tips (CPR Nos. 6, 7, 8) for use deep within root canals in challenging situations.

BOX 6-1

Ultrasonics in Nonsurgical Root Canal Preparation

Endosonics can shape curved canals, but overinstrumentation can occur if it is used in the canal too long. Therefore the clinician should keep in mind the following:
- The files need to be pre-curved.
- Small files (such as #15) should be used.

Ultrasonic files behave in a similar manner to hand instruments, but transportation of the canals does occur:
- It is less common in the apical region.
- It is greatest in the middle portion of the canal.

Root canal débridement depends on the following:
- Oscillation of the file to oscillate

- The choice of irrigant solution, sodium hypochlorite being the preferred choice
- The form of irrigation, with ultrasonic irrigation being superior to a needle and syringe*

Ultrasonic preparation produces cleaner canals because of the following:
- The synergistic relationship between the ultrasound and the sodium hypochlorite
- The increased temperature produced in the sodium hypochlorite

*Krell KV, Johnson R, Madison S: Irrigation patterns during ultrasonic canal instrumentation Part 1. K-type files, *J Endod* 14:65, 1988.

---

ing the smear layer and debris harboring bacteria and loosening aggregates of bacteria, thereby facilitating their mechanical removal.

The main advantage of ultrasonic files is that they move irrigant around the canal and penetrate to the most apical extent of the instrument (Figure 6-11).[12,13] The general conclusion is that acoustic microstreaming does occur around the oscillating file. To be effective in this action, the file must be kept moving at all times so that free oscillation can be maintained. In-

struments are generally moved circumferentially within the canal space. Box 6-1 provides a summary of the way ultrasonics can be used in conventional root canal treatment.

In addition to the use of endosonic files to clean and shape the root canal, numerous additional applications for ultrasonic activated instruments have been developed. Specifically, modified ultrasonic tips have been developed that play valuable roles in access refinement (Figure 6-12), root canal retreatment (Figure 6-13), and

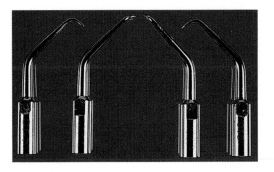

FIGURE 6-14 Examples of the original CT (Analytic, Sybron Dental Specialties, Orange, CA) ultrasonic tips that revolutionized apical root end cavity preparation.

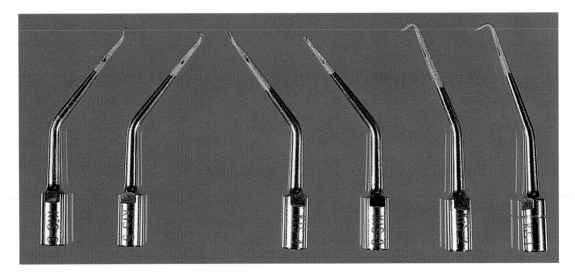

FIGURE 6-15 KIS (Obtura Spartan, Fenton, MO) ultrasonic surgery tips. The increased length offers improved visibility and cutting.

apical surgery (Figures 6-14 and 6-15). A variety of different tip designs are available for these clinical tasks.[14] Generally these tips are used with ultrasonic drivers because they have more power, but sonic drivers have been used as well.

ACCESS REFINEMENT

Ultrasonic tips offer a precise method of dentine removal and thereby facilitate canal location and identification. The narrow profile of these tips allows excellent visualization compared with that of conventional handpieces because no bulky head obstructs the path of vision.

RETREATMENT

During root canal retreatment the operator needs to gain access to the root canal system. The most important part

of the canal to be instrumented is the apical third, which may present many obstructions that complicate the procedure. Metallic posts often obstruct access. Ultrasonic energy is a useful tool in such cases to vibrate the post or chip away at the surrounding cement.

Metallic objects such as silver points and fractured instruments may also obstruct access to the apical third. The clinician must take particular care when vibrating silver points because the soft metal is easily abraded. Often silver points break into fragments, making retrieval more difficult. This difficulty may be overcome by using indirect ultrasonic vibration (e.g., grasping the point with a pair of Steiglitz pliers and applying ultrasonic energy to the pliers).

Sectioned silver points in the apical third of roots can be difficult to remove. Ultrasonic vibration can be used to chip away any remaining cement and provide access for a K-type and/or Hedström file to bypass the silver point and aid in retrieval.

FRACTURED INSTRUMENT REMOVAL

Ultrasonic vibration may be used to facilitate fractured instrument removal. The clinician must take care to ascertain the type of metallic obstruction because nickel-titanium (NiTi) and stainless steel respond differently to ultrasonic vibration. Direct ultrasonic vibration causes NiTi to fragment, so the clinician must work carefully around the fragment. Stainless steel is more resistant to vibration and responds to it by subsequently loosening.

Ultrasonic vibration is applied directly to stainless steel files. Fine inserts can be used to work counterclockwise around broken instruments. This technique often results in an "unscrewing" action that assists in removal.

USE OF ULTRASOUND IN APICAL SURGERY

Ultrasound offers considerable advantages in apical surgery. Rotary instrument heads are relatively bulky compared with ultrasonic tips. Ultrasonic tips allow better access and visibility because of their small size, and the unique bends incorporated in their design permit easy access to the root end.[15,16] The decreased size of ultrasonic tips enables small root-end preparations to be made parallel to the long axis of the root.

SUMMARY

The two main advantages of ultrasonic systems are the ultrasonically activated file and the action of irrigant passing over it. Although the ultrasonic system provides excellent irrigation, it depends on the proper technique and clinicians must use it with care if maximum benefit is to be obtained. Sodium hypochlorite is the irrigant of choice. Evidence supports the importance of keeping the file oscillating and moving freely within the canal.

Since the introduction of ultrasonics to endodontics, the application of the technology has evolved and expanded. The development of new instruments has led to the use of ultrasonics in access modification, removal of foreign objects, and apical surgery.

The introduction of piezoelectric ultrasonic units offers the clinician a more compact and powerful device compared with more traditional magnetostrictive units.[17,18] Both types of ultrasonic units are more powerful than sonic devices, which rely on air pressure to produce oscillation of the instruments. Piezoelectric units convert crystal deformation into mechanical oscillation, whereas magnetostrictive units convert electromagnetic energy into mechanical energy.[3]

Modern endodontic tools such as the operating microscope have allowed increased operative precision, and ultrasonic instrumentation has an important place in the armamentarium of the endodontic practitioner.

References

1. Richman RJ: The use of ultrasonics in root canal therapy and root resection, *J Dent Med* 12:12, 1957.
2. Martin H: Ultrasonic disinfection of the root canal, *Oral Surg Oral Med Oral Pathol Oral Radiol Endod* 42:92, 1976.
3. Walmsley AD: Endosonics: ultrasound and root canal treatment: the need for scientific evaluation, *Int Endod J* 20:105, 1987.
4. Walmsley AD, Williams AR: The effect of constraint on the oscillatory pattern of endosonic files, *J Endod* 15:189, 1989.
5. Lumley PJ, Walmsley AD: The effect of precurving on the performance of endosonic K-files, *J Endod* 18:232, 1992.
6. Walmsley AD, Laird WRE, Lumley PJ: Ultrasound in dentistry: II. Periodontology and endodontics, *J Dent* 20:11, 1992.
7. Briggs PFA et al: The dentine-removing characteristics of an ultrasonically energized K-file, *Int Endod J* 22:259, 1989.
8. Cunningham WT, Martin H, Forrest WR: Evaluation of root canal débridement with the endosonic ultrasonic synergistic system, *Oral Surg Oral Med Oral Pathol Oral Radiol Endod* 53:401, 1982.
9. Walmsley AD, Laird WRE, Williams AR: Dental plaque removal by cavitational activity during ultrasonic scaling, *J Clin Periodontol* 15:539, 1988.
10. Ahmad M, Pitt Ford TR, Crum LA: Ultrasonic débridement of root canals: acoustic streaming and its possible role, *J Endod* 13:490, 1987.
11. Ahmad M: Effect of ultrasonic instrumentation on *Bacteroides intermedius*, *Endod Dent Traumatol* 5:83, 1989.
12. Krell KV, Johnson R, Madison S: Irrigation patterns during ultrasonic canal instrumentation Part 1. K-type files, *J Endod* 14:65, 1988.
13. Druttman AC, Stock CJR: An in vitro comparison of ultrasonic and conventional methods of irrigant replacement, *Int Endod J* 22:174, 1989.
14. Ruddle CJ: Micro-endodontic non-surgical retreatment, *Dent Clin North Am* 41:429, 1997.
15. Carr GB: Endodontics at the crossroads, *J Calif Dent Assoc* 24:20, 1996.
16. Carr GB: Ultrasonic root end preparation, *Dent Clin North Am* 41:541, 1997.
17. Stamos DE et al: An in vitro comparison study to quantitate the débridement ability of hand, sonic, and ultrasonic instrumentation, *J Endod* 13:434, 1987.
18. Archer R et al: An in vivo evaluation of the efficiency of ultrasound after step-back preparation in mandibular molars, *J Endod* 18:549, 1992.

7

OBTURATION

FREDERICK R. LIEWEHR *and* **WILLIAM T. JOHNSON**

Since the end of the nineteenth century, dentists suspected that bacteria were responsible for pulpal and periapical disease, but in 1965 Kakehashi et al[1] published a study that conclusively demonstrated the role bacteria play in pulp pathosis. The authors created pulp exposures in rats maintained in a germ-free environment and in rats that lived in a conventional environment and allowed the teeth to remain open. Histologic evaluation of the tissues showed pulp necrosis with chronic inflammatory tissue and abscess formation in the animals maintained in a conventional environment. Pulp necrosis did not occur in the tissues from the germ-free animals, and histologic evaluation indicated minimal pulpal inflammation with no apical abscess formation. In addition, reparative bridge formation was evident as early as 14 days postexposure.

The implication of this definitive study is that in order for the pulp or periapical area to repair, minimal or no bacteria should be present. Therefore successful endodontic treatment is achieved by cleansing and shaping the root canal space and removing the pulp tissue, organic remnants, and bacteria and their by-products. Obturation after cleaning and shaping provides a seal that prevents re-infection of the canal and subsequent leakage into the periradicular tissues. Realistically, the clinician may not always be able to remove all bacteria from the canal and dentinal tubules to sterilize the canal, so obturation can have a second objective: that of sealing any remaining contaminants within the root canal where they will not escape to cause periapical disease.[2]

Currently no instrumentation technique completely cleans the radicular space.[3,4] Residual bacteria sequestered in fins and isthmuses within the canal system, as well as in the dentinal tubules, prevent complete sterilization by the cleansing and shaping process and thereby preclude healing. The persistence of bacteria within the root canal system after cleansing and shaping requires that any remaining bacteria be sealed within the root canal system for healing to occur. Some authors maintain that these sequestered bacteria will lose their viability,[2,5] but even if they are merely dormant, as long as neither the bacteria nor their by-products (e.g., lipopolysaccharides) can contact the periapical tissues, those tissues should heal.

Historically, the emphasis in endodontic treatment was on obtaining a good apical seal. The root canal was seen as a tube with an open end situated in the jawbone that simply needed to be sealed to prevent the ingress of tissue fluids and the egress of bacteria or their toxins. Today clinicians realize that no root canal filling material seals perfectly[6] and that some communication between the contents of the root canal and the periapical tissues is inevitable despite their best efforts at obturation. If biomechanical canal preparation eliminates most of the microorganisms, and the remainder are "entombed" and possibly destroyed by the obturation process, insufficient numbers of unimpeded bacteria may remain in the canal to trigger a periapical inflammatory response. However, if an inadequate coronal seal exists, microleakage that brings fresh bacteria or nutrients for residual bacteria from the oral cavity may penetrate through the obturated tooth and reach the periapical area within a few days, producing chronic periapical inflammation.[7] The radicular space is not a simple tube with two open ends, but rather a complex system with accessory, lateral, and furcation canals, along with millions of dentinal tubules, that are potential paths of entry into the radicular space. Therefore the focus of root canal treatment must be the complete, three-dimensional obturation of the entire root canal space, followed by placement of a coronal restoration that produces optimal sealing of the access opening.[8]

Since the early days of endodontic treatment, much discussion has taken place regarding the ideal location for the terminus of the root canal filling. This obsession with the apical extent of the fill is undoubtedly a result of the historical fact that dentists in the late nineteenth and early twentieth centuries were hindered by an inadequate armamentarium. Access openings were difficult because only belt-driven, low-speed handpieces using burs that dulled quickly were available. Files were likewise made of inferior alloys that did not remain sharp, corroded, fractured easily, and exhibited poor flexibility. Their manufacturing also lacked consistency. Local anesthesia was in its infancy and was infrequently employed. Patients were frequently uncomfortable and unwilling or unable to tolerate the cleaning and shaping procedures required to produce an ideal preparation. Therefore instrumentation was frequently discontinued when the procedure became too uncomfortable for the patient or when the dentist could instrument no further because of his own discomfort or the limitations imposed by his armamentarium. These numerous constraints meant that dentists had great difficulty reaching the apical portion of the root canal, particularly in posterior teeth, much less instrumenting it adequately. The only means early operators had to evaluate their progress was to expose a radiograph (the equipment for which was itself in its infancy and not universally available) and see whether they had succeeded in reaching the apex. If they were fortunate enough to have overcome all the procedural obstacles in their path and arrived at the root apex, filling could begin.

As one might suspect, not all endodontic treatment is successful. In an attempt to define important parameters in determining success or failure, a large-scale investigation was undertaken in the 1960s at the University of Washington.[9] The authors retrospectively observed radiographs of more than 1000 cases for 5 years and attempted to correlate their radiographic observations with clinical signs of success or failure. In their judgment, nearly 60% of the failures were caused by poor obturation. A more accurate way of expressing the findings would have been that more than 60% of the failures appeared radiographically to have been incompletely obturated, because the study design was incapable of demonstrating cause and effect. As a result of this semantic error, the impression was inadvertently created that obturation was more important than instrumentation, which is difficult to assess. In all probability, cases that were poorly obturated also exhibited inadequate cleaning and shaping.

Many prognosis studies have failed to emphasize the importance of cleaning and shaping, the quality of which is impossible to determine radiographically or clinically, while concentrating on the length of the obturation, which is more practical to measure. This resulted in numerous pronouncements regarding the importance of the exact length of the filling material in relation to the radiographic apex. Great importance was placed on whether a filling was "long" or "short."[10,11] This was the norm until Schilder[8] emphasized the fact that the objectives of endodontic instrumentation are to remove all organic debris (and bacteria) from the root canal and then produce a shape that is conducive to the placement of a three-dimensional root canal filling to fill the canal and all its ramifications, preventing the recontamination of the cleaned canal.

The earlier studies do, however, demonstrate that the difference in success depends on where the root canal filling ends. Root canal fillings that are long (i.e., those that extend beyond the radiographic apex) seem to be associated with a decreased chance of success.[12-14] Reasons for these findings are numerous and complex. The most favorable histologic responses to endodontic procedures are associated with working lengths short of the apical constriction regardless of the pulpal status (vital versus necrotic). This is also true when bacteria are present in the periapical tissues. Extrusion of sealer and/or core material results in a severe inflammatory response and foreign body reaction despite the absence of pain.[13]

First, a distinction must be made between the length of the instrumentation and the length of the obturation. Because the key to success is to eliminate bacteria from the root canal system, instrumentation must be carried throughout the length of the canal. When instrumentation was in its infancy, preparing the canal to receive gutta-percha was difficult, so other materials were sought that could be more easily introduced into a canal that was often inadequately prepared. Solid core materials such as silver points could be forced through residual bacteria and debris to the apex or beyond, which meant that despite the presence of obturating material in the apical area, the area was neither cleaned nor shaped and therefore the treatment was destined to fail.

A second distinction that must be made is between "overfilling" and "overextension." If a root canal is analogous to a pipe, then overfilling means that the pipe is filled to capacity and that any additional material must extrude from one end or the other (Figure 7-1). Overextension, which describes the presence of filling material in the periradicular bone, does not necessarily result only when the canal has reached maximum capacity (Figure 7-2). In the previous silver point example, a size 20 silver point could be pushed through a size 100 canal to exit through the apical foramen without approaching the dimension necessary to obturate the canal. Again, lack of an apical seal may result in the periapical area being infected by the contents of the root canal.

A third element that may portend success or failure is the toxicity of the contents of the root canal and/or the sealer used. One reason for overextension of a gutta-percha cone is poor adaptation. If the cone and the apical preparation are the same size and shape, the conical shape or resistance form should prevent overextension even in teeth with apical resorption where an adequate

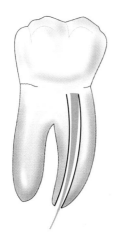

FIGURE 7-1   Note the overextension of gutta-percha and lack of adaptation to the canal walls.

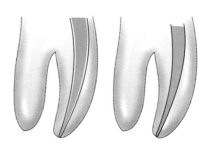

FIGURE 7-3   Diagram of two cones depicting the tapered canal and point adaptation. The taper developed in preparing the canal provides resistance form that prevents extrusion when the point is seated.

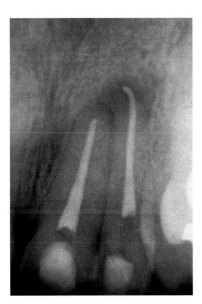

FIGURE 7-2   A radiograph of a failing maxillary left lateral incisor demonstrating an overextension.

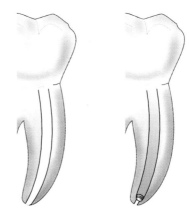

FIGURE 7-4   When the apical constriction has been lost because of inaccurate length determination or resorption, a stop can be prepared by deliberately creating a ledge within the canal space.

stop cannot be prepared (Figure 7-3). Overextension, then, may be indicative of a poor fit and a poor seal in the apical area. Bacteria and their toxins could continue to leak from the root canal, preventing apical healing. Additionally, although gutta-percha itself is relatively inert,[15] sealers are not. Sealers, even when confined to the root canal, are toxic and cause periapical inflammation that can last for years.[16] Overextension of sealer into the periodontal ligament and bone can preclude healing and promote chronic inflammation.

Therefore the goals of nonsurgical root canal treatment should be to clean the canal thoroughly, remove as much bacteria and debris as possible, shape the canal into a continuously tapering cone to accommodate the obturating material, and fill the space completely. The obturating material should fill the canal, but it should not extend beyond its confines. Respecting the apical constriction and preparing a stop for the obturating material is desirable when possible, but in many cases periapical inflammation has already caused resorption of the apex.[17] In this case, several alternative methods can be used to confine the material to the canal. Clinicians should carefully determine the length of the tooth to the apex, then step back 1 or 2 mm and deliberately create a circumferential ledge by reaming the canal several sizes larger. This technique can be used advantageously in some canals, but can also fracture the thin apical end of the root (Figure 7-4).

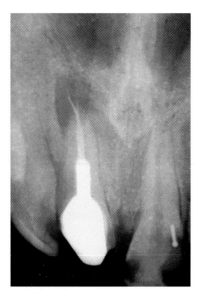

FIGURE 7-5 A radiograph of a maxillary right lateral incisor demonstrating an accessory cone extending into the periradicular tissues. This results when the master cone is not adapted circumferentially in the apical third of the root.

In reality, if the canal and the gutta-percha points are tapered, the point should enter the canal until it makes circumferential contact with the canal walls. The reason points are overextended or accessory points slide past a master cone that has stopped at the prepared length is that the master cone is making only partial contact with the canal walls (Figure 7-5). This problem can be circumvented by using solvent to customize the apical end of the point or by using a form of thermoplasticized gutta-percha.

Another method to prevent the overextension of gutta-percha is to use an apical plug. The plug can be formed of dentin removed from the canal walls; dentin packed into the apical portion of the canal can prevent extrusion.[18,19] The difficulty with dentin chips is that the clinician can never be certain exactly what is being packed into the apical portion of the canal—it seems to be a mixture of dentin, canal contents, and potentially bacteria and their by-products. This unknown mixture, if bacterially contaminated (teeth with infected, necrotic pulps frequently exhibit apical resorption), can lead to non-healing and chronic periapical inflammation.[20-22] A better choice may be to mix a nearly solid mass of calcium hydroxide and create a plug of that biocompatible material in the apex of the tooth.[23] Recently mineral trioxide aggregate (MTA) has become available and is a viable option.[24]

OBTURATING MATERIALS

Sealers

Regardless of the obturation technique employed, sealers are an essential component of the process. Sealers fill the space between the canal wall and core obturation material and may fill lateral and accessory canals, isthmuses, and irregularities in the root canal system. The ideal properties of an endodontic sealer were outlined by Grossman[25] and are provided in Box 7-1.

The most popular sealers are grouped by type: zinc oxide–eugenol formulations, calcium hydroxide sealers, glass ionomers, and resins. Regardless of the sealer selected, all are toxic until they set. For this reason, extrusion of sealers into the periradicular tissues should be avoided.[13]

Zinc oxide–eugenol and resin sealers have a history of successful use over an extended period. Zinc oxide–eugenol sealers have the advantage of being resorbed if extruded into the periradicular tissues.[26] Calcium hydroxide sealers were recently introduced for their potential therapeutic benefits. In theory these sealers exhibit an antimicrobial effect and have osteogenic potential. Unfortunately these actions have not been demonstrated, and the solubility required for release of calcium hydroxide and sustained activity is a distinct disadvantage. Glass ionomers have been advocated for use in sealing the radicular space because of their dentin bonding properties. A disadvantage is their difficult removal if retreatment is required.

Sealers containing paraformaldehyde are contraindicated in endodontic treatment. Although the lead and mercury components have been removed from the formulations over time, the paraformaldehyde content has remained constant and toxic. These sealers are not approved by the U. S. Food and Drug Administration.[27]

Controversy surrounds removal of the smear layer before obturation. The smear layer is created on the canal walls by manipulation of the files during cleaning and shaping procedures. It is composed of inorganic and organic components that may contain bacteria and their by-products. In theory remnants left on the canal wall may serve as irritants or substrates for bacterial growth or interfere with the development of a seal during obturation. Although fluid movement may occur in obturated canals, bacterial movement does not appear to take place.[28] Recent evidence suggests that removal of the smear layer can enhance penetration of the sealer into the dentinal tubules.[29,30]

Removal of the smear layer can be accomplished after cleaning and shaping by irrigation with 17% ethylenediaminetetraacetic acid (EDTA) for 1 minute. Irrigation should be followed with a final rinse of sodium hypochlorite.

The radiopacity of sealers can be increased by adding opacifiers such as barium sulfate or silver particles. Although these opacifiers can produce an esthetically pleasing result, claims of superiority of obturation based on radiographic appearance are inaccurate. The increased radiopacity may mask voids or imperfections in the compaction and is unrelated to the quality of seal obtained. In addition, sealers with silver particles may stain the tooth structure if they are left in the pulp chamber.

Acceptable methods of placing the sealer in the canal include the following[31]:

- Placing the sealer on the master cone and pumping the cone up and down in the canal
- Placing the sealer on a file and spinning it counterclockwise
- Placing the sealer with a lentulo spiral
- Using a syringe
- Activating an ultrasonic instrument

The clinician should use care when placing sealer in a canal with an open apex to avoid extrusion.

Core Obturation Materials

The ideal properties of an obturation material as outlined by Grossman[25] are listed in Box 7-2.

Historically, a variety of materials have been employed to obturate the root canal, falling into three broad categories: solids, semisolids, and pastes. In the early days of endodontics, because of the limitations of their equipment dentists found preparing canals to the size and shape necessary for the introduction of guttapercha points very difficult. In the 1940s, Jasper[32] introduced cones made of silver, which he claimed produced the same success rate as gutta-percha but were easier to use. Silver cones met many of the criteria for filling materials but suffered from several deficiencies. The rigidity that made them easy to introduce into the canal also made them impossible to adapt to the inevitably irregular canal preparation, encouraging leakage. When leakage occurred and the points contacted tissue fluids, they corroded, further increasing leakage[33] (Figure 7-6). The

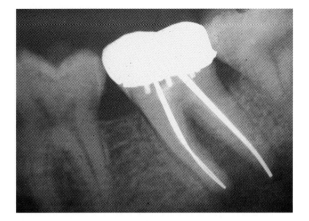

FIGURE 7-6   A mandibular left second molar treated with silver cones. Failure has occurred despite placement to the correct length.

BOX 7-2

Ideal Properties of an Obturation Material

1. It should be easily manipulated and provide ample working time.
2. It should be dimensionally stable and not shrink or change form after it is inserted.
3. It should seal the canal laterally and apically, conforming to its complex internal anatomy.
4. It should not irritate the periapical tissues.
5. It should be impervious to moisture and nonporous.
6. It should be unaffected by tissue fluids and not corrode or oxidize.
7. It should not support bacterial growth.
8. It should be radiopaque and easily discernible on radiographs.
9. It should not discolor tooth structure.
10. It should be sterile.
11. It should be easily removed from the canal if necessary.

---

corrosion products themselves were cytotoxic,[34] which impeded periapical healing.

At the opposite end of the rigidity spectrum are the pastes. Pastes also fulfill many of the criteria listed previously and can easily adapt to the most complex internal anatomy. However, their extreme flowability can be a negative factor, and overextension or underextension is a frequent result of using a paste technique.[35] The movement of the material occurs along the path of least resistance; pressure is required for the material to flow laterally to fill the anatomic variations of the canal. If less pressure is required to flow through the apex than to flow laterally, the material will flow through the apex. Unfortunately, the operator has no way of knowing where the material is

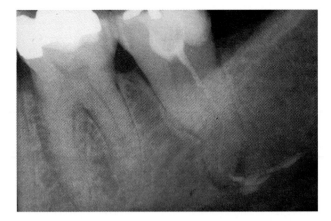

FIGURE 7-7 A mandibular left second molar treated with a Sargenti formulation paste. Note the unfilled mesial canals and the extrusion of material into the mandibular canal, which resulted in paresthesia.

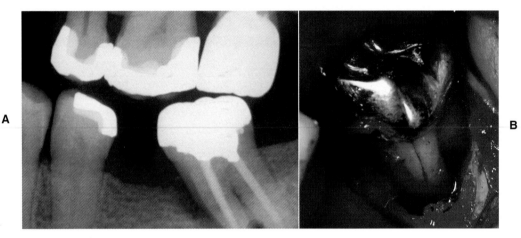

FIGURE 7-8 **A,** A treated mandibular left second molar exhibiting mesial bone loss. **B,** On flap reflection a vertical root fracture was detected.

flowing except by exposing a radiograph. By the time the radiograph develops, retrieval of overextended material becomes a surgical matter. Additionally, pastes have been associated with the addition of undesirable and toxic chemicals such as paraformaldehyde, which can produce irreversible tissue damage when extended beyond the confines of the root canal system (Figure 7-7).[36,37]

Currently gutta-percha, a semisolid material, is the most widely used and accepted obturating material.[38] Chemically, gutta-percha is the *trans* isomer of polyisoprene, a naturally occurring relative of rubber. In the production of dental obturating cones, approximately 20% gutta-percha is combined with approximately 65% zinc oxide, 10% radiopacifiers, and 5% plasticizers. Clearly, what clinicians refer to as *gutta-percha* is really a compound composed primarily of other substances. Unlike rubber, gutta-percha *cannot* be compressed by pressure, being less compressible than water,

which is considered incompressible.[39] Excessive condensation pressure cannot cause flow of gutta-percha and does not improve the seal of a root canal fill[40] but can fracture roots (Figure 7-8). Gutta-percha can be made to flow if it is modified by either heat or solvents. Gutta-percha exists in two distinctly different crystalline phases, which Bunn termed "alpha" and "beta" modifications.[41] The naturally occurring form is the alpha form, which melts when heated above 65° C. If it is cooled extremely slowly, the alpha form will recrystallize. If it is cooled routinely, the beta form recrystallizes, which is the form in which most gutta-percha exists. Although the mechanical properties of the two forms are the same, when alpha phase gutta-percha is heated and cooled, it undergoes less shrinkage than the beta form, making it more dimensionally stable for use with thermoplasticized techniques.

In addition to its ability to conform to canal irregularities, gutta-percha exhibits very low toxicity, being es-

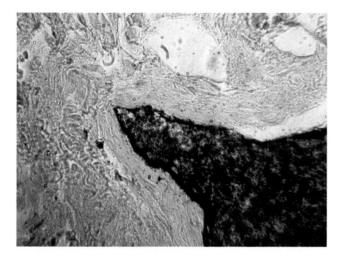

FIGURE 7-9 Gutta-percha is relatively inert in periradicular connective tissues.

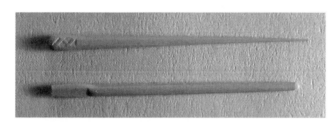

FIGURE 7-10 Nonstandardized *(top)* and standardized *(bottom)* cones.

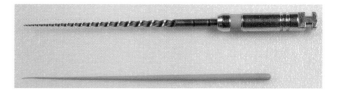

FIGURE 7-11 A .20 series GT file and a .04 gutta-percha cone.

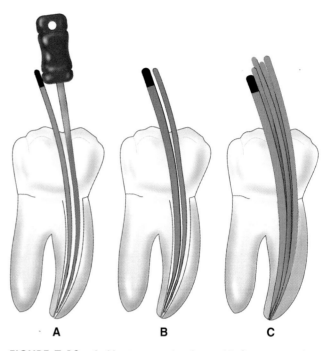

    A   **B**   **C**

FIGURE 7-12 **A,** Master cone in place with finger spreader. **B,** Accessory cone placed in space created by the finger spreader. **C,** Accessory cones in place, completing the obturation process.

sentially inert when in contact with the periapical tissues (Figure 7-9).[42,43] Additionally, it is easily removed if post space is needed or if retreatment becomes necessary. Gutta-percha does not adhere to the canal walls even when thermoplasticized and still requires a sealer to prevent leakage.[44,45]

    Gutta-percha cones are available in two forms: nonstandardized and standardized (Figure 7-10). The nonstandardized cones have relatively small diameter tips compared with their larger bodies. Their nomenclature refers to these two dimensions—a "fine-medium" cone has a fine tip and a medium body. Standardized cones are designed with an overall 0.02 mm / mm taper, to match the taper of endodontic files. Recently, as files of various tapers have been introduced, different tapers of gutta-percha cones are now being manufactured (Figure 7-11).

TECHNIQUES

Clinicians should be able to use a variety of obturation techniques because each case is unique and may require

modification of routine procedures for an optimal result. The following are common obturation techniques currently within the standard of care.

Lateral Condensation

Lateral condensation is the most common technique for obturating the root canal space. This technique can be used in most clinical situations and can be modified to facilitate unusual cases. Before performing obturation with lateral condensation, the clinician prepares the root canal in a continuously tapering manner to an endpoint that ideally coincides with the minor constriction,[46] often referred to as the *working length*. A standardized point (the "master cone") is selected with a diameter that is consistent with the largest file used in the canal at the working length (Figure 7-12).

    The clinician grasps the master cone with forceps at the point where the distance from the forceps to the tip is equal to the working length and inserts it into the canal. If the fit is correct, the point will exhibit "tugback," or resistance to removal at working length. A

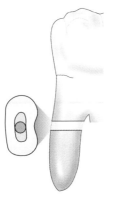

FIGURE 7-13 An ovoid distal canal of a mandibular molar with a master cone in place.

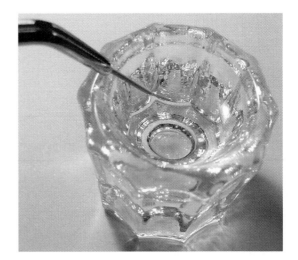

FIGURE 7-14 Adaptation of the master cone can be accomplished by softening the point in a solvent such as chloroform.

radiograph is exposed to verify that the point is correctly positioned in the canal. The cone is then removed, coated with sealer, and reinserted.

Nonstandard points are used to obliterate the remaining space. A spreader is selected that matches the length of the canal and the taper of the points. Finger spreaders provide better tactile sensation and are less likely to induce fractures in the root than the more traditional D-11T spreader.[47] Nickel-titanium spreaders provide increased flexibility, reduce stress, and penetrate deeper compared with stainless steel instruments.[48,49] The spreader is introduced into the canal to a depth that approaches within 1 mm of the working length[50] and rotated to create a space lateral to the master cone for placement of an accessory cone. The process is repeated, with the cones being condensed until the spreader can no longer penetrate the mass. Only light pressure is required because the gutta-percha is not compressible and because as little as 1.5 kg of pressure is capable of fracturing the root.[51] The excess gutta-percha in the chamber is then seared off and lightly vertically condensed with a heated plugger approximately 1 mm below the orifices to the canals or the cementoenamel junction in anterior teeth.

Apical Modification with Solvent

A disadvantage to lateral condensation of gutta-percha is that the material does not conform to the irregularities of the canal. Although lateral condensation reduces the space between the obturating cones, unfilled areas ("voids") remain as potential paths for leakage.[52] Because the preparation of a completely round canal is impossible and because the crucial apical area of the canal is likely to contain lateral canals, the tug-back experienced and the image displayed on a two-dimensional radiograph may give a misleading impression of a dense

fill. In reality only point contact may exist between the core and the walls of the canal (Figure 7-13). This situation is often discovered when an accessory point extends into the periapical area despite a seemingly well-placed master cone (see Figure 7-5).

To overcome this shortcoming, the clinician can temporarily soften the tip of the point by dipping the master cone in a solvent (chloroform, halothane, or eucalyptol) for several seconds and placing the softened point in the canal (Figure 7-14). This produces an impression of the apical portion of the canal in the material. The clinician then removes the cone from the canal for a few moments to allow the solvent to evaporate, applies the sealer, and replaces it so that it is oriented in the same direction as when the impression was made.[53] Although concerns have been raised about the use of chloroform in the dental operatory, evidence indicates that it is safe to use the material for fabricating custom cones and for retreatment.[54,55]

Although standardized cones are available from size 15 (0.15 mm) to 140 (1.40 mm), occasionally a canal is encountered that exceeds these dimensions. In such cases a customized gutta-percha point can be created by rolling several warmed gutta-percha points together with a cement spatula on a glass slab. The point is cooled with water and the size is tested in the canal and re-rolled until an approximate fit is achieved. Solvent dip may then be used to further adapt it to the walls of the canal. Sealer and accessory points can then be used as previously described (Figure 7-15).

Warm Lateral Condensation

Warm lateral condensation is a variant of traditional lateral condensation. A heated instrument is introduced into a tooth already obturated by lateral condensation to soften the gutta-percha mass and enhance adaptation to

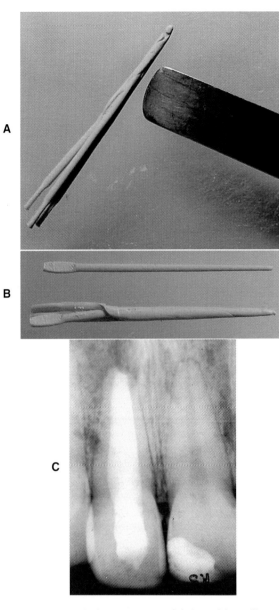

FIGURE 7-15   **A,** A master cone fabricated by rolling several gutta-percha cones together on a glass slab. **B,** A standardized cone compared with the fabricated cone. **C,** Obturation of a large canal in a maxillary right central incisor using a rolled gutta-percha cone.

the internal anatomy of the canal. This technique is useful to increase the adaptation and density of teeth obturated with lateral condensation, but it is especially indicated for teeth with internal resorptive defects and C-shaped canals. Liewehr et al[56] demonstrated a nearly 15% increase in weight after the use of the Endotec (Lone Star Technologies, Westport, CT) device (Figure 7-16). The Endotec is a battery-powered spreader, the tip of which heats to approximately 350° C when activated. One technique, called the "zap-and-tap" technique,[57] was devised to avoid the problems caused when accessory

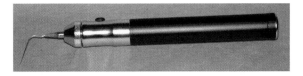

FIGURE 7-16   An Endotec instrument used for warm lateral condensation.

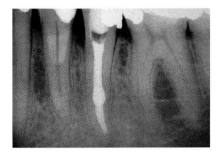

FIGURE 7-17   Obturation of a mandibular premolar with internal resorption using the zap-and-tap technique.

points placed during warm lateral condensation are heated and subsequently removed en masse when the Endotec spreader is withdrawn. In the zap-and-tap technique the canal is filled by lateral condensation and the excess gutta-percha removed. The Endotec instrument is then activated (the "zap") for 4 to 5 seconds and moved in short, continuous motions in and out of the gutta-percha mass. As the gutta-percha becomes warm, the tip of the Endotec instrument sinks further into the mass with each successive tap. When continued tapping fails to cause the tip to penetrate further or when the tip is within 2 mm of the working length, a cold spreader is introduced and rotated to condense the thermoplasticized gutta-percha into the canal anatomy. Accessory points coated with sealer are then added until the canal is completely obturated (Figure 7-17). The same technique can be used with the Touch 'N Heat (Kerr Division, Sybron Digital Specialties, Inc., Orange, CA) instrument or with the System B (Analytic Endodontics, Sybron Dental Specialties, Inc., Orange, CA) instrument using Touch 'N Heat tips.[58] Alternatively, an ultrasonically activated spreader may be used.[59]

Warm lateral condensation has many advantages. Since it follows cold lateral condensation, heat is not introduced to the apex of the tooth. The technique also allows precise length control in the placement of the gutta-percha and permits filling of voids, isthmuses, C-shaped canals, lateral and accessory canals, and internal resorptive areas. The potential for root fracture is reduced because the thermoplasticized gutta-percha mass flows easily into the anatomic variations with light spreader pressure. It is an easy technique to learn and requires only a relatively inexpensive addition to the armamentarium. Warm lateral condensation does not require preheating or special gutta-percha. In addition, cleaning and sterilization procedures are not complex.

Warm Vertical Condensation

In 1967, Schilder[8] advocated vertical condensation with warm gutta-percha as an alternative technique to cold lateral condensation or silver points. He recognized the importance of three-dimensional obturation of the entire root canal system and was concerned about the potential for voids and incomplete obturation occurring with other techniques.[52] The principal advantage of warm vertical condensation is its ability to adapt the warmed and softened gutta-percha to irregularities and accessory and lateral canals within the root canal system.[60,61]

Warm vertical condensation relies on the placement of a gutta-percha point, the removal of all but the apical portion of the cone with heat, and the addition of small segments that are heat-softened with a spreader and compacted vertically with a plugger. This produces a homogeneous mass throughout the root canal. Furthermore, because the hydraulic pressure forces gutta-percha and sealer into anatomic variations, the technique is noted for its demonstration of lateral and accessory canals radiographically.

The armamentarium needed consists of spreaders and pluggers. The spreaders are not used to condense the cold gutta-percha cones together, but rather serve as heat carriers to soften the gutta-percha mass before condensation with the cold plugger. The pluggers come in a variety of sizes (8 [0.4 mm], 8½ [0.5 mm], 9, 9½, 10, 10½, 11, 11½, 12) of increasing diameter and are marked at 5-mm intervals (Figure 7-18). After the root canal is ready for obturation, prefitted pluggers are selected that will enter the canal and descend to the desired depth. The clinician can mark the length by placing rubber stoppers on the cylindrical shaft of the instrument. Marking the pluggers in this manner allows the clinician to apply force to the gutta-percha mass while limiting the force applied to the canal walls.

A nonstandard gutta-percha point is selected and its tip cut away until it fits with tug-back approximately 2 or 3 mm short of the working length. The point is then coated with sealer and used to place and distribute sealer within the radicular space. A flame-heated red-hot carrier (spreader) is used to sear off the point at the orifice of the canal. Heavy vertical pressure is immediately applied with the largest cold plugger to force the cone apically. Because only the coronal 3 to 4 mm has been heated, the spreader is again heated and carried 3 to 4 mm further into the gutta-percha mass, followed by strong vertical condensation with the appropriate size plugger. This process softens and removes much of the gutta-percha, forcing it laterally and vertically into the irregularities of the canal. The procedure is repeated until the center of the canal is essentially empty except for the apical 5 mm. The clinician then refills the canal by touching the surface of the apical mass with the heat car-

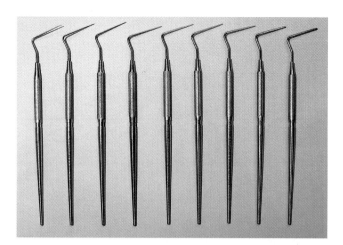

FIGURE 7-18 Schilder (Dentsply Maillefer, Ballaigues, Switzerland) pluggers used for warm vertical condensation. These instruments are manufactured from size 8 to size 12 with half sizes.

rier, placing a warmed 2- to 4-mm segment of gutta-percha in the canal, and condensing it vertically, repeating this process until the canal is filled (Figure 7-19).

Although the classic vertical condensation technique is capable of producing a dense, homogeneous root canal filling, there are several disadvantages. The technique is difficult to master and time consuming. It is particularly difficult to use in curved canals where the straight, rigid pluggers are unable to penetrate to the necessary depth. To allow the rigid carriers to contact the gutta-percha within 4 or 5 mm of the apex, the canals must be prepared larger and more tapered than in the lateral condensation technique, requiring the removal of additional dentin, which weakens the root. In addition, enormous pressures are created in the apical portion of the root, producing more fractures than lateral condensation.[62]

Because of these limitations, modifications to the technique have been suggested. One two-step technique consists of placing the sealer-coated initial gutta-percha point, then using a small spoon-shaped curette heated red hot to remove the coronal portion 8 to 10 mm inside the canal in anterior teeth. The portion of the point that was removed is set aside. A heat carrier is used to heat the apical portion, followed by heavy condensation with a plugger as before. The superficial part of the coronal apical gutta-percha mass is heated, and the reserved portion is warmed, reinserted into the canal, and condensed to fill the remainder of the canal. This simplified technique saves time but does not reduce the condensation pressures and may actually increase them.

A recent modification advocated by Ruddle[63] employs a similar technique for the placement and removal of the gutta-percha point, a process he terms "downpacking." With this technique a thermostatically controlled heat source, the Touch 'N Heat instrument (Figure 7-20), is used instead of flame-heated spreaders. The

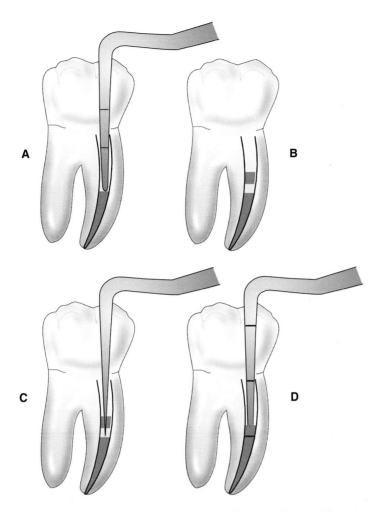

FIGURE 7-19   Diagram of the warm vertical condensation technique. **A,** After a heated spreader is used to remove the coronal segment of the master cone, a cold plugger is used to apply vertical pressure to the softened master cone. **B,** Obturation of the coronal portion of the canal is accomplished by adding a gutta-percha segment. **C,** A heated spreader is used to soften the material. **D,** A cold plugger is then used to apply pressure to the softened gutta-percha.

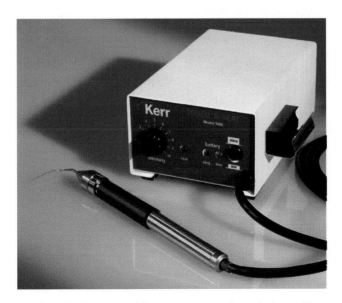

FIGURE 7-20   The Touch 'N Heat is used in warm gutta-percha techniques. (Courtesy Sybron, Inc. Orange, CA.)

second phase, refilling of the canal, is accomplished using the Obtura (Obtura Corporation, Fenton, Maryland) instrument, which is an electrically heated gutta-percha "gun" that heats gutta-percha to a flowable consistency and then expresses it into the canal through a 23-gauge needle. The canal is filled by injection and condensation of 4- or 5-mm segments. This step is referred to as "back-packing." The technique is somewhat faster and because it uses uniformly softened gutta-percha from the Obtura gun (Figure 7-21), it requires less pressure than the standard technique. Unfortunately, the down-packing portion produces the same pressures in the apical end as the Schilder technique, and because the same pluggers are used, identical amounts of tooth structure must be sacrificed for their introduction. Additionally, the technique is difficult to master and requires a considerable armamentarium to employ.

Continuous Wave Obturation

Buchanan recently introduced the continuous wave of condensation technique as a modification of the warm vertical compaction technique for canal obturation. This technique requires a smooth tapering funnel, an apical constriction, and appropriate master cone adaptation. The technique is often employed after cleaning and shaping procedures using nickel-titanium rotary files. GT

(Dentsply, Tulsa Dental, Tulsa, OK) gutta-percha points are now manufactured to mimic the dimensions of the GT files. The System B heat source is an electric device that supplies heat to a plugger on demand (Figure 7-22). Pluggers are available in standardized sizes, as well as nonstandardized sizes that match conventional gutta-percha cones. Cones and pluggers that match files of greater taper are also available (see Figures 7-11 and 7-23). Several hand pluggers are available.

Heat is applied using the System B heat source at the prescribed temperature (200° C) for a period of time determined by the operator. Applying a constant source of heat to a prefitted gutta-percha cone softens the gutta-percha so the clinician can apply hydraulic pressure in one continuous motion. As the plugger moves apically the cone adaptation is more precise and the hydraulic pressure increases, forcing the gutta-percha into canal irregularities and accessory canals.

With the continuous wave technique a master cone is adjusted to fit at the corrected working length and cut back 0.5 mm. The largest plugger that will go to a depth 5 to 7 mm from the apex is selected, and the reference point is marked with a stop. The master cone is coated with sealer and used to coat the canal walls. The System B heat source is set to 200° C and placed in touch mode. The master cone is severed at the canal orifice and re-

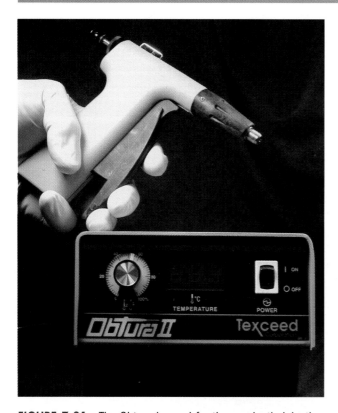

FIGURE 7-21 The Obtura is used for thermoplastic injection techniques and back-filling procedures with other techniques.

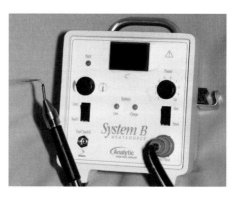

FIGURE 7-22 The System B unit.

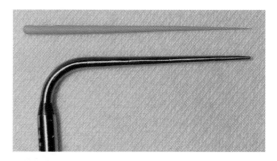

FIGURE 7-23 A System B plugger and a nonstandardized gutta-percha point.

moved. The clinician then places the cold plugger in the orifice with firm pressure and activates the heat source. The plugger is moved apically over a 1- to 2-second period until it is 3 mm short of the binding point. Care must be taken to ensure that the heat is never activated for more that 4 seconds. Pressure is maintained on the apical gutta-percha while the heat source is shut off for 5 to 10 seconds. After the gutta-percha has set the heat source is activated for 1 second to separate the plugger from the apical mass so the instrument can be removed. A hand plugger with a tip diameter of 0.4 mm is used to ensure the gutta-percha is not displaced and has set.

If no post space is required, a single cone backfill can be accomplished by placing a sealer-coated gutta-percha cone trimmed to a 0.5-mm tip diameter in the space vacated by the plugger. This cone is seared off at the orifice, and a final sustained pressure completes the condensation. An alternative method is back-filling with injectable thermoplasticized gutta-percha (Obtura).

As with all procedures, continuous wave obturation has inherent risks. The use of thermoplasticized gutta-percha techniques creates a potential for extrusion of materials into the periodontal structures as well as damage to the periodontal ligament and supporting alveolar bone from heat. An increase of 10° C above body temperature appears to be a critical threshold for injuring osseous tissues.[64] Evidence suggests that the use of flame-heated carriers poses a greater risk of injuring the periodontal structures.[65,66] Carriers heated in this manner can reach temperatures of 342° to 380° C.[67,68] The injectable gutta-percha technique[69] and the continuous wave condensation technique[66,70] appear to produce temperature changes below the critical threshold when used at the recommended temperatures.

Injection of Thermoplasticized Gutta-Percha

Instead of introducing gutta-percha into the root canal and applying heat to cause it to flow, the material can be heated outside the tooth and injected in a thermoplasticized state. The previously mentioned Obtura system (see Figure 7-21) consists of a handheld gun that contains a chamber surrounded by a heating element into which pellets of gutta-percha are loaded and heated. Silver needles are attached to deliver the thermoplasticized material to the canal. The gun is connected by a cord to a control unit that allows the operator to adjust the temperature and therefore the viscosity of the gutta-percha. To use the system, the clinician prepares the canal in the same manner as for lateral condensation. Because the needles are small and the thermoplasticized material flows readily, the clinician should not create too much flare in the preparation. The apical terminus must remain as small as possible to prevent extrusion. After preparing and drying the canal, the clinician loads the last file used with sealer and uses it to coat the canal

walls. The gutta-percha is preheated, and the needle is placed in the canal within 3 to 5 mm of the apical terminus. Gutta-percha is then gradually, passively injected by squeezing the trigger of the gun. The needle backs out of the canal as it is filled. The gutta-percha is then gently compacted with pluggers that have been dipped in alcohol to prevent the plugger from sticking to the softened gutta-percha. Alternatively, the clinician may use a segmental technique, in which 3- to 4-mm segments of gutta-percha are sequentially injected and condensed. In either case, condensation should continue until the gutta-percha cools and solidifies, which takes 3 to 5 minutes. This compensates for the contraction that takes place when it cools.

The difficulty with this system is the same as that of the other warm gutta-percha techniques and paste systems—lack of control. Both overextension and underextension are common findings (Figure 7-24). To overcome this drawback, the clinician may use a hybrid technique, beginning obturation using the lateral condensation technique. When the master cone and several accessory cones have been placed so that the mass is

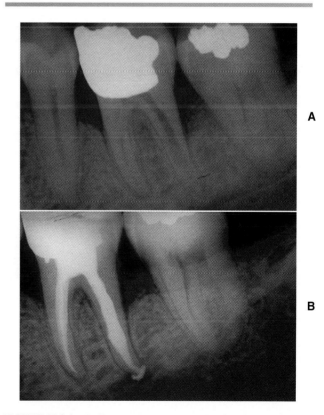

A

B

FIGURE 7-24 **A,** Preoperative radiograph of a mandibular left first molar exhibiting internal resorption in the distal root. **B,** Obturation with thermoplasticized gutta-percha reveals obliteration of the resorptive space and extrusion of material into the periradicular tissues, a potential complication of any of the warm gutta-percha techniques.

firmly lodged in the apical portion of the canal, a hot plugger is introduced, searing the points off approximately 4 to 5 mm from the apex. Light vertical condensation is applied to restore the integrity of the apical plug of gutta-percha, and no attempt is made to warm it. The remainder of the canal is then filled with thermoplasticized gutta-percha as described previously. This technique is similar to Ruddle's but avoids the down-packing step, which is time consuming, requires additional widening of the canal, and creates potentially fracture-producing apical pressure.

Carrier-Based Gutta-Percha

Originally the gutta-percha carrier systems (Thermafil, Dentsply, Tulsa Dental, Tulsa, OK) were manufactured with a metal core to which the manufacturer applied a coating of gutta-percha. When heated over an open flame, the gutta-percha would soften and could then be introduced into the root canal. The technique became popular because the central core provided a rigid mechanism to facilitate placement of the obturation material. This ease of placement often resulted in incomplete cleaning and shaping and an attendant decrease in prognosis. As with other obturation techniques, the quality of cleaning and shaping dictates success. In addition, the metallic core made placement of a post challenging.

Current advances in the carrier systems include the development of a plastic core coated with alpha-phase gutta-percha and a heating device that heats the carrier and controls the temperature (Figure 7-25). Thermafil offers another alternative to obturation with heated gutta-percha[71] (Figure 7-26). Recently Dentsply/Tulsa Dental (Tulsa, OK) introduced GT obturators designed to correspond to the sizes of the GT Profile nickel-titanium rotary files (Figure 7-27). Having obturators that are manufactured to correlate with the precise size of the prepared canal may enhance the quality of obturation. The traditional Thermafil obturators are manu-

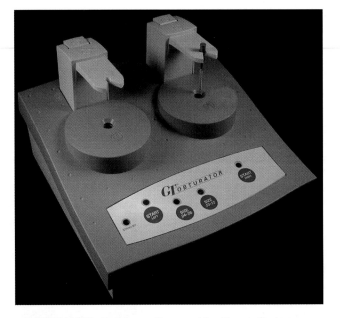

FIGURE 7-25   The Thermafil oven with a Thermafil obturator.

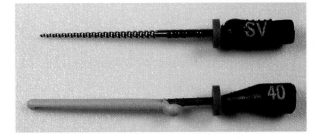

FIGURE 7-26   A Thermafil obturator and appropriate size verifier.

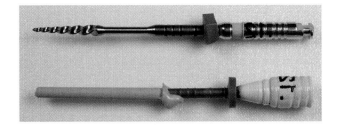

FIGURE 7-27   A size 50/.12 GT nickel-titanium file and the corresponding GT obturator.

factured consistent with International Standards Organization file sizes but may not adapt to the coronal position of the canal, which exhibits greater taper after preparation with Gates Glidden drills.

The carrier-based technique requires the use of a sealer, and the removal of the smear layer is recommended.[72] Grossman formulation sealers or resin sealers consistent with AH26 are acceptable. Tubliseal and Wach's Paste are not recommended. Size verifiers for the gutta-percha carriers are available for selecting the size of the obturator necessary for placement. The verifier should fit passively at the corrected working length. When the GT obturators are used the size should correlate with the shaping objective file.

After drying the canal and placing a light coat of sealer, the clinician marks a carrier with a rubber stop set at the predetermined length. This must be accomplished using the millimeter calibration markings on the carrier shaft. Markings are made at 18, 19, 20, 22, 24, 27, and 29 mm. A Bard-Parker blade can be used to remove gutta-percha on the shaft that may be obscuring the calibration rings. After the rubber stop is set, the carrier is disinfected with 5.25% sodium hypochlorite for 1 minute and rinsed in 70% alcohol.[73]

The carrier is then placed in the heating device. After it is heated to the appropriate temperature, the operator has approximately 10 seconds to retrieve the carrier and insert it into the canal. This is accomplished without rotation or twisting. The position of the obturation material is verified radiographically. After waiting 2 to 4 minutes for the material to set, the clinician can section the carrier several millimeters above the canal orifice. This is accomplished by applying stabilizing pressure to the carrier and cutting the device with an inverted cone, round bur, or specially designed Prepi bur. Heated instruments are not recommended for this process because they may result in displacement of the obturator. Vertical compaction of the coronal gutta-percha can be accomplished and when necessary gutta-percha can be added, heat softened, and condensed. A lubricant should be applied to the plugger to prevent adhesion and possible displacement.

If post space is required for restoration of the tooth, specially designed ProPost (Dentsply, Tulsa Dental, Tulsa, OK) drills are recommended. The unique eccentric cutting tip keeps the instrument centered in the canal while friction softens and removes the gutta-percha and plastic carrier. Evidence suggests that the seal is not altered if this procedure is accomplished immediately.[74,75]

If retreatment is required the plastic carrier has a groove along its length to provide an access point for placement of a file. Rotary .04 and .06 nickel-titanium files may facilitate complete removal of the obturation materials. When necessary, chloroform and hand files can be used to remove the gutta-percha surrounding the carrier.

The plastic carriers are composed of two materials. Sizes up to 40 are manufactured from a liquid crystal plastic. Sizes 40 to 90 are composed of polysulfone polymer. Both have similar physical characteristics, with the polysulfone carriers being susceptible to dissolution in chloroform.

THE CORONAL SEAL

Regardless of the technique used to obturate the canals, coronal microleakage can occur through seemingly well-obturated canals within a short time, potentially causing infection of the periapical area.[7,76-79] A method to protect the canals in case of failure of the coronal restoration is to cover the floor of the pulp chamber with a lining of glass ionomer cement after the excess gutta-percha and sealer have been cleaned from the canal. Glass ionomers have the intrinsic ability to bond to the dentin, so they do not require a pretreatment step. The resin-modified glass ionomer cement is simply flowed approximately 1 mm thick over the floor of the pulp chamber and polymerized with a curing light for 30 seconds. Investigators found that this procedure resulted in none of the experimental canals showing leakage.[79]

WHEN TO OBTURATE

In patients who are asymptomatic, obturation may be completed during the instrumentation appointment. In general, teeth exhibiting vital pulp tissue and normal periradicular structures are the best candidates for obturation at the instrumentation visit. Although there appears to be no difference in postoperative pain after single-visit endodontic treatment of teeth exhibiting pulp necrosis,[80] teeth exhibiting necrotic pulps as well as those exhibiting chronic apical periodontitis and chronic apical abscesses resulting from pulp necrosis may be best managed in two treatment visits. Recent clinical studies[81-83] indicate an improved prognosis for these cases if calcium hydroxide is placed as an intracanal medicament and obturation delayed until a second visit.[84] The calcium hydroxide serves as an antimicrobial dressing, reducing the bacteria present in the radicular space, as well as a temporary obturant.

Contraindications to single-appointment root canal treatment include the following:

1. Significant pain and/or swelling
2. Inability to dry the canal
3. Persistence of purulent drainage in the canal during instrumentation

Two additional considerations are esthetics and the ability to provide an adequate provisional restoration to prevent coronal leakage between visits. The clinician may need to obturate a tooth to facilitate placement of an esthetic temporary crown in the anterior region.

References

1. Kakehashi S, Stanley H, Fitzgerald R: Effect of surgical exposures of dental pulps in germ-free and conventional laboratory rats, *Oral Surg Oral Med Oral Pathol Oral Radiol Endod* 20:340, 1965.

2. Delivanis PD, Mattison GD, Mendel RW: The survivability of F43 strain of *Streptococcus sanguis* in root canals filled with gutta-percha and ProcoSol cement, *J Endodon* 9(10):407, 1983.

3. Walton RE: Histologic evaluation of different methods of enlarging the pulp canal space, *J Endodon* 2(10):304, 1976.

4. Peters OA, Barbakow F: Effects of irrigation on debris and smear layer on canal walls prepared by two rotary techniques: a scanning electron microscopic study, *J Endodon* 26(1):6, 2000.

5. Matsumiya S, Kitamura S: Histo-pathologic and histo-bacteriological studies of the relation between the condition of sterilization of the interior of the root canal and the healing process of periapical tissues in experimentally infected root canal treatment, *Bull Tokyo Coll* 1:1, 1960.

6. Seltzer S: *Endodontology*, Philadelphia, 1988, Lea and Febiger.

7. Swanson K, Madison S: An evaluation of coronal microleakage in endodontically treated teeth. Part I. Time periods, *J Endodon* 13(2):56, 1987.

8. Schilder H: Filling root canals in three dimensions, *Dent Clin North Am* 11:723, 1967.

9. Ingle JI: *Endodontics*, Philadelphia, 1965, Lea and Febiger.

10. Strindberg LZ: The dependence of the results of pulp therapy on certain factors. An analytic study based on radiographic and clinical follow-up examinations, *Acta Odontol Scand* 14:1, 1956.

11. Grahnen H, Hansson L: The prognosis of pulp and root canal therapy. A clinical and radiographic follow-up examination, *Odont Rev* 12:146, 1961.

12. Sjögren U, Sundqvist G, Nair PNR: Tissue reaction to gutta percha particles of various sizes when implanted subcutaneously in guinea pigs, *Eur J Oral Sci* 103:313, 1995.

13. Ricucci D, Langeland K: Apical limit of root canal instrumentation and obturation. Part 2. A histologic study, *Int Endod J* 31:394, 1998.

14. Smith CS, Setchell DJ, Harty FJ: Factors influencing the success of conventional root canal therapy—a five-year retrospective study, *Int Endod J* 26(6):321, 1993.

15. Spangberg L, Langeland K: Biologic effects of dental materials 1. Toxicity of root canal filling materials on HeLa cells in vitro, *Oral Surg Oral Med Oral Pathol Oral Radiol Endod* 35:402, 1973.

16. Pascon EA et al: Tissue reaction to endodontic materials: methods, criteria, assessment, and observations, *Oral Surg Oral Med Oral Pathol Oral Radiol Endod* 72:222, 1991.

17. Malueg LA, Wilcox LR, Johnson WT: Examination of external apical root resorption with scanning electron microscopy, *Oral Surg Oral Med Oral Pathol Oral Radiol Endod* 82:89, 1996.

18. Tronstad L: Tissue reactions following apical plugging of the root canal with dentin chips in monkey teeth subjected to pulpectomy, *Oral Surg Oral Med Oral Pathol Oral Radiol Endod* 45:297, 1978.

19. Oswald RJ, Friedman CE: Periapical response to dentin filings, *Oral Surg Oral Med Oral Pathol Oral Radiol Endod* 49:344, 1980.

20. Pascon EA et al: Tissue reaction to endodontic materials: methods, criteria, assessment, and observations, *Oral Surg Oral Med Oral Pathol Oral Radiol Endod* 72:222, 1991.

21. Holland R et al: Tissue reactions following apical plugging of the root canal with infected dentin chips, *Oral Surg Oral Med Oral Pathol Oral Radiol Endod* 49:366, 1980.

22. Brady JE, Himel VT, Weir JC: Periapical response to an apical plug of dentin filings intentionally placed after root canal overinstrumentation, *J Endodon* 11(8):323, 1985.

23. Pissiotis E, Spangberg LS: Biological evaluation of collagen gels containing calcium hydroxide and hydroxyapatite, *J Endodon* 16(10):468, 1990.

24. Torabinejad M, Chivian N: Clinical applications of mineral trioxide aggregate, *J Endodon* 25:197, 1999.

25. Grossman LI, Oliet S, Del Rio C: *Endodontics*, Philadelphia, 1988, Lea and Febiger.

26. Augsburger RA, Peters DD: Radiographic evaluation of extruded obturation materials, *J Endodon* 16(10):492, 1990.

27. The courts: FDA explains status of N2 material, *J Am Dent Assoc* 123:236, 1992.

28. Wu MK et al: Fluid transport and bacterial penetration along root canal fillings, *Int Endod J* 26(4):203, 1993.

29. Oksan T et al: The penetration of root canal sealers into dentinal tubules. A scanning electron microscopic study, *Int Endod J* 26(5):301, 1993.

30. Sen BH, Piskin B, Baran N: The effect of tubular penetration of root canal sealers on dye microleakage, *Int Endod J* 29(1):23, 1996.

31. Wiemann AH, Wilcox LR: In vitro evaluation of four methods of sealer placement, *J Endodon* 17(9):444, 1991.

32. Jasper EA: Adaptation and tissue tolerance of silver root canal fillings, *J Dent Res* 4:355, 1941.

33. Brady JM, del Rio CE: Corrosion of endodontic silver cones in humans: a scanning electron microscope and x-ray microprobe study, *J Endodon* 1(6):205, 1975.

34. Seltzer S et al: A scanning electron microscope examination of silver cones removed from endodontically treated teeth, *Oral Surg Oral Med Oral Pathol Oral Radiol Endod* 33:589, 1972.

35. Walton RE, Torabinejad M: *Principles and practice of endodontics*, Philadelphia, 2002, WB Saunders.

36. Langeland K et al: Methods in the study of biologic responses to endodontic materials, *Oral Surg Oral Med Oral Pathol Oral Radiol Endod* 27:522, 1969.

37. Fanibunda KB: Adverse response to endodontic material containing paraformaldehyde, *Bri Dent J* 157:231, 1984.

38. Nguyen NT: Obturation of the root canal system. In Cohen S, Burns RC, editors: *Pathways of the pulp*, ed 6, St Louis, 1994, Mosby.

39. Schilder H, Goodman A, Aldrich W: The thermomechanical properties of gutta-percha. I. The compressibility of gutta-percha, *Oral Surg Oral Med Oral Pathol Oral Radiol Endod* 37:946, 1974.

40. Hatton JF et al: The effect of condensation pressure on the apical seal, *J Endodon* 14(6):305, 1988.

41. Schilder H, Goodman A, Aldrich W: The thermomechanical properties of gutta-percha. II. The history and molecular chemistry of gutta-percha, *Oral Surg Oral Med Oral Pathol Oral Radiol Endod* 37:954, 1974.

42. Feldman G, Nyborg H: Tissue reactions of root canal filling materials. 1. Comparison between gutta-percha and silver amalgam implanted in rabbits, *Odontol Rev* 13:1, 1962.

43. Wolfson EM, Seltzer S: Reaction of rat connective tissue to some gutta-percha formulations, *J Endodon* 1(12):395, 1975.

44. Marshall FJ, Massler M: Sealing of pulpless teeth evaluated with radioisotopes, *J Dent Med* 16:172, 1961.

45. Kapsimalis P, Evans R, Tuckerman M: Modified autoradiographic technique for marginal penetration studies, *Oral Surg Oral Med Oral Pathol Oral Radiol Endod* 20:494, 1965.

46. Kuttler Y: Microscopic investigation of root apexes, *J Am Dent Assoc* 50:544, 1955.

47. Dang DA, Walton RE: Vertical root fracture and root distortion: effect of spreader design, *J Endodon* 15(7):294, 1989.

48. Berry KA et al: Nickel-titanium versus stainless-steel finger spreaders in curved canals, *J Endodon* 24(11):752, 1998.

49. Joyce AP et al: Photoelastic comparison of stress induced by using stainless-steel versus nickel-titanium spreaders in vitro, *J Endodon* 24(11):714, 1998.

50. Allison DA, Michelich RJ, Walton RE: The influence of master cone adaptation on the quality of the apical seal, *J Endodon* 7(2):61, 1981.

51. Pitts DL, Matheny HE, Nicholls JI: An in vitro study of spreader loads required to cause vertical root fracture during lateral condensation, *J Endodon* 9(12):544, 1983.

52. Brayton SM, Davis SR, Goldman M: Gutta-percha root canal fillings. An in vitro analysis. Part 1, *Oral Surg Oral Med Oral Pathol Oral Radiol Endod* 35:226, 1973.

53. Keane KM, Harrington GW: The use of a chloroform-softened gutta-percha master cone and its effect on the apical seal, *J Endodon* 10(2):57, 1984.

54. McDonald MN, Vire DE: Chloroform in the endodontic operatory, *J Endodon* 18(6):301, 1992.

55. Margelos J, Verdelis K, Eliades G: Chloroform uptake by gutta-percha and assessment of its concentration in air during the chloroform-dip technique, *J Endodon* 22(10):547, 1996.

56. Liewehr FR, Kulild JC, Primack PD: Improved density of gutta-percha after warm lateral condensation, *J Endodon* 19(10):489, 1993.

57. Liewehr FR, Kulild JC, Primack PD: Obturation of a C-shaped canal using an improved method of warm lateral condensation, *J Endodon* 19(9):474, 1993.

58. Nelson EA, Liewehr FR, West LA: Increased density of gutta-percha using a controlled heat instrument with lateral condensation, *J Endodon* 26:748, 2000.

59. Baumgardner KR, Krell KV: Ultrasonic condensation of gutta-percha: an in vitro dye penetration and scanning electron microscopic study, *J Endodon* 16(6):253, 1990.

60. DuLac KA et al: Comparison of the obturation of lateral canals by six techniques, *J Endodon* 25(5):376, 1999.

61. Wolcott J et al: Effect of two obturation techniques on the filling of lateral canals and the main canal, *J Endodon* 23(10):632, 1997.

62. Wollard RR et al: Scanning electron microscopic examination of root canal filling materials, *J Endodon* 2(4):98, 1976.

63. Ruddle CJ: Three-dimensional obturation: the rationale and application of warm gutta-percha with vertical condensation. In Cohen S, Burns RC, editors: *Pathways of the pulp*, ed 6, St Louis, 1994, Mosby.

64. Eriksson AR, Albbrektsson T: Temperature threshold levels for heat-induced bone tissue injury; a vital microscopic study in the rabbit, *J Prosthet Dent* 50:101, 1983.

65. Lee FS, Van Cura JE, BeGole E: A comparison of root surface temperatures using different obturation heat sources, *J Endodon* 24(9):617, 1998.

66. Silver GK, Love RM, Purton DG: Comparison of two vertical condensation obturation techniques: Touch 'n Heat modified and System B, *Int Endod J* 32(4):287, 1999.

67. Hand RE, Hugel EF, Tsaknis PJ: Effects of a warm gutta percha technique on the lateral periodontium, *Oral Surg Oral Med Oral Pathol Oral Radiol Endod* 36:872, 1973.

68. Marciano J, Michailesco PM: Dental gutta-percha: chemical composition, x-ray identification, enthalpic studies, and clinical implications, *J Endodon* 15(4):149, 1989.

69. Weller RN, Koch KA: In vitro radicular temperatures produced by injectable thermoplasticized gutta-percha, *Int Endod J* 28(2):86, 1995.

70. Floren JW et al: Changes in root surface temperatures with in vitro use of the System B HeatSource, *J Endodon* 25(9):593, 1999.

71. Gutmann JL: Adaptation of injected thermoplasticized gutta-percha in the absence of the dentinal smear layer, *Int Endod J* 26(2):87, 1993.

72. Behrend GD, Cutler CW, Gutmann JL: An in-vitro study of smear layer removal and microbial leakage along root-canal fillings, *Int Endod J* 29(2):99, 1996.

73. Glickman GN, Gutmann JL: Contemporary perspectives on canal obturation, *Dent Clin North Am* 36:327, 1992.

74. Rybicki R, Zillich R: Apical sealing ability of Thermafil following immediate and delayed post space preparations, *J Endodon* 20(2):64, 1994.

75. Saunders WP et al: An assessment of the plastic Thermafil obturation technique. Part 3. The effect of post space preparation on the apical seal, *Int Endod J* 26(3):184, 1993.

76. Torabinejad M, Ung B, Kettering JD: In vitro bacterial penetration of coronally unsealed endodontically treated teeth, *J Endodon* 16(12):566, 1990.

77. Saunders WP, Saunders EM: Assessment of leakage in the restored pulp chamber of endodontically treated multirooted teeth, *Int Endod J* 23(1):28, 1990.

78. Barrieshi KM, Walton RE, Johnson WT: Coronal leakage of mixed anaerobic bacteria after obturation and post space preparation, *Oral Surg Oral Med Oral Pathol Oral Radiol Endod* 84:310, 1997.

79. Chailertvanitkul P et al: An evaluation of microbial coronal leakage in the restored pulp chamber of root-canal treated multirooted teeth, *Int Endod J* 30(5):318, 1997.

80. Roane JB, Dryden JA, Grimes EW: Incidence of postoperative pain after single- and multiple-visit endodontic procedures, *Oral Surg Oral Med Oral Pathol Oral Radiol Endod* 55:68, 1983.

81. Sjögren U et al: Influence of infection at the time of root filling on the outcome of endodontic treatment of teeth with apical periodontitis [erratum appears in *Int Endod J* 31(2):148, 1998.], *Int Endod J* 30(5):297, 1997.

82. Katebzadeh N, Hupp J, Trope M: Histological periapical repair after obturation of infected root canals in dogs, *J Endodon* 25(5):364, 1999.

83. Trope M, Delano EO, Orstavik D: Endodontic treatment of teeth with apical periodontitis: single vs. multivisit treatment, *J Endodon* 25(5):345, 1999.

84. Sjögren U et al: The antimicrobial effect of calcium hydroxide as a short-term intracanal dressing, *Int Endod J* 24(3):119, 1991.

8

RETREATMENT

GEORGE A. BRUDER III *and* **ROBERT R. WHITE**

RETREATMENT

Endodontic retreatment comprises nonsurgical and surgical procedures performed on teeth that were previously subject to endodontic treatment. The American Association of Endodontists Glossary of Terms[1] states that these procedures revise the shape of canals, remove root canal filling materials, and obturate canals. Retreatment is usually initiated if the original treatment appears inadequate, if initial treatment has failed, or if microorganisms from the oral environment have contaminated the root canal. The goals of retreatment and subsequent restorative procedures are to return or maintain the comfortable function of a tooth in an environment that is free of inflammation and pathosis.

Considerations of endodontic retreatment have grown logarithmically in the past 15 years. Reasons supporting the increasing need for retreatment procedures include the following:

1. The increasing number of initial endodontic procedures and the biologic certainty that some of these will fail
2. Recognition of the potential effect of coronal to apical microbial leakage
3. Growing realization that "the best implant" is a healthy natural tooth

Practitioners who provide endodontic care should further orient themselves toward nonsurgical and surgical retreatment approaches.

SUCCESS AND FAILURE

Routine clinical and radiographic examinations at 6 months, 1 year, and 2 or more years after endodontic treatment are essential. These evaluation methods determine and attempt to predict the success and stability of endodontic treatment. Teeth that have received endodontic treatment must also be reevaluated if signs or symptoms manifest; reevaluation should also occur before any new restorative or complex periodontal procedure (Box 8-1).

With healing, successfully treated teeth should demonstrate an intact lamina dura, normal periodontal ligament space, and normal periradicular bone on radiographic examination. These teeth should function without signs or symptoms, and their endodontic and restorative procedures should demonstrate adherence to high standards of care.

Questionably successfully treated teeth can also function in a normal manner; they may demonstrate normal periradicular structures on radiographic examination. However, when the quality of the root filling or coronal restoration is considered, concerns may be noted that can eventually affect the long-term prognosis. Caries and open margins around restorative materials may lead to coronal apical leakage. Inadequate obturation and extrusion of endodontic obturating materials may also lead to failure.

Questionably failing teeth frequently demonstrate signs and symptoms, as well as partial or incomplete healing on radiographic examination. Substantial discrepancies are usually noted in the coronal and/or radicular fillings. Often the patient and dentist tolerate these situations until they fail or require further restoration.

Endodontic treatment failures demonstrate new or persistent pathosis. Patients can have symptoms and clinical signs, including radiographically demonstrable loss of the periodontal ligament space, lamina dura, and bone. Questionable or failing outcomes necessitate consideration for retreatment, further restorative procedures, or extraction.

BOX 8-1

Endodontic Treatment Concerns

Success (endodontic/restorative)	→ Recall		
Questionable success			
Adequate function and restoration	→ Recall		
Restoration or extensive periodontal therapy	→ Consider retreatment	→ Restore	→ Recall
	→ NSRCT* retreatment	→ Restore	→ Recall
	→ NSRCT retreatment, SRCT† (BX)‡	→ Restore	→ Recall
	→ SRCT (BX)	→ Restore	→ Recall
	→ Extraction (BX)	→ Recall	
Questionable failure and failure			
Adequate function	→ Recall		
Restoration or extensive periodontal therapy	→ NSRCT retreatment	→ Restore	→ Recall
	→ NSRCT retreatment, SRCT (BX)	→ Restore	→ Recall
	→ SRCT (BX)	→ Restore	→ Recall
	→ Extraction (BX)	→ Recall	

*Nonsurgical root canal treatment.
†Surgical root canal treatment.
‡Biopsy.

PLANNING, RESTORATION, AND CONSENT

Successful retreatment depends on accurate diagnosis and identification of the etiology of failure. The clinician begins by recording the patient's chief complaint and pertinent history. The causes of failure can almost always be found by looking for a source of microorganisms and nutrients (persistent or recurrent) associated with the root canal system. A thorough clinical and periodontal examination should be performed. At this time the type, angulation, and number of subsequent radiographs are determined. All sinus tracts and pockets greater than 6.0 mm should be traced on these films. Usually a bite-wing and several periapical radiographs are taken. The resulting information (Box 8-2) is then combined and synthesized to produce a mental three-dimensional reconstruction of the tooth. As the clinician performs the evaluation, he or she forms an impression that attempts to differentiate between previously inadequate treatment and treatment compromised by clinical limitations. When possible, the dentist who performed the original treatment should be contacted. Their records and radiographs may provide a valued perspective on the nature of the problem and the quality of care provided. Restorative dentists should also be involved at this time in anticipation of their role in retreatment.

As endodontic retreatment is considered, so too is the ability to restore the tooth after retreatment. Interdisciplinary treatment planning is as important as endodontic diagnosis. Realistically, almost any tooth can be retreated, but restoring it to biologic health and function may not always be possible. This treatment planning process focuses on periodontal conditions and remaining tooth structure

BOX 8-2

*Endodontic Considerations**

- Caries, open margins
- Natural anatomy versus crown contour (prosthetic realignment)
- Extent of previous access preparation and lateral perforations
- Floor to furcal distance, scoring, perforations
- Location, size, and number of orifices
- Root anatomy, missed canals
- Curves, dilacerations, calcifications, fractures, and resorptions
- Natural and dentistogenic anatomy
- Strips, ledges, transportations, zips
- Pins, posts, cores, and separated instruments
- Obturation: overfilling, underfilling, overextension, or underextension
- Periradicular anatomy for surgical endodontics
- Systemic health, patient expectations

*Each canal system in a multicanaled tooth must be considered separately.

(Boxes 8-3 and 8-4). Occlusal and orthodontic considerations may also influence the decision process (Box 8-5). With the new diagnosis, the clinician forms an impression as to how retreatment and restoration will benefit the patient.

What are the endodontic expectations to:

1. Improve the original débridement and canal shape.

Periodontal Considerations

- Active disease?
- Level of control
- Patient motivation, systemic health, habits
- Recurrent periodontal abscesses, furcation involvement
- Excessive mobility, occlusal stability
- Gingival margins, esthetics, lip lines
- Osseous height, defects, biologic width
- Implants: Suitability of location for implant, cost, medical history

Prosthetic Considerations

- Crown-root ratio
- Root width, depth, and proximity
- Amount and quality of remaining tooth structure
- Ability to place an adequate ferrule or margins
- Occlusal load and function
- Floor to furcal distance, perforations (repairs)
- Relationship to the entire restorative picture

Orthodontic Considerations

- Patient goals, desires, esthetics
- Overall control of inflammatory dental disease
- Occlusal stability: function and parafunction
- Periodontal disease and tooth position
- Abutment inclination
- Potential pontic or implant spaces

2. Débride newly accessed and contaminated regions of the canal system.
3. Improve on the radicular filling, restoration, and function.

Recently, critical abutments compromised in many respects have been considered for extraction and implant placement. The decision to retreat should also embrace the patient's financial and emotional considerations.

After pretreatment assessment and diagnosis the focus shifts to the operator, patient, and restoring dentist. For the operator, each retreatment procedure is unique, frequently testing his or her limits of ingenuity, flexibility, and persistence. Rather than a single magic "silver bullet" treatment, a deliberate, logical, stepwise approach is more successful. Treatment, which sometimes seems tedious and time-consuming, presents an exciting challenge to the retreating dentist. The operator should never underestimate the potential difficulty of the procedure. If doubt exists regarding professional ability, armamentarium, time apportionment, expectations, or compensation, referral to an experienced colleague is indicated.

After giving initial consent to treatment the patient must remain an informed partner as the prognosis evolves during retreatment. A mid-treatment complication may arise or the outcome may be less than anticipated. A surgical approach or extraction may be necessary. In all instances, ongoing forthright communication with the patient is essential. This intimate communication must also be maintained with the restoring dentist. After endodontic treatment the outcome must be appraised; the tooth must be restored and then evaluated on recall to confirm success. Root canal treatment is never complete until the tooth is restored to function.

CORONAL DISASSEMBLY: REGAINING ACCESS TO THE CHAMBER FLOOR

With a plan in place, retreatment procedures may commence. A common finding on initiation of retreatment procedures is that the original access preparation was too small and restrictive. If maximal straight-line access was not achieved, it probably contributed to subsequent deficiencies in instrumentation, débridement, and obturation. Physically and visually restricted access preparations make the search for additional canals more difficult. These considerations frequently lead to the removal of existing restorations. If a new restoration is planned or a temporary restoration is already in place, this procedure should be relatively uncomplicated. If a fracture is suspected, the clinician should remove the entire restoration, apply dye stain, transilluminate, and view with magnification. Active caries must always be removed, and faulty, leaking restorations should be replaced or repaired. If the existing restoration is to be maintained, consideration must be given to its removal or careful, nondestructive penetration (often without a rubber dam so the clinician can observe prosthetic realignment). Occasionally the existing restoration can be removed and then temporarily replaced for esthetics or function after treatment (Box 8-6).

Beneath the coronal restoration the operator should anticipate a filling, core material, or a post and core combination. With adequate provisional access, core and filling materials can be rapidly removed with burs. If canal filling materials such as carriers, silver cones, or posts extend into the chamber and core material, the clinician should attempt to work around them, preserving their coronal extensions. Methods to achieve this include changing the bur-cutting direction (Figure 8-1) and isolating posts by ultrasonics (Figure 8-2). Material on the walls and floor

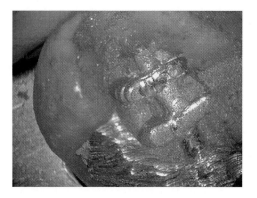

FIGURE 8-1   Bur-cutting directions.

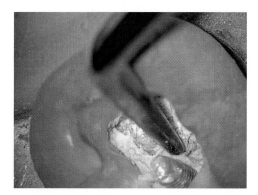

FIGURE 8-2   Post isolated using ultrasonics.

BOX 8-6

Advantages and Disadvantages of Removing the Existing Crown or Restoration

ADVANTAGES	DISADVANTAGES
· Easier to visualize and explore tooth and pulp morphology · Easier to evaluate for fractures, caries, and open margins · Easier to radiograph coronal structure · Easier to evaluate for further restoration · Shorter working distances and easier entry · Reduced from occlusion: Less risk of fracture or percussion sensitivity	· Loss of esthetics and/or function · Loss of interproximal and occlusal contact · Time necessary to remove and replace a temporary restoration · Increased difficulty of isolation · Increased difficulty of temporization

---

should be chipped free with ultrasonics, magnification, illumination, and preferably microscopy.

Careful observation and particular care are necessary to detect the presence of titanium alloy posts and carriers.[2] Their radiopacity is similar to that of most radicular filling materials. Clinically their dull gray color usually distinguishes them from surrounding materials.

As access is reestablished, microscopy and its attendant illumination permit visualization of anatomic landmarks and identification and location of the root canals. The "map" on a chamber floor or the color of the dentin further assists in localization of the canal orifices. Localization may be followed by occlusal access modifications for better straight-line access. Unless a post or radicular filling material is obviously loose or completely blocking exploration, the clinician should not attempt to remove it. This phase of retreatment should be limited to identification of orifices and exposure of the chamber floor. Copious irrigation and aspiration are invaluable. Organic material in an undiscovered orifice often demonstrates a "bubble trail" on the chamber floor as the sodium hypochlorite breaks down the tissues and effervesces.

Cast posts, cast interlocking posts, and Richmond crowns are initially exposed in a similar manner, with the clinician using a bur to remove coronal or core struc-

ture until the tooth-metal interface can be visualized near the orifice for each canal.

POST REMOVAL

In 1926, Kells[3] suggested using two strong magnets to remove cemented posts. Present techniques have given clinicians a far greater advantage. The clinician must consider all the factors that significantly influence post retention—length, shape, surface characteristics, cementation media, and active or passive placement—before attempting post removal. Large post diameters, likelihood of fracture, and the risk of removing too much tooth structure are other notable concerns. Occasionally, when a post seems adequate but difficult to remove and the endodontics for that root is questionable, the post may be retained and a surgical approach considered.

Pretreatment radiographs from various angles help identify posts that are close to or actually perforating a root. Sound practice frequently dictates the evaluation of a post with an apex locator before removal. After removal the clinician can use transillumination, microscopy, and paper points to evaluate the post space.[4,5] Even when perforation repairs are possible, structural losses may have excessively weakened the root, predisposing it to fracture.

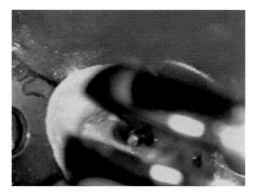

FIGURE 8-3   The clinician can use Steiglitz forceps to engage the post while applying ultrasonics.

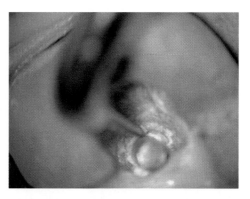

FIGURE 8-4   Troughing cement around post.

Unless the post is obviously loose, reduction of post retention should follow post isolation.[6] Ultrasonic vibration can be applied to the coronal extension of the post. Vibration applied in this manner has been shown to reduce post retention substantially and facilitate removal. If the post shows signs of disintegration when touched by ultrasonic tips, the clinician can clamp the post with a hemostat or Steiglitz and vibrate on the forceps (Figure 8-3). The first motion detected is usually rotational. A gentle drawing force on the hemostat, with continued ultrasonic vibration, should complete the removal process. Troughing the cement line around posts may also help reduce retention (Figure 8-4). Because canals are not perfectly round and no post fits precisely, a cement line or space that small, delicate ultrasonic tips can penetrate should be evident with magnification (Figure 8-5). When using these smaller ultrasonic tips, the clinician should lower the power setting to minimize instrument breakage. A primary objective is to preserve as much sound dentin as possible. Small hand files with solvents may also be used adjacent to recalcitrant posts. These files can be ultrasonically energized.[7] If ultrasonics and discrete troughing fail to dislodge a post, a variety of post removal devices may be used (Figure 8-6). These devices generally work using principles similar to that of a corkscrew. The post is engaged and pulled from the fulcrum, the tooth (Figure 8-7). When the use of a removal system is anticipated, reduction and tapping (threading) of the post should be accomplished before any signs of mobility occur.

CLINICAL TECHNIQUE—REMOVAL SYSTEM PROCEDURE

1. Isolate the tooth with a rubber dam.
2. Achieve straight-line access with coronal clearance for tapping.
3. Expose the post using previously described methods.

4. Prepare the post, reducing it to fit the coinciding tap size.
5. Tap the post in a counterclockwise (preferred) or clockwise direction, depending on the system
6. Remove the threading device, place a padded ring on the tap, and thread it back onto the post.
7. Place the extractor, engaging the tap between the padded ring and tap knob.
8. Activate removal device and turn removal knob or extractor clockwise in combination with ultrasonics delivered directly to the device.
9. Remove post, completing the first step of nonsurgical retreatment.

Occasionally clinicians must alternate between ultrasonically activating this assembly and incrementally increasing the drawing force. They must be patient and try to avoid excess tension that can lead to root fractures. Repeated, deeper troughing may also be necessary to further weaken and break cement bonds. If magnification and visualization are adequate, drilling a post out with a small, high-speed, long-shank round bur can be a tedious but effective last resort.

As radicular disassembly progresses, the clinician can cover other open canal orifices with cotton, especially when modifying the access preparation through a restoration. This will help minimize debris from becoming an additional canal obstacle.

THE REMOVAL OF RADICULAR FILLING MATERIAL OR OBSTRUCTIONS

The following basic principles must be considered as radicular filling materials are removed:

1. The hardness or consistency of a nonmetallic filling or the ability to remove an intracanal material cannot be determined radiographically.

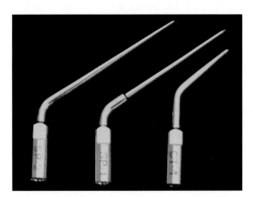

FIGURE 8-5 Ultrasonic tip assortment.

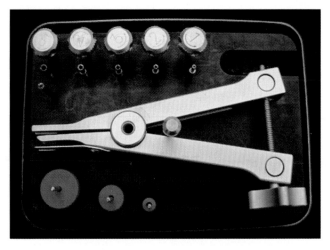

FIGURE 8-6 Post removal devices.

2. Removal of a previous filling material is usually easier if the root canal treatment is failing because of recurrent leakage.
3. No canal space is naturally round.
4. Access to the apex and patency are necessary to achieve the root goals of cleaning and shaping the canal system.
5. The philosophy behind the "crown-down" approach[8] is most applicable to the removal of radicular filling materials or obstructions.
6. All preparations increase in size during retreatment. Usually the coronal third demonstrates the greatest enlargement.[9]
7. Canals that initially deviate from their natural centerline tend to continue to deviate in the same direction during retreatment. Areas not instrumented during initial treatment are more difficult to contact during retreatment.
8. Irrigation and disinfection must be emphasized because all canals that are retreated should be considered contaminated with microorganisms.
9. Solvents, while useful, can interfere with débridement.
10. All methods of instrumentation and removal leave debris remaining in the canals.
11. Open canals not being treated should be protected or covered.
12. Patience is a virtue.

The three categories of materials most commonly considered during retreatment are pastes, semisolids with sealers, and solids placed with or without sealers (Box 8-7).

Removal of Paste Fillings

Injectable paste filling materials may be soft and penetrable or firm and resistant to entry. These materials may or may not extend to the apical portion of the canals. Soft materials, usually zinc oxide and eugenol base materials, may be removed using small hand files with gentle instrumentation (traditionally a reaming or balanced force action) and copious irrigation with sodium hypochlorite (NaOCl). The actual constituents of many pastes may remain a mystery because formulations are variable. Some may contain extremely toxic materials such as paraformaldehyde, lead, and arsenic. The clinician should take great care to remove as much of the previous filling material as possible before attempting to proceed with definitive apical instrumentation.

Pastes, which are not initially penetrable, should be exposed to solvents such as chloroform (Box 8-8). Any open canal should be covered before the chamber is flooded with solvent. A stiff instrument such as a DG-16 or a clipped #25 K-file[10] can be used to determine solubility. If the material is soluble, the clinician should continue using the solvent until the material has been bypassed and removed and then return to NaOCl irrigation as soon as practical. If the material is hard and insoluble, the operator may reconsider the value and risks associated with retreating that canal. How much material will be penetrated? Are the canals curved? Is surgery a better option? If the clinician should discuss all these risks with the patient. If the patient and clinician decide to continue, ultrasonics, magnification, and illumination can be used to progress through the material. Clipped files are most useful. Radiographs are appropriate to determine the direction of instrumentation. Once "through," the feel of the canal on "the other side" is most rewarding. If the clinician is not successful penetrating or removing all the material, he or she may fill the working space conventionally or use it as a post space. Root-end surgery may be indicated.

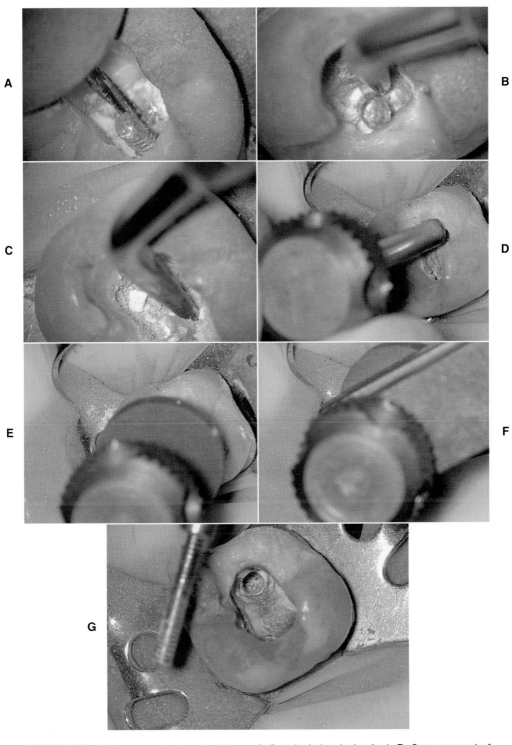

FIGURE 8-7   Post removal system technique. **A,** Post isolation (using bur). **B,** Gross removal of build-up (using large ultrasonic tip). **C,** Detailed removal of build-up (using small ultrasonic tip). **D,** Post tapping (counterclockwise). **E,** Screwing tap on with rubber cushion. **F,** Attachment of removal fork to tap and activation. **G,** Post removal.

BOX 8-7

Canal Filling Materials

PASTES (WITHOUT CORES)
· Zinc oxide and eugenol
· Medicated cements, N_2
· Zinc phosphate cements
· Copper cements
· Biocalyex

SEMISOLIDS (CEMENTED WITH SEALERS)
Gutta-percha cemented with:

· Zinc oxide and eugenol
· Calcium hydroxide sealers
· Epoxy resins
· Resin (polyvinyl ketones)
· Glass ionomer
· Thermoplastic and injectable gutta-percha techniques with sealer

SOLIDS (CEMENTED WITH SEALERS AS ABOVE)
· Silver cones
· Sectional silver cones
· Gutta-percha carriers:
Stainless steel
Titanium alloy
Liquid crystal plastic (up to size 30)
Polysulfone plastic (above size 35)

SOLIDS WITHOUT SEALERS (BROKEN INSTRUMENTS)
· Lentulo spirals
· Gates Glidden drills
· Post drills
· Stainless steel files
· Nickel-titanium files

BOX 8-8

Endodontic Solvents

· Endodontic solvents
· Chloroform
· Methyl chloroform
· Xylene
· Eucalyptol
· Tetrachloroethylene (Endosolv E)
· Formamid (Endosolv R)
· Rectified turpentine
· d-limonene (Hemo-De)

Removing Gutta-Percha Core Materials

Mechanical and/or solvent dissolution techniques can be used to remove gutta-percha and sealer. The preferred technique is mechanical because it allows for better debris removal. The use of solvents substantially complicates débridement. When solvents are used to remove gutta-percha or pastes, the dissolved infected debris from these materials is more likely to flow into and coat inaccessible canal irregularities and/or penetrate into the periradicular tissues.

The decision to use one or both techniques hinges on three factors:

1. *The existing condensation quality*—Densely filled canals may require a solvent to facilitate penetration. Poorly condensed fillings can usually be removed mechanically. Usually the coronal aspect of any canal is most densely compacted.
2. *The length of the existing filling material*—The use of solvents to dissolve filling materials in the apical third of the canal system risks pushing these materials into the periradicular tissues. The use of solvents in the apical third with an overextended cone all but ensures that the overextended segment will be severed and remain in the periradicular tissues.
3. *The tooth's root morphology, canal shape, size, and curvature*—Mechanical techniques remove more dentin than solvent approaches. With a comparatively straight and substantial root, the clinician may be able to remove all of the gutta-percha using rotary instrumentation. In contrast, a densely filled curved canal such as the mesiobuccal root of a maxillary first molar may require solvents to reduce the risk of apical transportation or furcal strip perforation.

A mechanical removal technique usually begins with rotary instrumentation (using Gates Glidden drills or nickel-titanium files) to rapidly remove the coronal portion of the gutta-percha. The canal is larger coronally and straight enough to tolerate these procedures. Minimal pressure is exerted as smaller sizes are used to progress apically in a crown-down manner. The clinician should promptly remove any material adherent to the rotary instrument and carefully cut away from furcal concavities. Alternatively, a heat source with diminishing sizes of heat carriers may be used to remove the gutta-percha.

As the coronal bulk of material is removed, penetration of the apical radicular filling becomes possible. Using an appropriately curved, short (21 mm) size 15 or 20 K-file with a repeated reaming action, the clinician should be able to instrument next to the previous filling material. He or she should not file, force, or push instruments apically. Frequently, the operator will sense that it is possible to almost "screw the file in." If this is feasible, the operator should be careful that the file is not placed so aggressively as to demonstrate "spring-back" when the handle is released. Ideally the entire gutta-percha filling will be bypassed with size 20 or larger K-files. The clinician can use an apex locator to estimate the file position if necessary. Frequent and generous irrigation with NaOCl is indicated. Old gutta-percha fillings are likely to be brittle. In such situations the gutta-percha will seem to shred and break into small pieces as the path alongside it is created and debris is removed. After establishing a path, the clinician chooses the next larger Hedström file (at least a size 20) and rotates it clockwise alongside the filling material, avoiding spring-back. Although this file will engage dentin, it will preferentially embed its flutes in the softer gutta-percha. With controlled force, the clinician removes the Hedström file as though it were a corkscrew, turning counterclockwise as necessary if too much resistance is encountered. The entire gutta-percha mass may release, but more often small fragments will be removed each time this process is repeated. The clinician may consider a larger file size if the canal anatomy permits but should be careful not to sever overextended segments. When working close to the estimated working distance, the clinician can take a radiograph with the file in place. Ideally, all apical filling materials should be removed. The value of removing materials that remain in the middle and coronal thirds must be carefully weighed against concerns for preservation of tooth structure.

Many solvents have been proposed to aid in retreatment of gutta-percha fillings. The authors of this chapter prefer chloroform, but less volatile solvents such as d-limonene (a xylene substitute)[11] are being investigated and may prove safer. A solvent dissolution approach usually begins, as does the mechanical approach, with the bulk of materials being removed by rotary instrumentation. This action creates a coronal space or reservoir where the solvent can be deposited. Initially, a 21-mm 15 or 20 K-file can be used to penetrate and remove the dissolving mass of filling material. The instrument flutes should be cleaned after each pass, with the solvent being replenished as it evaporates. As the material further softens, Hedström files may be used to expedite removal. Slowly and without forcing, the clinician can use precurved files to work through the previous filling. Unless it is necessary for visualization, irrigation is not indicated because it will dilute and diminish the solvent's effectiveness. As the apical extent of the filling is ap-

proached, the clinician may attempt to complete the process mechanically. If this is not possible, he or she may continue with the solvent while using files with a reaming action to minimize pushing debris apically. After the file has bypassed or is completely alongside the filling material, he or she can begin irrigating with NaOCl and follow the steps of mechanical removal.

Removal of Silver Cones

Once an extremely popular filling material, silver cones were used to fill canals for either their entire length or with an apical "sectional," "twist-off," or "plug" technique (Figure 8-8). To remove a silver cone that projects into the chamber from an orifice, the clinician begins by carefully exposing the coronal extent of the cone down to the level of the orifice. Gutta-percha or sealer surrounding the cone can easily be picked or chipped away with explorers, spoon excavators, and solvents. However, the clinician must exercise extreme care not to repeatedly bend or flex the free end of this soft metal, especially the smaller sizes. Bending often leads to breakage at or below the level of the orifice, further complicating removal. If the cones are embedded in amalgam, the clinician should remove the core as though it contained a post, leaving the silver cone surrounded by small amounts of alloy (Figure 8-9). Sometimes coronal portions of silver cones are folded to the chamber floor and covered with a zinc phosphate base. Ultrasonics, magnification, and illumination are most useful to expose these silver cones. The clinician should be careful to prevent direct contact between ultrasonic tips and silver cones because the soft silver will disintegrate. Unless the cone displays visible motion (not to be confused with flexure of the coronal free end), the initial urge to grasp the cone and pull on it should be resisted. Instead,

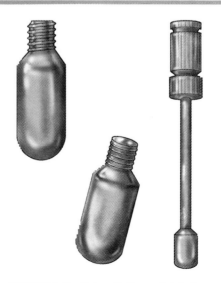

FIGURE 8-8   Twist-off silver point device.

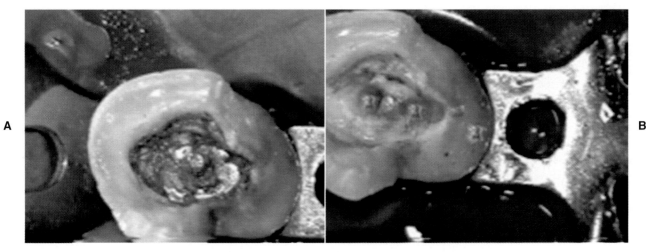

FIGURE 8-9   A, Silver cone with amalgam remnants. **B,** Amalgam removal using ultrasonics.

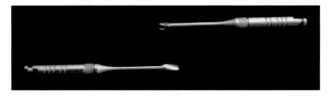

FIGURE 8-10   Modified Gates Glidden drills.

working with short-length, 21-mm 15 or 20 K-files and solvents, the clinician can begin to create a pathway alongside of the cone. If the cone remains secure, another path can be initiated, ideally on the opposite side of the cone. If possible, these paths should completely bypass the silver cone. The route of the path can be confirmed with a radiograph or an apex locator. In this classic approach, still using the solvent, the clinician selects a size 20 or larger Hedström file and turns it clockwise into the path, engaging both the cone and dentin. If spring-back is detected in the handle, the file must be turned counterclockwise until the perception is lost. The clinician then attempts to withdraw the Hedström file, hopefully engaging the silver cone. If the cone has not been dislodged, additional channels may be made alongside it. Frequently more than one Hedström file is placed and their coronal ends are braided before they are withdrawn. Many clinicians use ultrasonics to further loosen the cones as the pathways are created. The energy can be delivered in two ways, which prevents disintegration of the soft silver. The coronal free end of the cone can be grasped with a Steiglitz or similar forceps. The Steiglitz or forceps (not the silver cone) can then be energized with an ultrasonic tip while a gentle constant drawing force is exerted. Additionally, a small file and solvent or one of the smaller ultrasonic tips can be placed in the path and energized. Using lower power settings reduces the potential for breakage of these delicate

tips. Most silver cones yield to a combination of patience and repetition of these efforts. If the coronal free end breaks or the silver cone was placed by an apical method, it should be managed in the same way as a broken instrument. If an object is in the coronal third, the clinician may attempt to bypass it or engage and remove it with a Hedström file. Careful ultrasonic vibration is usually helpful. If the canal is straight and substantial root structure remains, an extraction tube technique can be used to regain attachment to the coronal free end. However, these devices cannot accommodate curves and are rarely used in the restricted confines of the apical third.

Staging

Metallic objects and apically placed silver cones may also be approached by *staging*. In this technique, files or modified Gates Glidden drills (Figure 8-10) are used to create a platform or stage at the coronal aspect of the object. From this location, with the use of magnification, micro-irrigation, and ultrasonics, the clinician may be able to trough around the coronal aspect of the object. This action may vibrate the object free, allowing for its removal or enabling it to be bypassed by an instrument. An extraction tube approach may also be possible. Accessory fiberoptic transillumination through the buccal soft tissues can substantially facilitate this tedious intracanal work.

The removal of fractured nickel-titanium instruments and gutta-percha carriers is further complicated by their predisposition to disintegrate on ultrasonic contact. More delicate ultrasonic tips used with lower power settings and controlled air flow through micro-irrigation syringes are used to facilitate the precise troughing necessary to remove nickel-titanium objects, which have the tendency to spring back toward the canal wall because of their material memory.

Removal of Gutta-Percha Carrier Devices

The first carrier devices[12] were made with stainless steel shafts and coated with gutta-percha. These carriers became available commercially in 1988 and have gained rapid acceptance in general dentistry. The manufacturers advocate their placement using either full-length or sectional filling techniques that allow for post spaces. In contrast to the more recently introduced gray-black nickel-titanium carriers, the original silver-colored stainless steel carriers are easily distinguished radiographically.[2] If the stainless steel carrier extends into the chamber it can be removed in a manner similar to that used for silver cones. The gutta-percha and sealer surrounding the coronal aspect of the carrier can initially be removed mechanically with small spoon excavators and Hedström files. If necessary a solvent can be used, but the dissolved gutta-percha will become runny and difficult to remove. After adequately exposing the carrier, the clinician can grasp it with a Steiglitz and heat the entire assembly while slowly drawing the carrier from the heat-softened gutta-percha. The remaining gutta-percha should be removed mechanically without a solvent. If a sectional technique has been used, removal efforts must follow the techniques used for broken instruments or apical silver cones. Root anatomy may necessitate the consideration of surgical retreatment.

More recently, manufacturers have begun to market two types of plastic carriers. Carrier sizes 30 or smaller are made of an insoluble liquid crystal plastic. Carrier sizes 35 and larger are made of polysulfone plastic, which is soluble in chloroform, and related solvents. Neither the plastic nor the nickel-titanium carriers can be distinguished radiographically from their gutta-percha coatings (Box 8-9). Because general dentists complete more than 90% of all endodontic procedures (many of them using carrier-filling techniques), the retreating dentist must always anticipate the potential for such a radiographically occult core material.

Removal of Plastic Core Materials

For canals containing plastic carriers, the clinician should initially attempt to remove the carrier in its entirety by grasping it with a Steiglitz or Peet's forceps and carefully drawing it coronally. If this is not successful, a solvent or heat source can be used to soften the coronal

---

> **BOX 8-9**
>
> *Detection of Titanium Posts and Radicular Filling Materials*
>
> ---
>
> 1. These materials may be occult on preoperative radiographs.
> 2. The retreating dentist should communicate with the treating dentist about these materials.
> 3. A parallel-sided surface pattern is possible.
> 4. A slight change in diameter at the post/root-filling interface may be evident.
> 5. These materials may be radiolucent laterally or at the post/root-filling interface.
>
> ---
>
> From Kleier DJ, Shibilski K, Averbach RE: Radiographic appearance of titanium posts in endodontically treated teeth, *J Endodon* 25(2):128, 1999.

gutta-percha. Plastic carriers in sizes 35 and larger are soluble in solvents such as chloroform. Next, using firm pressure the clinician turns one or more Hedström files clockwise alongside the plastic core, allowing the flutes to engage the carrier. Once they are engaged, the file and carrier are drawn coronally. If this is unsuccessful, the clinician uses a low-speed, high-torque handpiece to create a deeper channel alongside the plastic carrier and then carefully repeats the Hedström file/solvent technique until all the material is removed or anatomic limitations are encountered.

Another removal technique uses a .04 tapered size 30 file in a low-speed, high-torque handpiece rotating at approximately 600 RPM alongside the carrier. After removing the instrument, the clinician repeats the procedure with a file of even greater taper. If more aggressively tapered files are not available, .04 tapered 35 or 40 files may be used. The clinician can proceed with the wider tapered file at 300 RPM into the same channel preparation. The wider taper should engage the carrier and help dislodge it coronally. Generally, it does not remove the carrier in a single stroke. If one side is completed and the carrier is not loose, the clinician then proceeds with the same technique on the opposite side of the canal. After the carrier is dislodged, a working length film is obtained and the balance of the apical filling material is removed.

Removal of Nickel-Titanium Core Materials

The retreating dentist must remember that these carriers are radiographically difficult to discern and will shatter or disintegrate if excess ultrasonic energy is applied. If the gray-colored carrier extends into the chamber, removal is best accomplished in a manner similar to that used for its stainless steel counterpart, using heat to soften the surrounding gutta-percha. If the device is located in the middle or apical third of the canal, a sectional silver cone approach is necessary. Surgical treatment may need to be considered. In all instances a nonjudgmental, matter-of-fact approach is essential as the patient is advised of changes in prognosis and possible outcomes.

REGAINING ACCESS TO THE APEX: REINSTRUMENTATION, IRRIGATION, DÉBRIDEMENT, AND DISINFECTION

After removing previous filling materials and obstructions, the clinician must re-establish access to the apex along the path of the original canal. It is unusual to find a readily patent and negotiable canal "on the other side." If this were the case, the operator could proceed with the usual techniques of cleaning and shaping, while placing particular emphasis on irrigation to débride and disinfect. Working length radiographs are essential to evaluate length and preparation. Information provided by electronic measuring devices is complementary to these radiographs. As the final cleaning and apical shaping continues, the operator must recall that continued preparation naturally tends to deviate from the original centerline of the canal, especially in the coronal third.

If the previous filling materials were under-extended, the goal of apical instrumentation may be complicated by the following canal abnormalities:

1. Blockages with dentinal and/or pulpal debris
2. Dentistogenic complications such as ledges and transportation
3. Calcifications
4. Anatomic complexies

In the worst case scenario, a canal will feel solidly blocked and impenetrable. Recalling basic principles of endodontic instrumentation, the operator should choose a short (21-mm, size .08, .10, or .15) file size, irrigate, and gently feel for a "catch." Usually a small J hook is placed at the instrument's tip and a gradual bend is placed throughout the instrument's length. While exploring the canal, the clinician should resist the natural tendency to push more aggressively, which will only complicate a blockage or ledge. Frequent irrigation should be employed to remove debris. If no catch is detected, the canal should be dried and irrigated with a chelating agent such as 17% ethylenediaminetetraacetic acid (EDTA) in aqueous solution. As gentle exploration continues, the clinician should curve and recurve the file, while ascertaining that no coronal or radicular access restrictions impede the motion of the file. Irrigation should not be performed with NaOCl because it will neutralize the effect of the chelating agent. If several canals are being re-entered and the first yields no initial signs of progress, the clinician should leave EDTA in place and proceed to work on another canal. Without rushing, the clinician continues to explore each canal for even the slightest catch and gently pursues it with the smallest file sizes when a catch manifests. This gentle but persistent effort rarely results in perforation, even with EDTA. The clinician should conscientiously discard worn instruments while replenishing the EDTA. After the estimated distance has been achieved, it can be enlarged to a size 15 file and a working radiograph can be taken to confirm length and file position. If a previously blocked canal continues to resist apical instrumentation, a clipped file approach may carefully be attempted.[10] Typically about 1 to 2 mm are clipped from the tip of a 21-mm size 15 file. This procedure leaves the tip with sharp cutting edges that can be used with a back-and-forth, auger-like motion.[13] With this technique the clinician may be able to work through the resistant blockage. Discretion normally dictates that only 1 to 2 mm of length should be attempted in this manner before the clinician gently feels for the natural canal again with a small, unclipped, curved file. Radiographs are essential to monitor the files' progress, especially around curves. After the original canal has been re-established, hand or rotary instrumentation techniques can be used to finish shaping the preparation.

Considerable emphasis must be placed on débridement, irrigation, and finally disinfection. The retreating dentist must remove as much of the contaminated previous materials as possible, as well as debris created by new instrumentation. Any motion that might push this debris apically should be avoided. As the preparation nears completion, the clinician must undertake a focused search for any additional untreated canals. The operating microscope offers ideal illumination and visibility to accomplish all of these goals. Anatomic grooves and dentin coloration can also guide the operator in locating additional canals. In the apical area, bubble trails and careful tactile exploration with appropriately curved small files may reveal patent apical ramifications. The radiographic file position (centered or not) within the root is also an excellent indicator of additional canals.

All authors concede that complete débridement of the root canal system is impossible. During retreatment, remnants of previous filling materials will always remain out of reach of reasonable instrumentation. The operator must assume that these uninstrumented areas and their adjacent dentinal tubules are contaminated with microorganisms. To date, the consensus of most authors[14,15] suggests that a conscious effort at further canal disinfection must follow cleaning and shaping and precede the filling appointment. At this time, placement of an intracanal dressing such as calcium hydroxide[14] (CaOH)[14] or an antibiotic-containing fiber[15] for a period of at least 1 week seems most appropriate. A temporary restoration at least 4 to 5 mm thick is then placed against the sound walls of the access preparation.[16]

FILLING, PROGNOSIS, AND POSTTREATMENT RESPONSIBILITIES

All filling techniques attempt to prevent recurrent leakage and seal in or entomb debris that cannot be removed from the root canal system. The clinical conceptualization of a root canal filling should be that of a maze on a micrometer scale. No ionic or covalent bonds come into play, only physical interfaces among dentin, sealer, and gutta-percha. All obturation techniques leak.[17] As long as clinicians continue to fill canals in a manner that facilitates nonsurgical retreatment, they will never measurably improve on existing obturation techniques. The time-honored adage, "It's what you take out, not what you put in," is as true today as it was 100 years ago (see Chapter 7). The reader is left to choose an appropriate filling technique.

The completion of canal obturation leaves the clinician with a sense of prognosis. As part of the ongoing process of consent, treatment outcomes must be conveyed to the patient. Additional referrals for periodontal or related procedures must be arranged if they were not anticipated preoperatively. For the patient, filling is usually perceived as completion, the end of the root canal treatment. They have survived, and usually their worst fears have passed uneventfully. They are also comfortable and all too frequently complacent, wishing to take a break from treatment. Beyond providing any required postoperative management (e.g., pain and/or infection control), the clinician also has a responsibility to ensure that the patient returns promptly for definitive restorative procedures. When a specialist provides treatment, this process may begin as a phone call and/or a referral acknowledgment and a radiograph.

Posttreatment follow-up is as essential as retreatment planning. If any delays in the restorative process are anticipated, a more definitive temporary restoration such as reinforced zinc oxide and eugenol or a light-cured intermediate composite should be placed. Application of an orthodontic band to reduce the possibility of fracture or placement of the core build-up and a temporary crown is frequently indicated. Loss of a temporary restoration requires immediate replacement. Treatment must never be considered complete until the tooth is restored to function. Endodontic recall examinations should be scheduled at any time if signs or symptoms develop and planned routinely at 1 and 2 or more years.

SURGICAL RETREATMENT

Surgical endodontic retreatment procedures may be considered if nonsurgical retreatment approaches fail or are unable to resolve treatment concerns or if a biopsy is indicated (see Chapter 10). Accurate diagnosis and the understanding that root-end surgery is never superior to proficiently accomplished nonsurgical treatment are fundamental to the best possible outcome.

Even though few medical or anatomic contraindications to surgical retreatment exist, this does not diminish the value of accurate diagnosis and careful treatment planning. These preparations must be approached with extreme care and substantial empathy for the patient.

Although periradicular surgical retreatment is the most common approach, replantation may also be considered. Alternative treatment plan options, including the use of three-unit bridges or the placement of implants, must be addressed before a surgical procedure is recommended. The etiology of failure must be identified when possible. The persistence of microorganisms or their toxic products must be considered in light of the potential to remove or entomb these irritants. Operators must always consider vertical root fractures when apparently well-done nonsurgical and surgical endodontic procedures fail repeatedly. Other possibilities include unfilled sections of canal. In this instance, if a surgical approach is indicated, instrumentation through the root-end and filling of these canals should be considered in addition to resection and root-end filling.[18]

From an operative perspective, significant fibrosis from previous healing may complicate flap elevation in cases previously treated surgically. A biopsy of the periradicular tissues is essential. With careful respect to the crown-to-root ratio, further root resection is usually appropriate. When a root-end filling material needs to be removed, appropriate crypt management is essential to prevent scattering of the filling material. After the root end has been prepared, dye staining and detailed microscopic examination are required before root-end instrumentation, root-end filling, and closure. Postoperative care must be timely and appropriate. It is axiomatic that recalls are essential.

References

1. American Association of Endodontists: *AAE glossary, contemporary terminology for endodontics,* ed 8, Chicago, 1998, American Association of Endodontists.
2. Kleier D, Shibilski K, Averbach R: Radiographic appearance of titanium posts in endodontically treated teeth, *J Endodon* 25:128, 1999.
3. Kells CE: *Three score years and nine,* Chicago, 1926, Lakeside Press.
4. Bruder G et al: Perforation repairs, *NY State Dent J* 65:26, 1999.
5. Nahmias Y, Aurelio JA, Gerstein H: Expanded use of the electronic canal length measuring devices, *J Endodon* 9:347, 1983.
6. Johnson WT, Leary JM, Boyer DB: effect of ultrasonic vibration on post removal in extracted human premolar teeth, *J Endodon* 22:487, 1996.
7. Krell KV, Fuller MW, Scott GL: The conservative retrieval of silver cones in difficult cases, *J Endodon* 10:269, 1984.
8. Morgan L, Montgomery S: An evaluation of the crown-down pressureless technique, *J Endodon* 10:491, 1984.
9. Wilcox LR, van Surksum R: Endodontic retreatment in large and small straight canals, *J Endodon* 17:119, 1991.
10. Fachin EVF, Wenckus C, Aun CE: Retreatment using a modified-tip instrument, *J Endodon* 21:425, 1995.

11. Metzger Z, Marian-Kfir V, Tamse A: Gutta-percha softening: Hemo-De as xylene substitute, *J Endodon* 25:385, 2000.
12. Johnson WB: A new gutta percha technique, *J Endodon* 4:184, 1978.
13. Roane J, Sabola C, Duncanson M: The "balanced force" concept of instrumentation of curved canals, *J Endodon* 11:203, 1985.
14. Sjorgen U et al: Influence on infection at the time of root filling on the time of teeth with apical periodontitis, *Int Endod J* 30:297, 1997.
15. Gilad JZ et al: Development of a clindamycin impregnated fiber as an intracanal medication in endodontics, *J Endodon* 25:722, 1999.
16. Webber RT et al: Sealing quality of a temporary filling material, *Oral Surg Oral Med Oral Pathol Oral Radiol Endod* 46(1):123, 1978.
17. Wesselink WM: Endodontic leakage studies reconsidered. Part I. Methodology application and relevance, *Int Endod J* 26:37, 1993.
18. Serota KS, Krakow AA: Retrograde instrumentation and obturation of the root canal space, *J Endodon* 9:448, 1983.

9

RESTORATION OF THE ENDODONTICALLY TREATED TOOTH

DEBRA R. HASELTON

*T*eeth that have been treated endodontically may continue to contribute to the overall function of the dentition (Figure 9-1). Endodontic success depends not only on the quality of the root canal treatment, but also on timely coronal restoration of the compromised tooth.[1] Restorative techniques have evolved from the placement of wooden posts in the 1800s to the advanced ceramic and polymer fiber technologies currently available. Restoration techniques for these teeth can range from the use of a conservative composite resin to seal the access opening to the application of complex multiple component casting.

Endodontically treated teeth often exhibit minimal tooth structure after treatment. These teeth should be restored in a manner that will provide a coronal seal, adequate retention, and a ferrule to ensure optimal success. Many techniques and materials are available to restore the pulpless tooth (Table 9-1). Each tooth is unique and empirical opinions abound regarding the best system or technique to be used. The clinician must choose carefully because many of the more recent materials have not been validated scientifically through independent laboratory research and clinical trials. This chapter presents several techniques that are effective for the restoration of various endodontically treated teeth.

TREATMENT GOALS

1. Maintain the coronal and apical seal of the root canal filling material.
2. Protect and preserve remaining tooth structure.
3. Provide a supportive and retentive foundation for the placement of a definitive restoration.
4. Restore function and esthetics.

TREATMENT PLANNING

Before a definitive restoration can be placed, the following conditions must exist:

1. Adequate obturation of the root canal system
2. No sensitivity to percussion or biting pressure
3. No sensitivity to palpation
4. No sinus tract
5. No periodontal probing deeper than 3 mm
6. No evidence of active inflammatory disease

The clinician should consider the function of the tooth in the dental arch. An extremely debilitated tooth may compromise the treatment plan, and in such cases extraction should be considered. However, a greater effort is often warranted to retain a key tooth such as a first molar or canine. The endodontically treated tooth should be restored as soon as possible to prevent coronal leakage that could compromise the endodontic outcome and to prevent fracture, which may render the tooth unrestorable.[1] Saunders[2] states that root canal treatment failure is usually caused by incomplete preparation or infection that enters through a poor coronal seal. After providing root canal treatment, the clinician should remove all caries and/or defective restorations if this cannot be accomplished before treatment. If a final restoration cannot be placed within a few weeks of treatment, a durable, leak-resistant provisional restoration should be placed. In treating structurally compromised teeth the clinician may use core build-ups, orthodontic bands, or provisional crowns to help prevent fracture; these techniques should be used if a delay in crown placement is anticipated[1] or if the endodontic prognosis is questionable and future reassessment is desirable.

If a crown cannot encircle a minimum of 1.5 to 2 mm of tooth structure, the clinician should consider

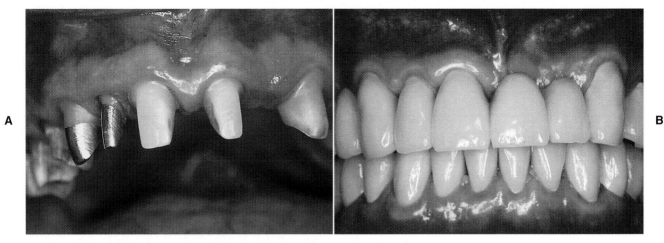

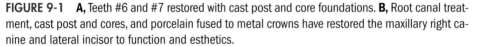

FIGURE 9-1   A, Teeth #6 and #7 restored with cast post and core foundations. **B,** Root canal treatment, cast post and cores, and porcelain fused to metal crowns have restored the maxillary right canine and lateral incisor to function and esthetics.

crown lengthening, orthodontic extrusion, or extraction. Key abutment teeth in a patient with extensive fixed reconstruction should have a good endodontic prognosis before a definitive restoration is placed. The clinician should also consider the need for elective root canal treatment and retreatment before placing the definitive restoration. Endodontically treated teeth should probably not be used as abutments for fixed partial dentures with more than one pontic because the greater load placed on the prosthesis may render them more likely to fracture.[3] Anterior endodontically treated teeth used as abutments for fixed partial dentures should be restored with cast post and core restorations. Endodontically treated teeth should not be used as abutments for distal extension partial dentures because they are more than four times as likely to fail than pulpless teeth not serving as abutments.[3] Nyman and Lindhe noted that fractures occurred more frequently in teeth treated endodontically and then used as abutments for free end segments.[4] Other studies support this finding as well and caution against the use of endodontically treated teeth as distal extension abutments.[5,6]

Structure of Endodontically Treated Teeth

Papa and others[7] found no significant difference in the moisture content between matched pairs of endodontically treated and vital teeth. Vital dentin exhibited a moisture content of 12.35%, whereas dentin from endodontically treated teeth had a moisture content of 12.10%. Huang et al[8] compared the mechanical properties of human dentin from treated pulpless teeth with dentin from normal vital teeth and noted an insignificant effect of endodontic treatment on compressive and tensile strength of the dentin. Research by Reeh and colleagues[9] compared the reduction in tooth stiffness in en-

dodontic and restorative procedures. The relative tooth stiffness as a result of endodontic procedures was reduced by 5%; however, restorative procedures generated stiffness loss between 20% and 63%. Many operative preparations result in larger amounts of tooth structure loss when compared with endodontic access preparations. The volume of tooth loss is perhaps the primary factor in the decreased strength of endodontically treated teeth.

Restoration of Endodontically Treated Teeth

ANTERIOR TEETH. With only a conservative access opening, anterior teeth can be restored with a resin restoration. Placement of a post is not necessary when a complete coverage restoration is not indicated. Post installation may inhibit attempts to bleach a discolored endodontically treated tooth. Moreover, a post does not strengthen the root. A retrospective study by Sorensen and Martinoff[10] showed no improvement in prognosis for endodontically treated anterior teeth restored with a post. Lovdahl and Nicolls[11] found that endodontically treated maxillary central incisors with intact natural crowns exhibiting access openings were stronger than teeth restored with cast posts and cores or pin-retained amalgams. Large interproximal restorations, incisal edge fractures, or esthetic concerns may necessitate the placement of a post and core, as well as full coronal coverage.[1]

POSTERIOR TEETH. A significant improvement is noted in the clinical success of endodontic treatment of maxillary and mandibular premolars and molars when coronal coverage restorations are present. Full-coverage crowns prevent fracture when occlusal forces act to separate the cusp tips.[10] Crowns should generally be used

TABLE 9-1

Restorative Options for the Endodontically Treated Tooth

OPTION	ADVANTAGES	DISADVANTAGES	INDICATIONS	CONTRAINDICATIONS
Resin restoration in access opening	· One appointment · Cost · Preserves tooth structure · Esthetics	· Potential for microleakage	Intact anterior tooth with only an access opening or very small Class III restorations	Numerous or large restorations in tooth resulting in extensive destruction; most posterior teeth
Amalcore foundation	· One appointment · Cost less than casting · Demonstrated clinical effectiveness · High compressive and tensile strength	· Large foundations may not be able to be prepared for a crown at the same appointment · Potential for corrosion and discoloration at gingival margin	Posterior teeth that are to receive crowns; cuspal coverage can be considered for strength as an option to crown	Teeth in which a bulk of amalgam cannot be obtained
Prefabricated post and direct resin core	· One appointment · Cost less than cast post · May be more esthetic under all-ceramic crown · Decreased need for undercut removal; may conserve tooth structure	· Strength less than amalgam · Failure of the core component may render the tooth unrestorable	Small teeth that would require considerable removal of tooth structure to use a cast post	Teeth in which high functional forces are likely to cause breakage of the core from the post
Prefabricated post and amalgam core	· One appointment	· Tooth may not be able to be prepared for crown at same appointment · May be challenging to matrix · Not one integral unit	Posterior teeth that cannot retain an amalgam core alone	Posterior teeth that are able to retain an amalgam core alone

Continued

TABLE 9-1

Restorative Options for the Endodontically Treated Tooth—cont'd

OPTION	ADVANTAGES	DISADVANTAGES	INDICATIONS	CONTRAINDICATIONS
Cast metal post and core (indirect or direct pattern)	· Strength: post and core are one integral unit · Relatively easy to incorporate anti-rotation features	· Numerous appointments · Cost · Undercuts may necessitate more tooth removal than a prefabricated post and core build-up · May be unesthetic under some types of all-ceramic crowns	Teeth in which minimal tooth structure remains; a tooth that is to be used as an abutment for a fixed partial denture; situations in which optimal strength is required	Teeth requiring some types of very translucent all-ceramic crowns
Ceramic post and core (direct or indirect pattern)	· Esthetics	· Numerous appointments for indirect post and core · Cost · Long-term data are limited · Ceramic materials may have a tendency to fracture · Conventional retreatment not likely an option	Teeth requiring some types of very translucent all-ceramic crowns	Teeth for which a metal-ceramic crown is planned
Crown placement	· Protection of remaining tooth structure by encirclement	· Removal of more tooth structure · Cost	Enhancement of esthetic outcome; situations in which existing restorations combined with the endodontic access undermine the structural integrity of the natural crown	Anterior teeth that have only a conservative endodontic access opening

on all endodontically treated posterior teeth.[10,12] If significant tooth structure has been retained, a crown may be all the coverage required. If minimal structure remains, a post may be necessary to help retain a foundation before crown placement. If a crown cannot be placed because of a patient's financial limitations, the clinician should provide some other form of cuspal coverage such as an amalgam onlay.

The Role of Posts in the Restoration of Endodontically Treated Teeth

Most in vitro laboratory studies that have tested endodontically treated teeth by applying force with a mechanical testing machine have shown that placement of a post and core does not increase fracture resistance. Researchers are in general agreement that posts do not reinforce endodontically treated teeth and actually weaken the root.[1,13-17] The primary purpose of a post is to retain a core that is used to retain the definitive restoration.

Types of Posts

Posts can be made of a variety of materials (Figure 9-2). Prefabricated posts are generally made of stainless steel, platinum-gold-palladium, or titanium, but newer compositions include ceramic and carbon fiber. Cast custom posts are usually cast from Type II or III gold alloy. Posts can be categorized by mode of retention (active or passive) or shape (parallel or tapered). Laboratory studies indicate that threaded (active) posts are the most retentive, followed by cemented, serrated, parallel-sided posts.[18] Cemented, tapered posts are the least retentive. Although threaded posts are the most retentive, they place insertion stress on the root and can cause root

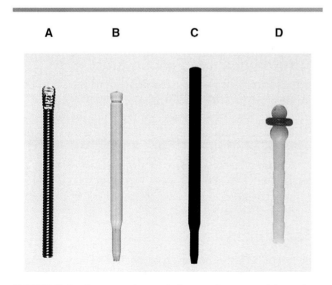

FIGURE 9-2 Posts can be made from various materials such as stainless steel **(A)**, esthetic carbon fiber **(B)**, carbon fiber **(C)**, and ceramic **(D)**.

fracture. The tapered post has a wedging effect that also places stress on the root. Parallel serrated posts have the advantage of good retention with uniformly distributed functional stresses.[1] A study by Felton,[19] however, demonstrated no statistical effects of post design on the potential for root fracture and concluded that the amount of remaining dentin and existing root morphology may be determining factors for fracture resistance during dowel placement in endodontically treated teeth. Although retention is often evaluated in comparisons of post and core systems, clinical experience indicates that a post placed to adequate length is not likely to fail regardless of the design. Intact, adequately placed posts are difficult to remove when necessary.

Failure of Post and Cores

Failures occur in several ways. The post may loosen, the post and core complex may fracture or separate, or the root may fracture. Approximately 3% to 10% of post and core failures are attributable to root fractures. This may be more likely in teeth that have lost some periodontal support (Figure 9-3). A parallel, serrated (passive) post places less stress on the tooth root than tapered or threaded (active) posts. Split and threaded flexible posts do not reduce stress concentration during function because the post is not flexible in three dimensions. Cemented posts produce the least root stress.[18] Turner found that post loosening was the most common type of failure among 100 failures examined.[17] Sorensen's study of the records of 1273 endodontically treated teeth yielding 246 total failures concluded that 36% of the failures were caused by post dislodgment, 33% were related to nonrestorable tooth fractures, 5% were related to restorable tooth fractures, and 8% were related to post perforations.[10]

Post Size and Length

Post length is unique and individualized for each case. The clinician should have a thorough knowledge of root morphology before placing a post. The effect of the embedded depth of posts on retentive capacity has been shown to be significant.[20] The longer the post, the greater the retention. A guideline of one half to three quarters of the root length is often followed but may not be reasonable for extremely long, short, narrow, or curved roots. At a minimum, research has established that the post length should be equal to or greater than the crown length of the restored tooth (see Figure 9-3). Retrospective clinical data on 1273 endodontically treated and restored teeth demonstrated few failures for posts that were as long as the crown or longer.[10] At least 4 to 5 mm of gutta-percha should be left in the apical portion of the canal to ensure an adequate seal. If this guideline cannot be followed and the post is shorter than the crown, extraction should be considered. The width of the post should not be greater than one third of the

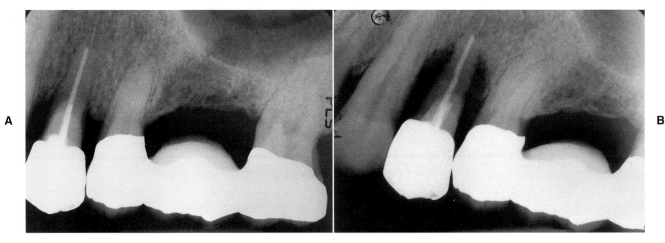

FIGURE 9-3 **A,** Tooth #12, which exhibited loss of periodontal support, was restored with a post to a level unsupported by bone. **B,** The maxillary premolar eventually demonstrated a root fracture at the apex of the post.

width of the root at any point along the dowel. Maintaining a minimum of 1 mm of sound dentin around the post is also advisable. Tjan[21] demonstrated that root walls with 2 or 3 mm of buccal dentin were less likely to fracture than those having only 1 mm. Because of the two-dimensional nature of radiographs, buccal-lingual dimensions cannot be assessed and therefore the actual amount of dentin present in the mesio-distal direction may be smaller than the amount perceived. The clinician should keep this in mind and carefully consider teeth that have roots with fluting or depressions along the mesial and distal surfaces. Smaller posts not only conserve tooth structure, but also provide increased resistance to fracture compared with larger posts.[22]

Preparation of the Post Space As It Relates to the Apical Seal and Microleakage

The post space may be prepared immediately after root canal treatment is completed.[2,23] This procedure is a two-step process. Gutta-percha should be removed incrementally with a heated instrument or solvents before canal enlargement. This method reduces the chance of root perforation and microleakage[23] (Figure 9-4), a common sequela of gutta-percha removal during post space preparation. The use of a heated instrument results in significantly less leakage at both the 3 and 5 mm levels of remaining gutta-percha, compared with rotary instrument removal.[23] Whenever possible, post space should be prepared with rubber dam isolation to prevent bacterial contamination of the root space. If the space becomes contaminated during post space preparation or before cementation, an antibacterial solution such as 2.5% sodium hypochlorite can be used to disinfect the space before treatment continues.

Excessive removal of gutta-percha may contribute to failure of the root canal treatment (Figure 9-5). A retrospective study of 200 patients concluded that the increased apical periodontitis associated with teeth with posts may result from the loss of the apical seal or the improper removal of root canal obturating material.[24] Observation of teeth with less than 3 mm of remaining root filling indicated a statistically significant increased frequency of periapical radiolucencies than teeth where more than 3 mm of root filling remained.[25] An in vitro study by Nixon[26] also demonstrated that leaving more than 3 mm of filling material greatly decreases the level of leakage; 5 mm or more is optimal. Numerous other authors support leaving 4 to 5 mm of undisturbed gutta-percha after post preparation.[1,27-34]

Anti-Rotation and Positive Stop

Anti-rotation features are required in all post and core restorations. Techniques for applying these features include using pins or keyways or preparing the remaining coronal tooth structure. In a ribbon-shaped canal anti-rotation is achieved in the core. The rounder the canal, the greater the need to provide anti-rotation in the preparation.[3] A positive stop of the core onto sound dentin is required to prevent a wedging effect that could contribute to root fracture.

Ferrule Effect

The ferrule effect is achieved by encircling the remaining tooth structure with a cast band of metal. This effect has been shown to significantly increase the fracture resistance of an endodontically treated tooth by counteracting functional stresses such as lever forces and wedging

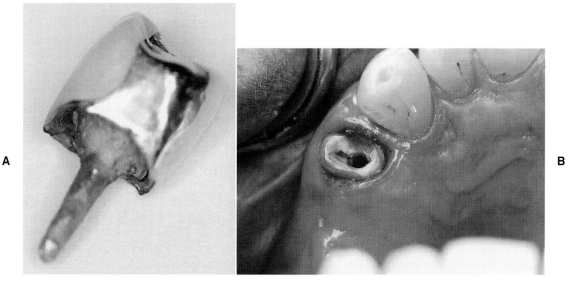

FIGURE 9-4   **A,** The inadequate length of this post, which was shorter than the crown, may have contributed to the failure of the restoration. **B,** The prepared tooth exhibits a lack of ferrule on the mesial side of the tooth.

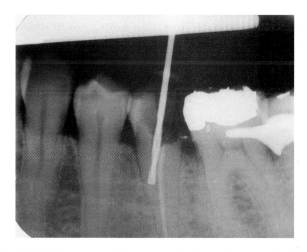

FIGURE 9-5   A rotary drill was used instead of a heated instrument to remove gutta-percha. This technique resulted in perforation of the root.

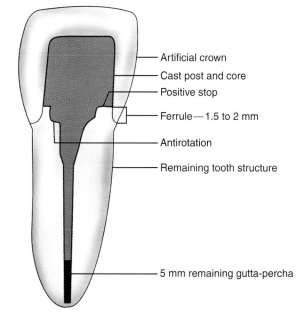

— Artificial crown
— Cast post and core
— Positive stop
— Ferrule—1.5 to 2 mm
— Antirotation
— Remaining tooth structure
— 5 mm remaining gutta-percha

FIGURE 9-6   Key features of an endodontically treated incisor restored with a crown include antirotation, ferrule, positive stop, and a minimum of 5 mm of remaining gutta-percha.

effects (Figure 9-6).[28] Opinions vary regarding the amount of ferrule needed,[35,36] but 1.5 to 2 mm should be considered the clinical minimum.[28] Surgical crown lengthening is often used to increase ferrule. This option should be considered with caution. Gegauff[37] demonstrated that decoronated premolar teeth that received surgical crown lengthening to provide a 2-mm ferrule were more likely to fracture because of the altered crown-to-root ratio than teeth receiving no crown lengthening. Orthodontic extrusion can be used to increase ferrule without compromising the crown-to-root ratio.[38] Incorporation of a ferrule is perhaps the single most important factor in maintaining the endodontically treated tooth restored with a crown.

Core Materials

The core should provide an ideal preparation form for the final restoration. Similar to a preparation in natural tooth, the core provides retention and a resistance form for the fabricated crown. A number of direct core materials are commercially available for use with prefabricated posts. Categories of core materials include amalgam alloy, reinforced resins, and glass ionomer. Advantages of alloy include its strength and stability. However, it requires a bulk of material and therefore is more frequently applicable to molars and larger premolar teeth. Amalgam demonstrated no microleakage in a study of various core materials placed under crowns and should therefore be considered for a core material whenever the crown margin cannot be extended more than 1 mm from the core junction.[39] Resin cores are often placed in anterior teeth because of their ability to mimic natural tooth color, which can be advantageous under all-ceramic crowns. This matching color can be a disadvantage if it makes detecting the location of the resin with respect to the crown margin difficult. An opaque white resin core material precludes a graying effect and allows detection of its location by the clinician. In vitro research on glass ionomer has demonstrated low strength compared with other core materials. Glass ionomer cements should probably be reserved for use in very selected anterior and posterior teeth because of their insufficient adhesion when used alone with pins or posts and their questionable long-term fatigability.[1]

PREPARATION AND FABRICATION TECHNIQUES

Corono-Radicular Amalgam Foundations

The corono-radicular amalgam foundation, also called an *amalcore* or *chamber-retained amalgam,* is condensed into the pulp chamber and occasionally the coronal root canal space to gain retention. It can be used for posterior teeth with adequate coronal structure (two remaining walls) that exhibit undercut chambers large enough to receive a bulk of amalgam. This foundation can be placed in one visit and can be as strong as other types of foundations provided adequate bulk is created.[40,41] Kane[42] demonstrated that 4 mm of remaining pulp chamber height negated the need to place amalgam into the canals. Amalgam cores placed in the chamber can easily be removed if retreatment becomes necessary. Removal is more difficult if the amalgam has been placed into the radicular space.

CLINICAL TECHNIQUE

1. Place a rubber dam if possible.
2. Remove the provisional restoration and all remaining coronal restorative materials, caries, and unsupported tooth structure.
3. Plan for at least a 2-mm thickness of amalgam over tooth structure that is going to be covered by amalgam.
4. Remaining gutta-percha in the pulp chamber can be removed with a warmed endodontic plugger.
5. Remove 2 mm of gutta-percha from each root canal only if this is necessary for additional retention (i.e., retention in chamber is less than ideal [4 mm]).
6. Inspect chamber for undercuts, and enhance retention if necessary by placing additional undercut areas into the chamber walls. An inverted cone or diamond bur is useful for this step.
7. Place a stainless steel or copper matrix band if needed. An existing provisional crown can be converted to a matrix by creating a large opening in the occlusal surface through which amalgam can be condensed.
8. Incrementally condense amalgam into the pulp chamber, then continue to fill the matrix to the level dictated by remaining tooth structure and predetermined height.
9. Begin to carve the alloy to the appropriate height while the matrix is in place.
10. Remove the matrix after initial setting has occurred and carefully check occlusion if the tooth has not already been prepared for a crown.
11. If the tooth has already been prepared for a crown, the amalgam may be carved to the contours of the desired crown preparation. In this situation the clinician should select a fast set amalgam alloy that will allow careful preparation of the core at the same visit.
12. The final prepared core should be well condensed and exhibit good retention and resistance form (Figure 9-7).
13. The clinician must take care when fabricating or relining a provisional crown not to fracture the newly placed core.

Prefabricated Posts

The tooth type, root length, and root morphology dictate the type of post to be used. Two basic categories of prefabricated posts are available: passive and active. Active posts primarily gain their retention by threads that engage the intraradicular tooth structure. Passive posts gain their retention from the luting agent.

A large number of prefabricated posts are available in lengths ranging from 8 to 22 mm and diameters ranging from 0.5 to 1.9 mm. A majority of current prefabricated posts are a passive design, are just as likely to be parallel as tapered, and tend to be made of stainless steel or titanium. Newer compositions include the carbon fiber post (C-Post, Bisco Dental Products, Schaumburg, IL). The manufacturer of the C-post claims that it has the same elasticity as dentin and prevents the root fractures associated with cast and prefabricated metallic posts. The newer zirconium oxide posts (CosmoPost, Ivoclar North America, Inc., Amherst, NY) are tooth-shaded posts to

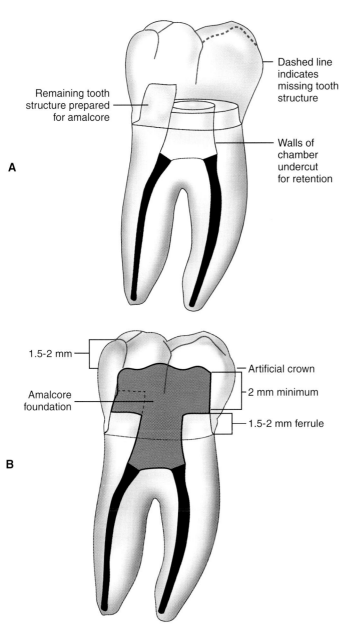

A

Dashed line indicates missing tooth structure

Remaining tooth structure prepared for amalcore

Walls of chamber undercut for retention

1.5-2 mm

Artificial crown

Amalcore foundation

2 mm minimum

1.5-2 mm ferrule

B

FIGURE 9-7   A, Preparation for an amalcore foundation. **B,** Restoration with an amalcore foundation.

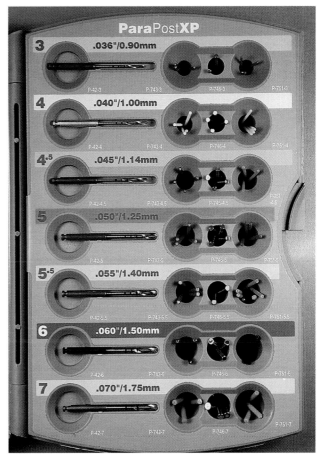

ParaPostXP

3	.036"/0.90mm
4	.040"/1.00mm
4·5	.045"/1.14mm
5	.050"/1.25mm
5·5	.055"/1.40mm
6	.060"/1.50mm
7	.070"/1.75mm

FIGURE 9-8   Preformed post systems usually contain calibrated drills to assist with post space preparation.

which a tooth-colored resin or ceramic core may be attached. Zirconium oxide posts are becoming popular because of the increased use of all-ceramic crowns. They are advocated for use with the more translucent all-ceramic crowns (such as IPS Empress) where a metallic post and core may render a graying effect.[43]

Prefabricated post systems often come with calibrated drills that correspond to the available diameters; these allow for ease of final post space shaping and remove minimal tooth structure (Figure 9-8). The following method is used for preparation and placement of a parallel-sided prefabricated post (ParaPost XP, Coltène/Whaledent, Mahwah, NJ).

CLINICAL TECHNIQUE

1. Prepare remaining tooth structure. Undercuts do not need to be removed.
2. Plan for the length and diameter of the post using a parallel, distortion-free radiograph as a guide.
3. Remove gutta-percha to the planned length desired for the post using a heated instrument or solvents. Adequate removal can be confirmed by exposing a radiograph.
4. Using Gates Glidden drills, enlarge the post space according to the size ParaPost desired, ending with the size that corresponds to the size of the planned ParaPost (Table 9-2).

TABLE 9-2

Approximate Diameter Comparisons for Whaledent ParaPost Drills and Gates Glidden Drills

	WHALEDENT DRILL			ISO D2 INSTRUMENT MEASUREMENT	GATES GLIDDEN MEASUREMENT (mm)*
#	INCHES	mm	COLOR		
3	0.036	0.90	Brown	55	#3–0.90
4	0.040	1.00	Yellow	60	#4–1.10
4.5	0.045	1.14	Blue	70	#4–1.10
5	0.050	1.25	Red	90	#4–1.10
5.5	0.055	1.40	Purple	100	#5–1.30
6	0.060	1.50	Black	110	#6–1.50
7	0.070	1.75	Green	140	#7–1.75

*#1 (0.50) and #2 (0.70) drills may be used to enlarge a small canal to accommodate a #3 drill.

5. To parallel the post space, select a ParaPost X drill that is smaller than the last Gates Glidden drill used in step 4. Place a rubber stop on the drill to the desired depth or use the drill markings as a guide. (ParaPost X drills can be used manually with the Universal Hand Driver or with a slow-speed contraangle [750 to 1000 rpm]. A new drill is indicated when manual drilling is performed.)

6. Sequentially step up to the next larger ParaPost X drill until the predetermined diameter and depth are achieved.

7. Select the ParaPost XP post that corresponds to the last drill used to prepare the post space.

8. Before cementing the post, confirm that the length of the post corresponds to the depth of the newly created post space. Reinsert the last drill used into the post space to confirm the depth of the preparation. Place the post next to the drill so the base of the post head is slightly above the final depth measurement identified on the drill. Using a cutting disc, remove the portion of the post that extends beyond the apical end of the drill. Re-chamfer the end of the post to its original shape. A radiograph can be made to confirm complete seating of the post before cementation.

9. Use a cylindrical diamond or carbide bur to prepare an anti-rotational box.

10. Place the post into the post space. Check for occlusal clearance. Remove the post and further adjust the length by trimming the apical end if needed. Re-chamfer the apical end to its original shape and débride the post.

11. Air abrade the post with 50 micron aluminum oxide before cementation to enhance micro-mechanical retention.

12. Use the dental cement of your choice, according to the manufacturer's instructions, to cement the post. Place the cement in the canal with a lentulo spiral. This results in an even coating of cement. However, this technique should be avoided when using a cement that sets by oxygen inhibition such as Panavia 21 (Kuraray America, Inc., New York, NY). For this type of cement, the luting agent should be placed only on the post.

13. Remove excess cement and fabricate the rest of the amalgam or composite core. This is most easily done with the aid of a matrix (Figure 9-9).

Cast Post and Core

The cast post and core has been considered the gold standard in restoration of the root canal treated tooth when a post must be placed to retain a core. This is particularly true for anterior teeth, where occlusal forces are oblique and not directed along the long axis of the tooth. Additionally, with a cast post and core the core will not separate from the post.

Fabrication of the Direct Cast Post and Core Pattern

A method for fabricating a custom cast post and core pattern using the ParaPost casting system is described in the following Clinical Technique. It allows the creation of a pattern that has the retentive features of a parallel, serrated post (apical portion) and the custom fit of a tapered post (coronal portion).

CLINICAL TECHNIQUE

1. Prepare the remaining coronal tooth structure, removing any unsupported or weakened tooth structure and all previous restorative material.

2. Plan for the diameter and depth of the post using a radiograph as a guide.

3. Remove gutta-percha to the length desired for the post using a heated instrument or solvents.

4. Using Gates Glidden drills, enlarge the post space according to the size ParaPost desired, ending with the size that corresponds to the size of the planned ParaPost (see Table 9-2).

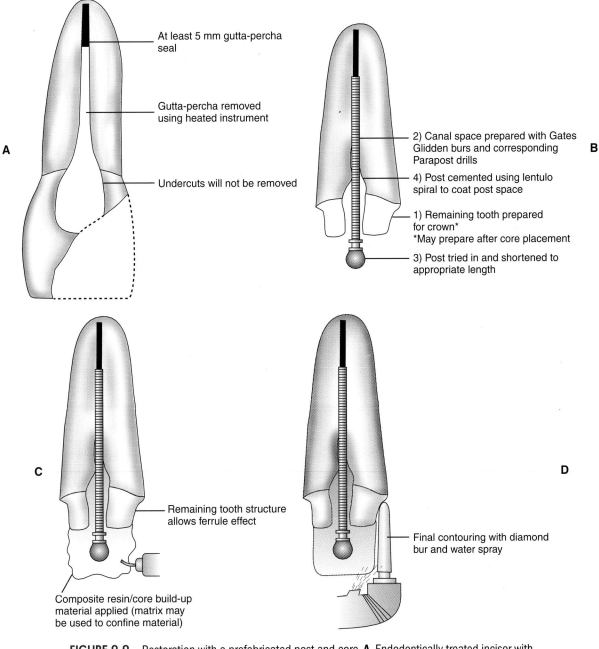

A

At least 5 mm gutta-percha seal

Gutta-percha removed using heated instrument

Undercuts will not be removed

B

2) Canal space prepared with Gates Glidden burs and corresponding Parapost drills

4) Post cemented using lentulo spiral to coat post space

1) Remaining tooth prepared for crown*
*May prepare after core placement

3) Post tried in and shortened to appropriate length

C

Remaining tooth structure allows ferrule effect

Composite resin/core build-up material applied (matrix may be used to confine material)

D

Final contouring with diamond bur and water spray

FIGURE 9-9   Restoration with a prefabricated post and core. **A,** Endodontically treated incisor with 5 mm of gutta-percha remaining; undercuts may persist. **B,** Canal space prepared with Gates Glidden burs and corresponding ParaPost drills. **C,** Composite resin build-up of direct core material. **D,** Final contour using a diamond bur and high-speed handpiece.

5. To parallel the post space, select the ParaPost X drill that is smaller than the last Gates Glidden drill used in step 4. Place a rubber stop at the desired depth or use the drill markings as a guide. (ParaPost X drills can be used manually with the Universal Hand Driver or with a slow-speed contra-angle [750 to 1000 rpm].)

6. Sequentially step up to the next larger ParaPost X drill until the predetermined diameter and depth are achieved.

7. Use a cylindrical diamond or carbide bur to prepare an anti-rotational box without undercuts.

8. Place into the prepared post space a ParaPost XP burnout post (P-751) that corresponds to the largest ParaPost X drill used to prepare the post space. If necessary, shorten the post from the apical end.

9. Build up the core pattern with pattern resin, then shape and finish the coronal mass of resin using medium and fine diamonds with water spray while

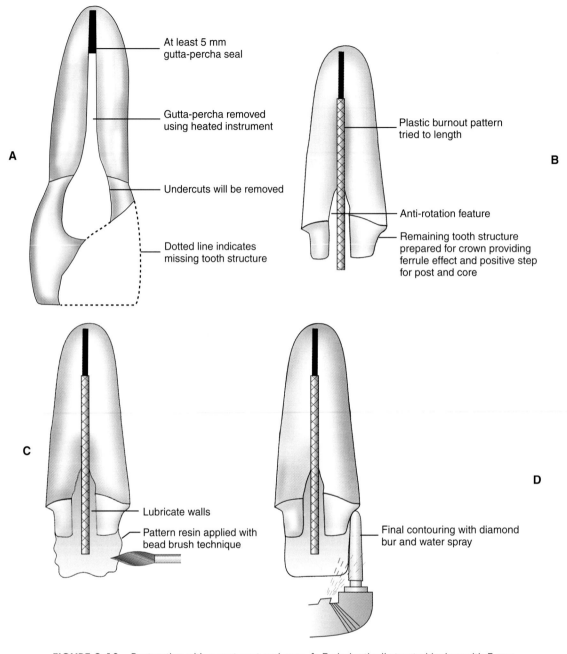

At least 5 mm
gutta-percha seal

Gutta-percha removed
using heated instrument

Undercuts will be removed

Dotted line indicates
missing tooth structure

Plastic burnout pattern
tried to length

Anti-rotation feature

Remaining tooth structure
prepared for crown providing
ferrule effect and positive step
for post and core

Lubricate walls

Pattern resin applied with
bead brush technique

Final contouring with diamond
bur and water spray

A

B

C

D

FIGURE 9-10 Restoration with a cast post and core. **A,** Endodontically treated incisor with 5 mm of gutta-percha remaining; undercuts must be removed. **B,** Canal space prepared with Gates Glidden burs and corresponding ParaPost drills. **C,** The tooth is lubricated and pattern resin is placed using a bead-brush technique. **D,** The coronal portion of the pattern is contoured using a fine diamond bur and high-speed handpiece with water spray.

holding the pattern firmly in the tooth. (Lubricate the tooth with a water-soluble lubricant such as SurgiLube [Figure 9-10].)

10. Building the pattern should be a two-step process. Build the internal portion of the pattern first and ensure that it can be removed before creating the entire pattern (Figure 9-11).

11. The finished pattern should be smooth and free

from voids and exhibit good resistance and retention form (Figure 9-12).

12. Sprue, invest, and cast with Type III dental alloy (Figure 9-13).

13. Perform try-in and cementation.

14. The post and core restored tooth should exhibit all the features of an ideal crown preparation (Figure 9-14).

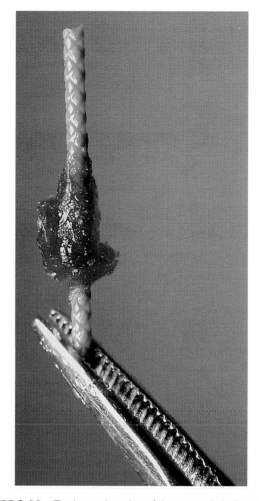

FIGURE 9-11   The internal portion of the pattern is built and easy removal ensured before the entire core is completed.

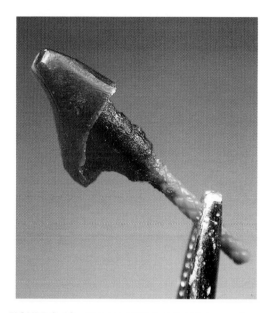

FIGURE 9-12   The completed post and core pattern.

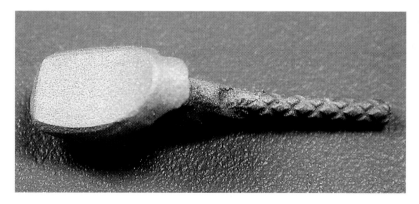

FIGURE 9-13   The post and core pattern has been cast with Type III gold and air abraded with 50-micron aluminum oxide.

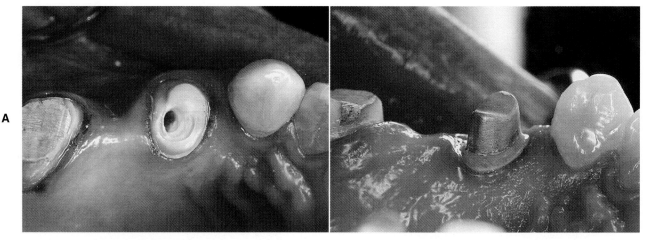

FIGURE 9-14 Tooth #5, an abutment for a fixed partial denture, was restored using a cast post and core. **A,** Prepared tooth. **B,** Cemented cast post and core; note the 360° of remaining tooth structure for ferrule.

Fabrication of an Indirect Cast Post and Core Pattern

▌ CLINICAL TECHNIQUE

Follow steps 1 through 7 described previously for fabrication of a direct cast post and core pattern, then perform the following steps:

8. Place into the prepared post space the ParaPost XP impression post (P-743) corresponding to the last drill used. If necessary, adjust the length of the impression post so the post does not contact the impression tray.
9. Take an impression with an elastomeric impression material. Make sure the anti-rotational box is filled with impression material.
10. Pour a model and fabricate a precision removable die.
11. Place the corresponding ParaPost XP burnout post into the post space of the model.
12. Complete the core pattern and remove it from the model. The finished pattern should be smooth and free from voids and exhibit good resistance and retention form.
13. Sprue, invest, and cast with Type III dental alloy.

The Provisional Post Crown

The temporary post crown is a potential weak link in the restoration of endodontically treated teeth because it may permit bacteria to enter the radicular space. Therefore a temporary post crown should be used for as short a time as possible.[15] A temporary post crown may be fabricated from a variety of provisional crown materials but should always have well-fitting margins to hinder leakage.

Fabrication of the Provisional Post Crown

After the custom post and core pattern is made, a provisional post such as the one provided in the ParaPost system can be used. This type of post provides good adaptation to the prepared canal and prevents leakage. The steps for fabricating a direct pattern are outlined in the following Clinical Technique.

▌ CLINICAL TECHNIQUE

1. Lubricate the tooth and adjacent teeth with a water-soluble lubricant such as SurgiLube.
2. Place a ParaPost XP aluminum temporary post (P-746) that corresponds with the planned final post size into the prepared canal space.
3. If a provisional crown was made previously, check that it fits over the post and seats fully into the proper occlusion. If it does not seat fully, remove material from the inside of the provisional crown or shorten the provisional post at the apical end.
4. Flow provisional crown reline material around the post, allowing it to fill any existing space.
5. Flow reline material into the provisional crown as well and seat it onto the post, allowing it to set but removing it before the final set to prevent it from locking into adjacent tooth undercuts.
6. When the provisional crown is removed, the post is incorporated into the internal surface.
7. Trim away excess reline material and evaluate margins for adequate seal and fit.
8. If discrepancies are evident, reline the margins to correct them. The finished provisional restoration should mimic the planned definitive restoration in contour and fit.

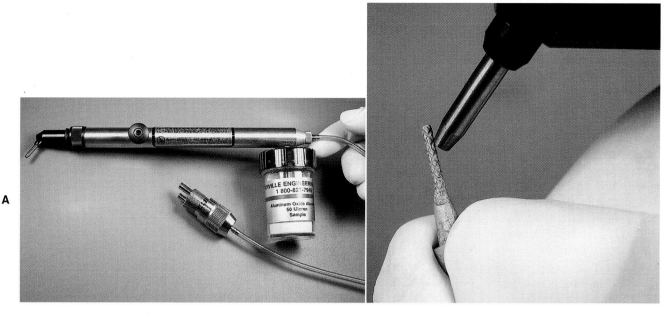

FIGURE 9-15   A, A Micro-Etcher allows air abrasion surface treatment with 50-micron aluminum oxide. **B,** The clinician should air abrade the entire surface of the cast post and core before cementation to increase retention.

9. Cement the provisional post crown with provisional cement. The use of non-eugenol cement such as TempBond NE (Kerr USA, Romulus, MI) is recommended because the provisional post crown will need to be relined after cementation of the cast post and core. Eugenol has been demonstrated to inhibit the set of some provisional crown materials. To preserve the integrity of the post space, apply temporary cement only to the margins of the crown; do not place any cement into the post space or on the post.

10. If a provisional crown was not made previously, a similar technique using some type of matrix such as a vacuum-formed polystyrene matrix or polyvinyl-siloxane putty matrix may be used to create a crown form around the post and remaining tooth.

11. A large endodontic file can be substituted for the provisional ParaPost post.

Post Cementation

Prefabricated posts and custom cast posts may be cemented with a variety of luting agents. Zinc phosphate has a long history of clinical effectiveness and is still frequently employed. Although it is more time consuming to mix and proper technique is essential, it has been reported to be least affected by eugenol compared with other cements.[44] An additional advantage to zinc phosphate is the potential for removal of the post with ultrasonic instrumentation if the tooth requires retreatment

or the post fractures. Eugenol has been shown to significantly reduce the retention of posts cemented with some resin cements and recommendations have been made to irrigate the post space with ethyl alcohol or etch with 37% phosphoric acid gel to remove the eugenol residue.[45] Other choices include glass ionomer and composite resin cements. When using glass ionomer, the clinician should consider the capsulated form instead of the hand-mixed variety. Because of its consistent powder-to-liquid ratio the capsulated glass ionomer has been shown to contribute to significantly increased retention compared with the hand-mixed form.[46] Resin ionomer hybrid cements should probably be avoided for post cementation because their tendency to expand may place undue pressure on the tooth root. One study evaluating the retention of posts with resin, glass ionomer, and hybrid cements revealed disappointing results for the hybrids compared with the resin and glass ionomer cements.[47] Composite and glass ionomer luting agents are not easily removed when retreatment is required.

To enhance retention, the surface of the post can be micro-roughened before cementation with 50-micron aluminum oxide and a micro air abrasive unit (Micro-Etcher, Danville Engineering Inc., Danville, CA) with 60 p.s.i. air pressure (Figure 9-15).[48] Before cementation of the definitive crown, the cast custom core may be treated with the micro abrasive unit intraorally. This removes residue from the temporary cement and leaves a clean, micro-roughened surface for final cementation. The tooth should be irrigated and dried with paper points before cementation to remove residue from the canal space preparation. The EndoEze System by Ultradent (South Jordan, Utah) features small capillary tips that can be attached to high-volume suction to remove irrigant from the post space efficiently and effectively. This system removes excess moisture but does not desiccate dentin, which is important particularly when resin cement is used (Figure 9-16). A single paper point can then be used to verify the absence of irrigant.

Installation stress during cementation should be minimized. Although tapered posts tend to be self-venting, placement of a parallel post can generate hydrostatic backpressure. Venting of the post should be considered to allow excess cement to escape during the cementation process, thereby relieving cementation pressure. Some post systems have vents incorporated into the post design. Alternatively, a vent may be placed along the side of the post using a ¼ round carbide bur. The clinician should also consider hydrostatic pressure when selecting a cement for the post. A study by Morando et al[49] examined posts cemented with three different luting agents: resinous cement, glass ionomer cement, and zinc phosphate cement. The mean hydrostatic pressures (p.s.i.) were recorded. Zinc phosphate cement created substantially greater hydrostatic pressure than either the resinous or glass ionomer cements. Therefore, venting may be particularly important during use of zinc phosphate cement.

Restoration of Endodontic Access through Full-Coverage Crowns

Endodontic treatment occasionally needs to be performed through an existing crown. In this situation, root canal treatment is more challenging. The restorative dentist must replace tooth structure removed during access opening and repair the void left in the crown. A decision must be made regarding whether the crown should be restored or replaced. Although endodontic access preparation can decrease retention of a crown, retention can be regained by subsequent placement of an appropriate restoration.[50,51] Amalgam is generally used to restore endodontic access through a cast gold crown. The current trend to place all-ceramic crowns on posterior teeth creates an esthetic dilemma. If the crown does not fracture during the access procedure, the patient probably will not want an alloy in the access cavity. In this situation, alloy may be still placed in the chamber, much as an amalcore would be placed. The last 2 mm of coronal opening is then treated as a porcelain repair. The porcelain is etched and receives a silane application, and composite is placed to restore the occlusal surface in a manner that mimics the original ceramic crown material. With this technique, amalgam provides a coronal seal over the root canal filling and the patient receives an esthetic restoration.

SUMMARY

Endodontically treated teeth do not appear to exhibit physical and mechanical properties that are significantly different from those of vital teeth. Loss of coronal structure is a major concern. Numerous techniques are available to restore the endodontically treated tooth. A significant factor in any technique is incorporation of a 1.5 to 2 mm ferrule. Success does not totally depend on the technique employed. Numerous factors such as remaining tooth structure, occlusal forces, and the function and periodontal status of the tooth are important. The clinician must consider all these factors when choosing a method for restoration.

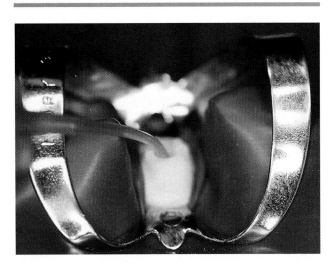

FIGURE 9-16 The capillary suction tip in the EndoEze System allows efficient and effective removal of irrigant from the post space.

References

1. Gutman JL, Tidwell E: Restoring endodontically treated teeth, *Texas Dent J* 114:14, 1997.
2. Saunders WP, Saunders EM: Coronal leakage as a cause of failure in root-canal therapy: a review, *Endod Dent Traumatol* 10:105, 1994.
3. Bateman LA: *Fundamentals of fixed prosthodontics,* Carol Stream, IL, 1997, Quintessence.
4. Nyman S, Lindhe J: A longitudinal study of combined periodontal and prosthetic treatment of patients with advanced periodontal disease, *J Periodontol* 50:163, 1979.
5. Sorensen JA, Martinoff JT: Endodontically treated teeth as abutments, *J Prosthet Dent* 53:631, 1985.
6. Hatzikyriakos AH, Reisis GI, Tsingos N: A 3-year postoperative clinical evaluation of posts and cores beneath existing crowns, *J Prosthet Dent* 67:454, 1992.
7. Papa J, Cain C, Messer HH: Moisture content of vital vs. endodontically treated teeth, *Endod Dent Traumatol* 10:91, 1994.
8. Huang TJ, Schilder H, Nathanson D: Effects of moisture content and endodontic treatment on some mechanical properties of human dentin, *J Endod* 18:209, 1992.

9. Reeh ES, Messer HH, Douglas WH: Reduction in tooth stiffness as a result of endodontic and restorative procedures, *J Endod* 15:512, 1989.

10. Sorensen JA, Martinoff JT: Intracoronal reinforcement and coronal coverage: a study of endodontically treated teeth, *J Prosthet Dent* 51:780, 1984.

11. Lovdahl PE, Nicolls JI: Pin-retained amalgam cores vs. cast-gold dowel-cores, *J Prosthet Dent* 38:507, 1977.

12. Goodacre CJ, Spolnik KJ: The prosthodontic management of endodontically treated teeth: a literature review. Part I. Success and failure data, treatment concepts, *J Prosthod* 4:243, 1994.

13. Leary JM, Aquilino SA, Svare CW: An evaluation of post length within the elastic limits of dentin, *J Prosthet Dent* 57:277, 1987.

14. Lu YC: A comparative study of fracture resistance of pulpless teeth, *Chin Dent J* 6:26, 1987.

15. Guzy GE, Nicholls JI: In-vitro comparison of intact endodontically treated teeth with and without endo-post reinforcement, *J Prosthet Dent* 42:39, 1979.

16. Trope M, Maltz Do, Tronstad L: Resistance to fracture of restored endodontically treated teeth, *Endod Dent Traumatol* 1:108, 1985.

17. Turner CH: Post-retained crown failure: a survey, *Dent Update* 9:221, 1982.

18. Newburg RE, Pameijer CH: Retentive properties of post and core systems, *J Prosthet Dent* 36:636, 1976.

19. Felton DA et al: Threaded endodontic dowels: effect of post design on incidence of root fracture, *J Prosthet Dent* 65:179, 1991.

20. Standlee JP, Caputo AA, Hanson EC: Retention of endodontic dowels: effects of cement, dowel length, diameter, and design, *J Prosthet Dent* 39:401, 1978.

21. Tjan AH, Whang SB: Resistance to root fracture of dowel channels with various thicknesses of buccal dentin walls, *J Prosthet Dent* 53:496, 1985.

22. Trabert KC, Caputo AA, Abou-Ross M: Tooth fracture—a comparison of endodontic and restorative treatments, *J Endod* 4:341, 1978.

23. Haddix JE et al: Post preparation techniques and their effect on the apical seal, *J Prosthet Dent* 64:515, 1990.

24. Eckerbom M, Magnusson T, Martinson T: Prevalence of apical periodontitis, crowned teeth and teeth with posts in a Swedish population, *Endod Dent Traumatol* 7:214, 1991.

25. Kvist T, Rodin E, Reit C: The relative frequency of periapical lesions in teeth with root canal-retained posts, *J Endod* 15:578, 1989.

26. Nixon C, Vertucci FJ, Swindle R: The effect of post space preparation on the apical seal of root canal obturated teeth, *Todays FDA* 3:1C, 1991.

27. McClean A: Criteria for the predictably restorable endodontically treated tooth, *J Can Dent Assoc* 64:652, 1998.

28. Sorenson JA, Engelman MJ: Ferrule design and fracture resistance of endodontically treated teeth, *J Prosthet Dent* 63:529, 1990.

29. Goodacre CJ, Spoolnik KJ: The prosthodontic management of endodontically treated teeth: a literature review. Part II. Maintaining the apical seal, *J Prosthod* 4:51, 1995.

30. Mattison GD et al: Effect of post preparation on the apical seal, *J Prosthet Dent* 51:785, 1984.

31. Schnell FJ: Effect of immediate dowel space preparation on the apical seal of endodontically filled teeth, *Oral Surg* 45:470, 1978.

32. Madison S, Zakariasen KL: Linear and volumetric analysis of apical leakage in teeth prepared for posts, *J Endod* 10:422, 1984.

33. Zmener O: Effect of dowel preparation on the apical seal of endodontically treated teeth, *J Endod* 6:687, 1980.

34. Camp LO, Todd MJ: The effect of dowel preparation on the apical seal of three common obturation techniques, *J Prosthet Dent* 50:664, 1983.

35. Cohen S, Burns RC: *Pathways of the pulp,* ed 4, St Louis, 1987, Mosby.

36. Trabert KC, Cooney JP: The endodontically treated tooth: restorative concepts and techniques, *Dent Clin North Am* 28:923, 1984.

37. Gagauff AG: Effect of crown lengthening and ferrule placement on static load failure of cemented cast post-cores and crowns, *J Prosthet Dent* 84:169, 2000.

38. Rosenstiel SF, Land MF, Fujimoto J: *Contemporary fixed prosthodontics,* ed 3, St Louis, 2001, Mosby.

39. Tjan AHL, Chiu J: Microleakage of core materials for complete cast gold crowns, *J Prosthet Dent* 61:659, 1989.

40. Nayyar A, Walton R, Leonard L: An amalgam coronal-radicular dowel and cone technique for endodontically treated posterior teeth, *J Prosthet Dent* 43:511, 1980.

41. Clark J: *Clinical dentistry,* Philadelphia, 1983, Harper and Row.

42. Kane JJ, Burgess JO, Summitt JB: Fracture resistance of amalgam coronal-radicular restorations, *J Prosthet Dent* 63:607, 1990.

43. Kakehashi Y et al: A new all-ceramic post and core system: clinical, technical, and in vitro results, *Int J Periodont Restor Dent* 18:586, 1998.

44. Dilts WE et al: Effect of zinc oxide eugenol on shear bond strengths of selected core/cement combinations, *J Prosthet Dent* 55:206, 1986.

45. Tjan AHL, Nemetz H: Effect of eugenol-containing endodontic sealer on retention of prefabricated posts luted with an adhesive composite resin cement, *Quintessence Int* 23:839, 1992.

46. Mitchell CA, Orr JF, Russell MD: Capsulated versus hand-mixed glass-ionomer luting cements for post retention, *J Dent* 26:47, 1998.

47. Love RM, Purton DG: Retention of posts with resin, glass ionomer and hybrid cements, *J Dent* 26:599, 1998.

48. Williamson RT: Cast core pre-cementation preparation, *J Prosthet Dent* 73:320, 1995.

49. Morando G, Leupold RJ, Meiers JC: Measurement of hydrostatic pressures during simulated post cementation, *J Prosthet Dent* 74:586, 1995.

50. McMullen AF, Himel VT, Sarkar NK: An in vitro study of the effect endodontic access preparation has upon the retention of porcelain fused to metal crowns of maxillary central incisors, *J Endod* 15:154, 1989.

51. Yu YC, Abbott PV: The effect of endodontic access cavity preparation and subsequent restorative procedures on incisor crown retention, *Aust Dent J* 39:247, 1994.

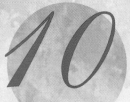

ENDODONTIC SURGERY

JAMES L. JOSTES *and* WILLIAM T. JOHNSON

Although conventional nonsurgical endodontic treatment has a high degree of clinical success, in certain cases surgical intervention is necessary. Before suggesting or undertaking surgical intervention, the clinician must identify the etiology of periradicular pathosis and develop a diagnosis and treatment plan. In many cases nonsurgical retreatment is the intervention of choice. Success rates for retreatment are high if the etiology of failure can be identified and corrected, and success rates for surgical procedures are enhanced if the root canal system has been properly cleaned and shaped.[1,2] Surgical treatment is indicated if retreatment would not improve the result or eliminate the etiology.

Surgical procedures include root end resection and root end filling, root amputation and hemisection, perforation repair (dentistogenic [iatrogenic] or pathologic), intentional replantation, transplantation, surgical repositioning, endosseous implants, incision and drainage, trephination, decompression, and limited periodontal procedures (e.g., crown lengthening, guided tissue regeneration, grafting). The most common of these procedures are root end resection and root end filling, root amputation, intentional replantation, and incision and drainage.

Common indications for root end surgery include calcified canals; a separated instrument; a tooth with a post; an unretrievable silver point; severe apical curve; incomplete apical development; external resorption; furcal and lateral perforations; gross overfill; procedural errors such as ledging, transportation, and apical zipping; persistent pain; retreatment failure; and biopsy. Adequate radiographs, including multiple views when necessary, are of paramount importance for determining accurate location, as well as for etiologic, treatment planning, and prognosis factors.

Before a surgical intervention begins, the patient's medical history should be reviewed and his or her vital signs recorded. Because endodontic surgical procedures are invasive and often require removal of bone, proper presurgical preparation can prevent serious medical complications.[3] Patients with hypertension, bleeding disorders, liver disease, or diabetes, as well as those who are immunocompromised or are undergoing anticoagulant therapy, may not be good candidates for surgery. At the very least they require medical consultation before treatment. In addition, a complete review of the medical history provides data regarding drugs the patient may be taking and any allergies the patient may have.

Informed consent must be obtained before treatment.[4] This entails explaining the procedure to the patient, discussing treatment alternatives, describing the postoperative care required, outlining potential complications, and reviewing the prognosis. These elements must be explained in language the patient can understand, and the patient should be given the opportunity to ask questions. A written informed consent form signed by the patient is the ideal method for documenting patient communication.

ANATOMIC AND PHYSIOLOGIC CONSIDERATIONS

The success of a surgical procedure depends on the establishment of adequate access and visibility. Factors affecting access and visibility include proximal anatomic structures, the thickness of bone, root anatomy and morphology, flap design, and hemostasis. Of these factors, the only ones the clinician can control are flap design and, to some degree, hemostasis.

Anatomic structures that play a role in surgical treatment planning include the interincisal opening, vestibular depth, palatal vault, maxillary sinus, inferior

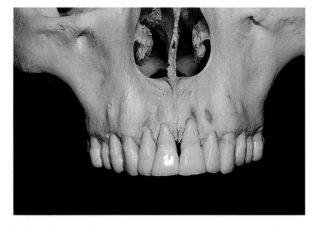

FIGURE 10-1 Skull specimen demonstrating the maxillary anterior osseous structures.

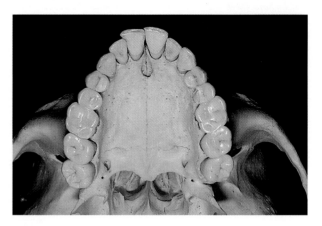

FIGURE 10-3 Palatal view demonstrating the incisive canal and the greater palatine foramen.

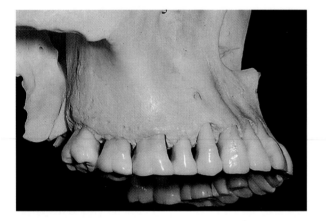

FIGURE 10-2 Skull specimen demonstrating the maxillary posterior region. Note the relationship of the zygomatic process and the maxillary first and second molars.

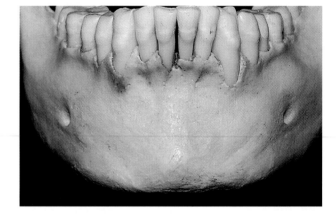

FIGURE 10-4 The mandibular anterior region of the mandible. Note the labial inclination of the incisors and the tendency for convergence of the roots.

alveolar nerve, and mental nerve. In addition, the thickness of bone in the maxillary and mandibular posterior areas can make access difficult.

Surgical procedures involving the maxillary anterior teeth are not usually complicated by the proximity of the roots to vital structures such as nerves and major vessels; moreover, the facial cortical bone is often thin. Root morphology is not complex because the teeth have only one canal (Figure 10-1). In the premolar and molar regions, the root anatomy becomes more complicated and the bone thickens. The premolars may exhibit one, two, or three roots that are often divergent. Even teeth with only one root may have more than one canal. In the posterior region the zygoma may prevent access to the buccal roots of the molars (Figure 10-2). This is especially important in treatment decisions regarding the mesiobuccal root, which is often broad and has a significant extension toward the palate. Often the roots of the maxillary molars are in proximity to the sinus. Strategic structures of the palate include the incisive neural vascular bundle and greater palatine nerve and vessels (Figure 10-3).

The cortical plate is significantly thicker in the mandible than it is in the maxilla (Figure 10-4). In the anterior area the teeth are often inclined facially, with the roots tipped lingually in the alveolar process. In addition, the roots tend to converge apically, placing them in close proximity (see Figure 10-4). Surgery in the premolar region is complicated by the presence of the mental foramen and nerve. The root canal anatomy of these teeth is often complex, with one, two, or three canals present. In the posterior region the buccal shelf becomes prominent, increasing the thickness of bone (Figure 10-5). As the bone thickness increases, access to the broad buccal-lingual roots of the mandibular molars becomes more difficult. Moreover, the roots may approximate the mandibular canal, and flap reflection must take into consideration the location of the mental foramen (see Figures 10-4 and 10-5). Mandibular second

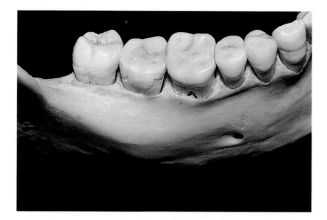

FIGURE 10-5   A mandible demonstrating the external oblique ridge and the mental foramen. Note the way the thickness of the osseous tissues on the buccal aspect increases in the second and third molar region.

TABLE 10-1

Blood Flow to Oral Mucosa and Skin Measured by Radiolabeled Microspheres

TISSUE REGION	MEAN BLOOD FLOW (±SEM)* ml/min PER 100 g OF TISSUE
Maxillary free gingiva	121.98 (23.99)
Mandibular free gingiva	114.71 (27.36)
Buccal mucosa	20.25 (2.48)
Maxillary attached gingiva	20.24 (4.33)
Mandibular attached gingiva	18.84 (5.83)
Alveolar mucosa	12.88 (3.58)
Skin	9.42 (2.04)

Modified from Squier CA, Nanny D: Measurement of blood flow in the oral mucosa and skin of rhesus monkey using radiolabeled microspheres, *Arch Oral Biol* 30:313, 1985.
*SEM, Standard error of mean.

molars are closest to the mandibular canal, followed by the second premolars. The mesial root of the mandibular first molar is farthest from the canal. The path of the mandibular canal follows an S-shaped curve in one third of the cases: lying buccal to the distal root of the second molar, crossing to the lingual below the mesial root of the second molar, and then running lingual to the first molar before crossing back to the buccal apical to the second premolar.[5]

Oral tissues are highly vascularized and have significantly greater blood flow than skin tissues (Tables 10-1 and 10-2).[6-9] Within the oral tissues, high blood flow is correlated with the thickness of the epithelium.[8] The primary blood supply for the gingival tissues comes from vertically oriented vessels in the alveolar mucosa.[10,11]

TABLE 10-2

Blood Flow to Osseous Tissues Measured by Radiolabeled Microspheres

TISSUE REGION	MEAN BLOOD FLOW (±SEM)* ml/min PER 100 g OF TISSUE
Cancellous rib	22.70 ± 4.66
Cortical rib	10.88 ± 1.11
Maxillary posterior whole bone	10.69 ± 2.65
Mandibular anterior whole bone	9.98 ± 2.36
Mandibular posterior whole bone	6.24 ± 1.60
Mandibular posterior cancellous bone	4.13 ± 0.97
Mandibular posterior cortical bone	3.71 ± 0.81

Modified from Johnson WT et al: Measurement of blood flow to osseous tissue in dogs using the radiolabeled microsphere method, *Comp Biochem Physiol* 106A:649, 1993.
*SEM, Standard error of mean.

Knowledge of the microvasculature permits the placement of vertical releasing incisions that do not compromise blood supply to the reflected tissue and that decrease bleeding by running parallel with the vessels.

Blood flow to the anterior and posterior maxilla and anterior mandible does not appear to have significant differences; however, blood flow to the posterior mandible is less than that to the other structures.[9]

ARMAMENTARIUM

Surgical treatment requires a unique set of instruments and materials (Figures 10-6 through 10-13). The basic tray set-up is as follows:

Mouth mirror
Explorer
Periodontal probe
Millimeter ruler
Cotton tip applicators
Gauze
Cotton forceps
Surgical blades and handle
Spoon excavator
Periosteal elevators
Surgical suction tip and stylet
Hemostat
Micro amalgam carrier
Condenser and carver
Aspirating syringe, needle, and anesthetic
Irrigating syringe bowl and sterile saline
Needle holder

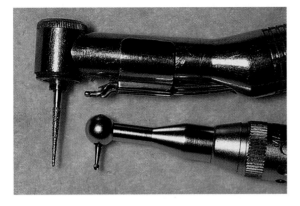

FIGURE 10-6 A conventional high-speed handpiece and a slow-speed microsurgical handpiece.

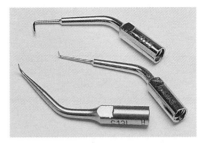

FIGURE 10-7 Ultrasonic tips.

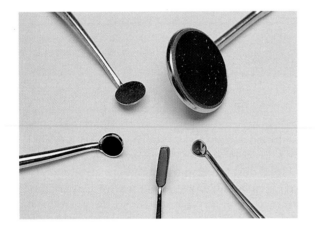

FIGURE 10-8 A conventional mouth mirror and various microsurgical mirrors.

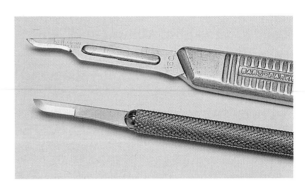

FIGURE 10-9 Microsurgical blades.

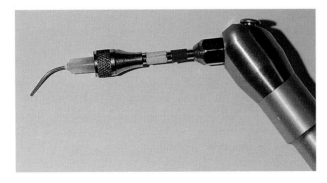

FIGURE 10-10 A Stropko irrigating device (EIE/Analytic Technology, San Diego, CA).

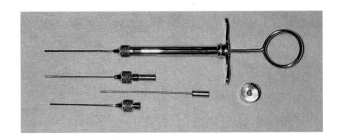

FIGURE 10-11 A Messing gun (Produits Dentaires, S.A., Vevey, Switzerland).

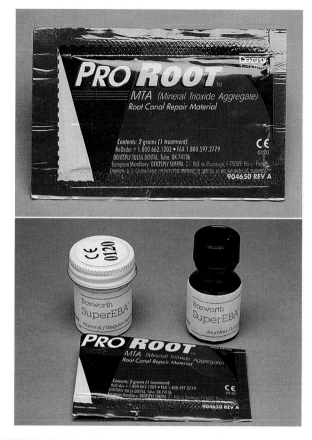

FIGURE 10-12   Mineral trioxide aggregate (ProRoot) and Super EBA cement.

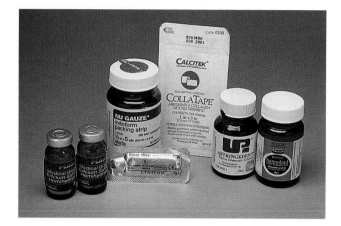

FIGURE 10-13   Various hemostatic agents (bone wax, CollaTape [Integra Life Sciences, Plainsboro, NJ], Nugauze [Johnson & Johnson Medical, Inc., Arlington, TX], Astringident [Ultradent Products, Inc., South Jordan, UT], Hemodent [Stone Pharmaceuticals, Philadelphia, PA], calcium sulfate [Surgi Plaster, Class Implant SRL, Rome, Italy]).

Scissors
Suture material

The following instruments are recommended:

Minnesota retractor
Messing gun (Produits Dentaires, S.A., Vevey, Switzerland)
Root tip elevators
Ultrasonic unit and surgical tips
Microsurgical blades
Microsurgical mirrors
Stropko irrigator (EIE/Analytic Technology, San Diego, CA)
Air impact handpiece (45 degrees)
Microsurgical scissors
Surgical operating microscope

ANESTHESIA

Local anesthesia is important in surgical procedures for pain control and hemostasis. The hemostatic action of vasoconstrictors is essential in the highly vascularized oral tissues, and the duration of action of the anesthetic solution is important for pain control. To maximize the benefits of these agents, the clinician's initial injections should include a long-acting local anesthetic agent such as bupivacaine or etidocaine. Long-acting anesthetic agents provide profound anesthesia for 2 to 4 hours and analgesia for as long as 10 hours.

The best method of controlling hemorrhage is to establish hemostasis before flap reflection. This is accomplished by injecting lidocaine with 1:50,000 epinephrine at various sites in the alveolar mucosa and near the root end. The slow injection of the solution in numerous sites within the localized operative field should be accomplished even with block anesthesia because the localized effect of the vasoconstrictor is more pronounced. Epinephrine that is administered slowly poses little risk to the patient and provides effective hemostasis.[12] Infiltration into the loose alveolar connective tissue produces predominantly vasoconstriction because of the action of epinephrine on the alpha-1 receptors associated with vessels of the microvasculature. The clinician should exercise care

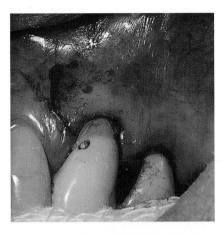

FIGURE 10-14 Initial incisions for a full-thickness mucoperiosteal flap for surgical treatment of the maxillary left first premolar. Note the initial oblique incision that preserves the papilla.

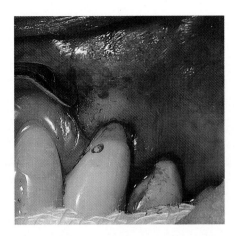

FIGURE 10-15 Tissue reflection involves an undermining technique initiated from the vertical releasing incision. The elevator is used laterally to lift the periosteum and associated tissues from the alveolar process. This prevents crushing of the crestal bone.

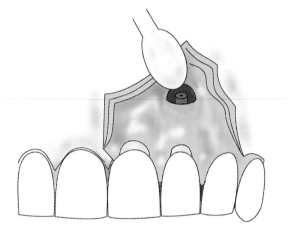
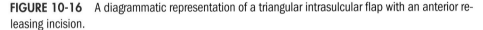

FIGURE 10-16 A diagrammatic representation of a triangular intrasulcular flap with an anterior releasing incision.

during the injection to avoid delivering the anesthetic into muscles, where beta-2 receptors are located. This action results in vasodilation and increases bleeding. In posterior periodontal surgery, 1:50,000 epinephrine significantly reduced blood loss compared with 1:100,000 epinephrine.[13]

FLAP DESIGN

General principles of flap design include the following:

1. The flap should provide for adequate access and vision.
2. The flap design should provide for adequate blood supply to the reflected tissues.
3. The flap design should provide for soft tissue closure over solid bone.
4. The flap used in periapical surgery should involve reflection of both mucosa and periosteum.

Additional considerations in flap design choice include the importance of locating incisions away from anatomic structures, awareness of any pathologic defects, and evaluation of the projected bony window. The integrity of the papilla should be maintained (Figure 10-14), reflection of the soft tissues should be performed with an undermining technique (Figure 10-15), sharp angles should be avoided, and the flap should permit passive tissue retraction. Horizontal incisions in the attached gingiva and alveolar mucosa may result in scar formation.

Most endodontic surgical procedures require a reflection of a full-thickness mucoperiosteal flap. The intrasulcular and submarginal flaps are each described by the location of the horizontal incision. Vertical releasing incisions can be used with either intrasulcular or submarginal flaps. These incisions can be made one or two teeth proximal to the tooth being treated and can be placed both mesial and distal to the operative site.

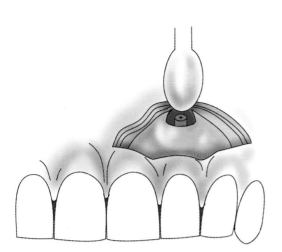

FIGURE 10-17   A diagrammatic representation of a submarginal flap.

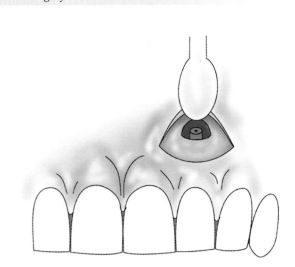

FIGURE 10-18   A diagrammatic representation of the seldom-used semilunar flap.

Flaps are described by their shape (triangular or rectangular). Triangular flaps are often employed in anterior areas, whereas the rectangular shape is more common in posterior areas. When a rectangular flap is used, the base should be as wide as the coronal portion of the reflected tissue to ensure an adequate blood supply to the reflected tissue. Vertical incisions should be made between the root eminences and parallel to the vasculature and the collagen fibers present in the tissue. This reduces hemorrhage, enhances healing, and discourages scar formation.

Intrasulcular Flap

The intrasulcular flap (Figure 10-16) involves an incision in the gingival sulcus. Advantages to the intrasulcular flap include good access and visibility. Because the supraperiosteal vessels are not cut and remain in the reflected tissue, bleeding is controlled and the reflected papilla provides a reference for closure. A disadvantage of this flap design is the potential for recession.[14] This disadvantage becomes crucial when esthetic restorations are present. To reduce the possibility of recession, the operative area should be free of inflammation and abnormal probing depths. The connective and epithelial tissues remaining on the root and cortical bone must be kept vital.[15] Incisions should sever the periodontal ligament fibers to the crestal bone, and the papillae should be incised in the midcol area because collateral circulation from the lingual aspect appears to be limited. The tissue should be reflected with an undermining technique initiated from the vertical releasing incision.[16] Working an elevator laterally, the clinician frees the periosteum and associated tissues from the alveolar process apical to the attached gingiva (see Figure 10-15). The intact attached marginal gingiva is then lifted from around the teeth. This undermining methodology minimizes damage to periodontal fibers

by eliminating direct crushing pressure of the elevator on the attachment apparatus and crestal bone. In the presence of healthy tissues and careful tissue management, the intrasulcular flap can be used without producing recession.[15]

Submarginal Flap

The submarginal flap (Figure 10-17) entails a scalloped horizontal incision placed in attached gingiva at least 2 mm apical to the attachment.[17] The main advantages with this flap are that the marginal gingiva and crestal bone are not disturbed. The submarginal incision allows both access and visibility. Disadvantages include the severing of vessels providing blood supply to the crestal tissues, as well as the lack of reference for closure. The horizontal incision also cuts across the collagen fibers, resulting in shrinkage and scar formation.[18] Contraindications to this flap include limited attached gingiva, periodontal defects in the operative site, short roots, and large periradicular lesions if the horizontal incision is made over the osseous defect.

Semilunar Flap

A third flap, the semilunar flap (Figure 10-18), is rarely used in contemporary root end surgery. With this flap a horizontal incision is made in the alveolar mucosa over the root to be treated. Although this flap does not disturb the periodontal attachment, it has the disadvantages of limited access and visibility, encroachment on and closure over osseous defects, increased potential for hemorrhage, and healing with scar formation.

Regardless of the flap selected for a surgical procedure, ensuring the health of the operative site is an important consideration. The use of 0.12% chlorhexidine as a presurgical mouth rinse can decrease the bacterial count and enhance the response to treatment. Patients should use the rinse the day before surgery,

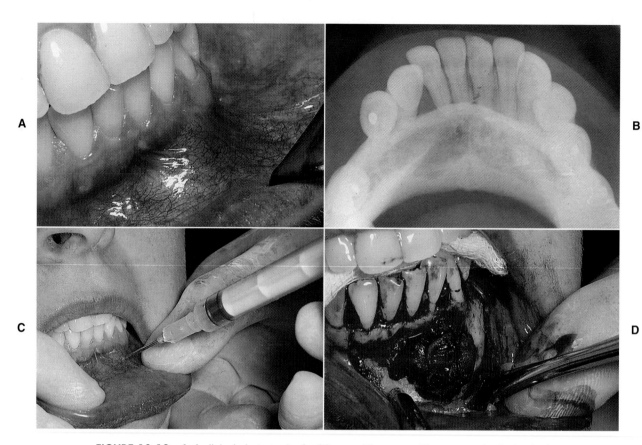

FIGURE 10-19 **A,** A clinical photograph of a 36-year-old woman with an expansive lesion in the anterior mandible. **B,** An occlusal radiograph revealing a radiolucent area in the mandible with associated tooth displacement. **C,** Aspiration of the lesion. **D,** Flap reflection reveals a soft tissue lesion that has eroded the buccal cortical plate. Histopathologic examination revealed the lesion to be a central giant cell granuloma.

immediately preceding surgery, and for the week after surgery.[19]

Before performing initial flap resection, the clinician can employ an aspiration technique as a diagnostic procedure. Aspiration is performed by inserting a 19-gauge needle into the lesion. Aspiration of significant amounts of blood may indicate a vascular lesion, aspiration of straw-colored fluid may indicate a cyst, and a nonproductive aspiration may indicate a neoplasm (Figure 10-19).

ROOT END RESECTION AND ROOT END FILLING

Before performing root end resection, the operator must have adequate access to the root end (Figures 10-20 through 10-22). After initial flap reflection the facial or buccal cortical plate should be inspected for perforation by the lesion. Often this inspection aids in locating the root end. The perforation may be small and appear similar to the surrounding bone. Tactile and close visual inspection should be performed to determine the presence of any defects. When a defect in the bone is noted, the clinician expands the area using a rotary bur in a high-speed handpiece. Light, intermittent pressure and a water coolant is essential to reduce frictional heat. If no perforation is noted, the clinician can estimate length by subtracting several millimeters from the length of the tooth on a distortion-free parallel preoperative radiograph. Accurate length estimation ensures that the operator will contact the root and not remove excessive amounts of bone apical to the root end. In areas with strategic anatomic structures, preparation of the osseous window should begin at mid-root and be carried apically. Because bone and root tissues appear similar, identification of the root may be difficult if no lesion is present. The yellow color of dentin and the presence of a bleeding periodontal ligament between bone and dentin are two clinical clues that distinguish root from bone. Application of methylene blue to the osseous crypt preferentially stains the periodontal ligament. On occasion, bone removal may occur without root visualization. In

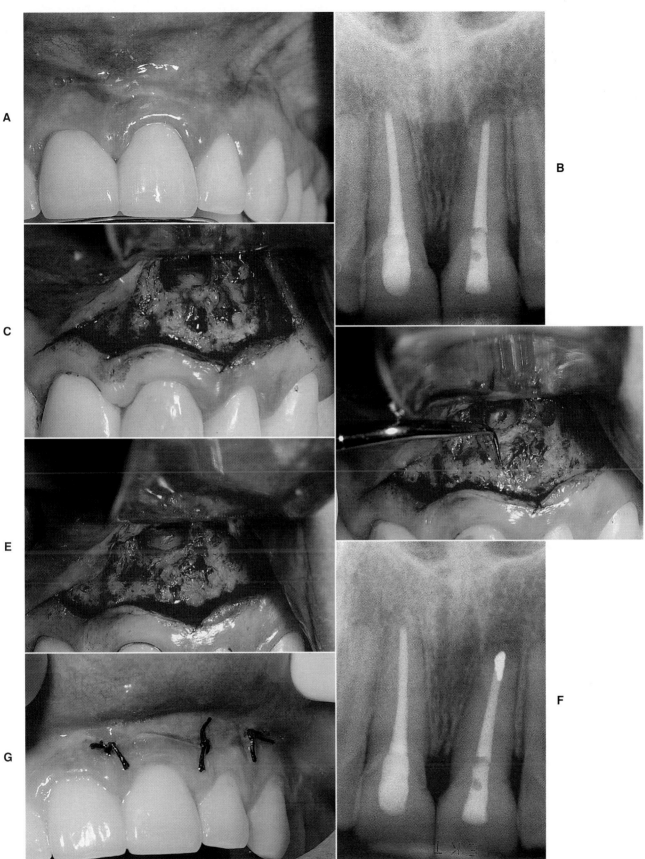

FIGURE 10-20 **A,** A clinical photograph of a 24-year-old female patient with a history of pulp necrosis of her maxillary central incisors after traumatic injury. Root canal treatment was performed on the maxillary left central incisor, resulting in an overfill. Root end resection was performed by an oral surgeon who failed to place a root end filling. The tooth has remained sensitive to biting pressure. **B,** A preoperative radiograph demonstrates previous root canal treatment and root end resection. **C,** A submarginal flap was used to gain access to the root end. **D,** Root end preparation was accomplished using an ultrasonic handpiece and tip. **E,** A root end filling was placed. **F,** Postoperative radiograph of the completed root end filling. **G,** Healing at 2 days after surgery.

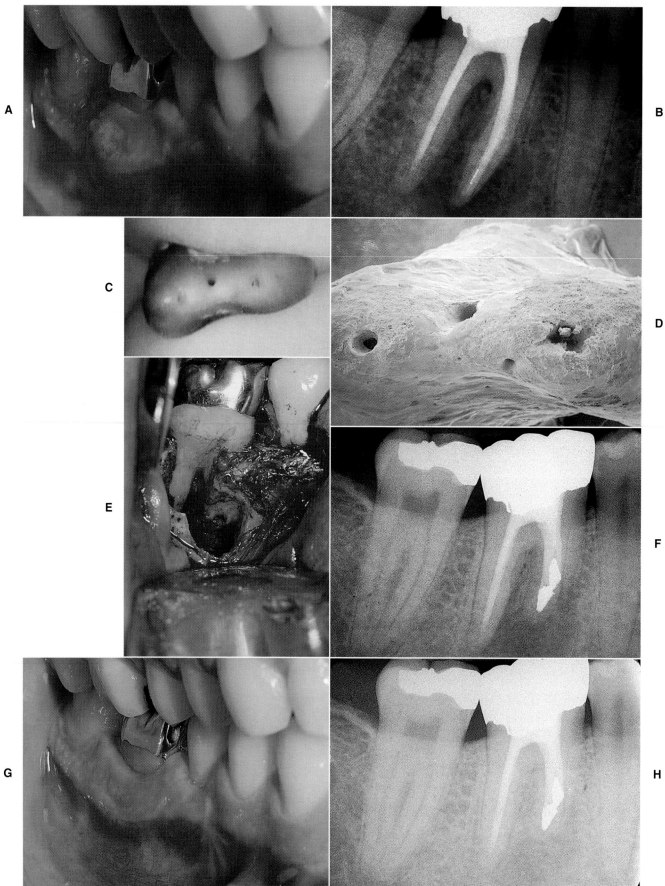

FIGURE 10-21 For legend, see opposite page.

FIGURE 10-21   A, A clinical photograph of a 34-year-old man with swelling in the buccal furcation area of his mandibular right first molar, tooth #30. He gives a history of previous root canal treatment with silver cones that required retreatment. **B,** A preoperative radiograph. Note the metallic-appearing material in the mesial root and associated radiolucent area. **C** and **D,** After root resection, inspection of the root and root tip is important. Note the accessory canals associated with the root tip. **E,** A clinical photograph taken after root end resection and filling. Note the perpendicular resection as well as the pathologic defect. **F,** A radiograph of the completed root end filling demonstrates inclusion of the isthmus. **G** and **H,** A 1-year recall photograph and radiograph demonstrate resolution of the lesion and osseous regeneration.

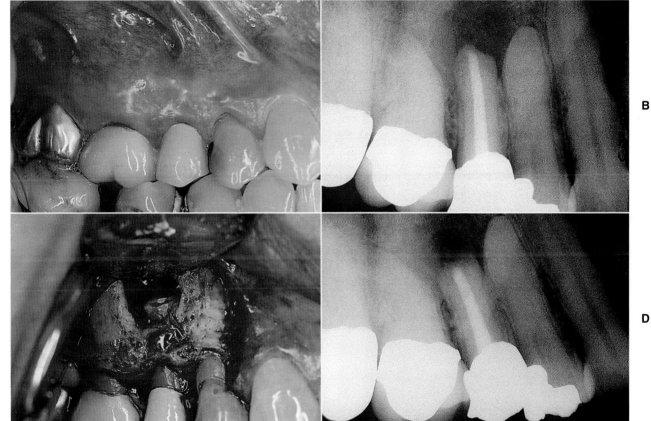

FIGURE 10-22   A, Preoperative clinical photograph of a draining sinus tract opposite the maxillary right second premolar, tooth #4, 6 months after retreatment. The adjacent teeth were responsive to pulp testing with CO_2. **B,** Preoperative radiograph demonstrates a periradicular radiolucent area. **C,** A clinical photograph of the resected root end demonstrates placement of a root end filling consisting of Super EBA cement. **D,** A postoperative radiograph.

these situations the clinician may place a small, sterile, radiopaque object in the area and expose a radiograph. Awareness of radiographic relationships and knowledge of the orientation of the osseous window and root end assist in location of the appropriate root apex.

After obtaining access, the clinician curettes the lesion and collects a specimen for histopathologic examination. Although complete removal of the lesion is ideal, it is not essential as long as the etiology for the lesion can be identified and eliminated. This concept is important when lesions extend to adjacent teeth and complete removal may compromise the blood supply to these teeth or other vital structures.[20,21]

Periradicular curettage is followed by inspection of the root for lateral and accessory canals, overextension of the obturating materials, vertical root fractures, and variations in tooth anatomy and morphology. This inspection is facilitated by the use of a surgical operating microscope. Root resection is accomplished by sectioning the apical 2 to 3 mm or by gradually shaving the root end to the desired length. Although an ideal resection should be perpendicular to the canal, resection may be oblique because placement of a bevel facilitates access for root end preparation. Root end resection removes the area where accessory canals are most likely to occur, provides a surface area for root end preparation, and promotes visualization of the entire periphery of the root. In general, the greater the root resection, the more surface area is available for root end preparation. A common error in root end resection is the failure to cut completely through the root. Because roots frequently exhibit a lingual orientation (maxillary lateral incisors, mesiobuccal roots of maxillary molars, mandibular anterior teeth), an oblique resection may fail to remove the root end. In addition, bevels expose more dentinal tubules on the root surface compared with perpendicular resections. The resected portion and the root surface should be inspected after completion of root resection.[22] In addition, the portion of the root that is removed should also be examined. When viewing the root end, the clinician should be able to visualize and follow the periodontal ligament circumferentially. The root should be inspected for fractures and anatomic variations such as the presence of an isthmus. Irrigation with sterile saline and application of methylene blue dye can assist this process. Transillumination is also an effective method of inspecting the root end. Visualization of the resected root end is best accomplished with a surgical operating microscope.[23]

After preparing the osseous window and resecting the root, the clinician should prepare the root end to receive an apical filling. Because visual inspection cannot confirm an apical seal, a root end filling should be placed where possible to ensure that the seal is adequate.[23] Historically the root end was prepared with a micro-handpiece or a small bur in a high-speed handpiece (see

Figure 10-6). Preparations were often round and large and seldom parallel with the canal. The recent introduction of ultrasonic tips permits root end preparations that mimic the shape of the canal (see Figures 10-7 and 10-20). These instruments exhibit a variety of tip designs, are small, and permit greater access in difficult locations. Tips with a zirconium nitride coating are also available. Ultrasonic preparations are parallel, can be extended to the recommended 3-mm depth, can include anatomic variations such as the isthmus between two canals in a single root, and are generally cleaner because of the irrigation used with the system.[23,24] Because an isthmus may not be visually detectable, roots with two canals should be prepared as though an isthmus is present.[23]

Root end preparation using ultrasonic instrumentation has been shown to produce preparations that are cleaner, smaller, deeper, and more parallel; they also accurately follow the root canal space.[25-31] An additional advantage to the use of ultrasonics is the decreased bevel required to perform the preparation. Evidence suggests that more leakage occurs with a beveled root compared with a perpendicular root end resection.[25,32]

A disadvantage to ultrasonic preparation is the potential for cracks and chipping. Although the production of cracks is controversial, the power setting used and the remaining thickness of dentin may be significant factors in their etiology.[33-35]

Regardless of the risks, ultrasonic root end preparation has a higher clinical success rate than use of the micro-handpiece.[36] An alternative to ultrasonic preparation is preparation with a sonic handpiece and diamond coated retro-tips. The success rate of this technique appears similar to that seen with ultrasonics.[37]

On completion of root end preparation the osseous crypt should be irrigated with sterile saline, dried, and inspected. The depth of the preparation should be assessed to ensure that it extends 3 mm into the root and follows the long axis of the root. The preparation should extend apical to the facial or buccal level of the resected surface.

Control of hemorrhage and management of the osseous crypt are essential components of placing a root end filling.[38-40] Hemostasis can be achieved in a number of ways (see Figure 10-13). The use of epinephrine-impregnated pellets has been advocated.[41] After removing the granulomatous tissue from the osseous site, the clinician places an epinephrine-impregnated pellet, as well as several sterile cotton pellets. Pressure is applied for several minutes. The sterile cotton pellets are then removed, leaving the epinephrine pellet in place. The vasoconstriction produced by this technique is synergistic with the application of pressure. Racemic epinephrine pellets are available commercially as Racellets (Pascal Co, Bellevue, WA). The #2 size pellet averages 1.15 mg of epinephrine, whereas the #3 pellets average 0.55 mg of epinephrine. Although the pellets are effective, their fibers may remain in the surgical site. Impeccable technique and thorough attention to removal should eliminate foreign body responses and healing impairment.

Ferric sulfate is an effective solution for hemostasis. Coagulation occurs rapidly after direct application to the osseous tissue. The solution is caustic and can be placed on a cotton pellet or Telfa pad for application to the crypt. Use of the solution should be limited to the crypt. After the procedure the coagulated material should be curetted from the osseous site.[42] Viscostat (Ultradent Products, Inc., South Jordan, Utah) is a commercially available ferric sulfate solution that is somewhat viscous.

Additional materials that can be used to control hemorrhage include CollaTape and CollaCote (Integra Life Sciences, Plainsboro, NJ), as well as Avitene (Davol, Inc., Cranston, RI). These microcrystalline collagen substances are biocompatible, trigger platelet aggregation, and activate the intrinsic clotting pathway. After their application, the osseous defect can be packed with cotton pellets, Telfa pads, Gelfoam (Pharmacia and Upjohn Company, Kalamazoo, MI), or Surgicel (Johnson & Johnson, Somerville, NJ). Although it is understood that cotton pellets and Telfa pads *must* be removed, Gelfoam and Surgicel also must be removed because they retard healing.[43]

Bone wax has been advocated as a mechanical hemostatic agent in periapical surgery.[44] The material is packed to fill the entire osseous defect. Excess material is then removed to expose the root end. After placing the root end filling, the clinician must remove the bone wax. Evidence indicates that inadequate material removal can elicit a foreign body reaction.[43]

Calcium sulfate is a biodegradable agent that may be used as a hemostatic agent. As with bone wax it mechanically plugs the vascular channels. Long used as a bone void filler in orthopedic surgery, the material is mixed to a putty-like consistency and placed in the bony crypt. Pressure is applied with a wet cotton pellet. The material is biocompatible and resorbs over time.

One factor that has been promoted to enhance healing involves demineralization of the resected root end before root end filling. Citric acid burnished on resected surfaces removes the smear layer, exposes collagen, and enhances cementogenesis.[45] Discussion remains regarding the advantages of using this technique. No significant improvement in long-term success rates may occur using this or other demineralization agents.

Root end filling can be accomplished after establishment of a dry operating field. Materials that are acceptable include amalgam, Diaket, super ethoxybenzoic acid (Super EBA), Intermediate Restorative Material (IRM), and Mineral Trioxide Aggregate (Pro Root MTA, Dentsply/Tulsa Dental, Tulsa, OK).[46-51] Although controversy regarding the use of amalgam has existed for many years because of concerns about toxicity, leakage, and long-term success, the majority of studies indicating

poor long-term success were done before the advent of new technologies that have improved visualization, crypt management, and root end preparation techniques.[50] These significant variables may have a greater effect on successful treatment than the material used as the root end filling. Currently amalgam is being replaced with alternative materials. Super EBA and IRM are similar in that both are zinc oxide and eugenol materials, Super EBA having less eugenol. Super EBA consists of a powder composed of zinc oxide, silicone dioxide, and a resin and a liquid made up of ethoxybenzoic acid and eugenol. Both materials appear to have higher clinical success rates than amalgam.[48] Mineral trioxide aggregate is a new material that has been advocated as a root end filling material. The principal components of MTA are tricalcium silicate, dicalcium silicate, bismuth oxide, tricalcium aluminate, tetracalcium aluminoferrite, and calcium sulfate dihydrate. Advantages include a superior seal compared with Super EBA, low toxicity, and healing of the periapical tissues with cementum forming over the material.[51]

Regardless of the material chosen for the root end filling, the field should be dry. The material is placed in the preparation and condensed. Because preparations with ultrasonic instrumentation are considerably smaller than those required with traditional methods, smaller condensers are required to compact the material. The preparation is overfilled and, as in the use of amalgam, the excess is removed. Super EBA and IRM should be allowed to set before finishing. When setting is complete, the excess can be removed and the material smoothed with a carbide finishing bur. MTA does not adhere well and sets slowly, so after placement a damp cotton pellet can be used to remove the excess and clean the root surface.

After placement of the root end filling, an interim radiograph or radiographs should be exposed to ensure that the root tip has been totally removed, no excess material is present in the osseous crypt, and the placement of the root end filling is adequate.[52]

The osseous defect can be irrigated with sterile saline and the tissues re-approximated after an interim radiograph has been exposed. Blood loss during apical surgery is minimal.[53] Closure is accomplished in most cases with placement of interrupted sutures. Continuous, vertical mattress, and sling suturing techniques are also used. Suturing is performed by engaging the reflected flap and suturing it to the attached mucosa. The size and type of sutures are variable. Diameters range from 3-0 to 8-0. Nonabsorbable silk or absorbable collagen-derived materials such as gut and chromic gut are commonly employed. Synthetic absorbable materials containing polyglycolic acid and polyglactin have also been developed. After suturing the flap should be compressed with digital pressure and a moist gauze for 5 to 10 minutes. This decreases the thickness of the coagulum and enhances healing.[54]

Recently the use of guided tissue regeneration techniques has been advocated in periapical surgery where large lesions are present.[55] Large lesions appear to heal quicker and with a higher quality and quantity of bone when a membrane is placed before closure. The routine use of guided tissue regeneration in periradicular surgery remains controversial. The technique adds cost to the procedure and may not improve results in treatment of lesions of average size.[56]

Postoperative instructions should be given to the patient orally and in writing. The patient should be advised to apply an ice pack extraorally the day of surgery. Ice should be placed intermittently, 10 minutes on and 10 minutes off. A soft diet is recommended and hot liquids are to be avoided. The patient should be advised to limit physical activity for the rest of the day. The patient should be informed that oozing may occur for the first 24 hours and that some swelling and tissue discoloration is possible. The majority of patients exhibit very little discomfort after the procedure.[57] Ibuprofen, acetylsalicylic acid, and acetaminophen are effective in controlling pain in most patients. Narcotic analgesics can be considered if over-the-counter remedies are ineffective. Antibiotic therapy is not indicated unless signs and symptoms consistent with systemic infection occur or the patient's medical status dictates antibiotic use. In addition, oral hygiene instructions should be given. Generally patients are instructed to brush and floss their teeth as they normally would, except at the surgical site. The patient is instructed to rinse the surgical site with warm salt water three or four times a day, beginning the day after surgery. If the patient was placed on a chlorhexidine rinse before surgery, this should be continued. Sutures are removed after 3 or 4 days.

Recent advances in surgical techniques and materials have improved the success rates for root end surgery.[36,37,58,59] Factors that influence the success rate include improved visualization, enhanced methods of hemorrhage control, ultrasonic preparation techniques, and the use of new root end filling materials. Because many of these techniques and materials are incorporated in various combinations in patient treatment procedures, identification of which factor or factors is most significant is impossible.

ROOT AMPUTATION AND HEMISECTION
Root Amputation
Root amputation is a procedure designed to remove an entire root of a multirooted tooth while leaving the crown intact. *Hemisection* is a term frequently applied to the removal of one root of a mandibular molar. In this procedure both the root and associated portion of the crown are removed. *Bicuspidization* is a term that applies to the surgical separation of the roots of a mandibular molar without removal of the roots. Each root is then restored with a separate crown.

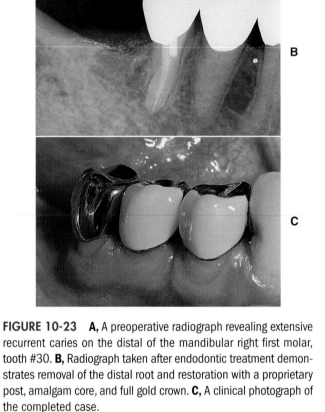

FIGURE 10-23 **A,** A preoperative radiograph revealing extensive recurrent caries on the distal of the mandibular right first molar, tooth #30. **B,** Radiograph taken after endodontic treatment demonstrates removal of the distal root and restoration with a proprietary post, amalgam core, and full gold crown. **C,** A clinical photograph of the completed case.

Root amputation can be considered if severe isolated bone loss occurs around an individual root; if caries, resorption, or vertical root fracture make a root nonrestorable; if endodontic treatment cannot be performed; or if perforation occurs during endodontic treatment (Figure 10-23). Contraindications to root removal include fused roots, roots that are in close proximity, inability to perform endodontic treatment on the retained segment, inability to restore or clean the retained segment, and poor oral hygiene. "Restorability" of the retained segment, maintenance of biologic width, and strict home care are crucial considerations often overlooked in the treatment planning process. Removal of a root requires an interdisciplinary approach with endodontic, periodontic, and restorative components.

ANATOMIC CONSIDERATIONS.   The anatomy and morphology of the tooth have significant implications for restorability, periodontal maintenance, and prognosis during treatment planning. The shape of the retained root may be difficult to restore and for the patient to maintain adequate oral hygiene.

MAXILLARY MOLARS.   In maxillary molars the mesiobuccal root generally curves distally, is broad in the buccal lingual dimension with the furcation toward the lingual, and exhibits mesial and distal concavities. The root alignment is similar to that of the maxillary premolars, and the root exhibits a large surface area for support. In cross-section the root may have an hourglass appearance. This may complicate the restorative plan and make oral hygiene difficult. In addition, the presence of one or two small canals makes post placement difficult. The distobuccal root is relatively straight, but may exhibit an apical curvature. The root is round in cross-section. The palatal root is the most divergent, extending lingually in relationship to the crown. The root is wider in the mesiodistal dimension than it is buccolingually.

MANDIBULAR MOLARS.   In mandibular molars the mesial root curves toward the distal, is wider in its buccolingual dimension than in its mesiodistal dimension, and exhibits the greatest surface area. The root has concavities on both the mesial and distal surfaces, giving the root an hourglass configuration in cross-section. The distal root is also wider in its buccolingual dimension than in its mesiodistal dimension. A concavity on the mesial surface gives the root a kidney bean configuration in cross-section.

Root Resection

When feasible, endodontic treatment should precede root removal. This permits adequate isolation for cleaning and shaping, assessment of the remaining tooth structure, and placement of a definitive restorative material in the coronal portion of the root to be resected. In addition, the tooth can be evaluated for occlusal interferences and a plan can be developed for provisional stabilization. To provide access and visibility and maintain adequate biologic width, flap reflection and osseous recontouring should be performed in conjunction with the root resection procedure.

Two primary methods are used for root removal (Figure 10-24): the horizontal cut and the vertical cut. A third, less popular, method involves presurgical crown contouring. The initial cut should be made in a manner that sacrifices tooth structure from the root to be removed while maintaining as much structure as possible on the segment to be retained. The retained segment can always be recontoured. After making the initial cut, the clinician should verify complete separation of the root before placing an elevator between the two segments and gently moving the two pieces apart. The root

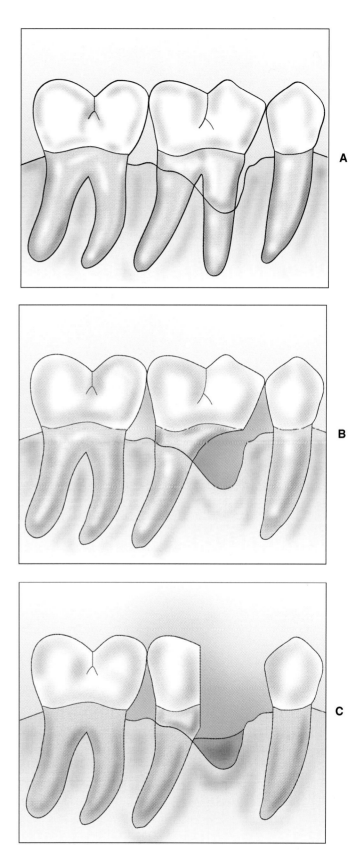

FIGURE 10-24   A, A diagrammatic sketch of a mandibular first molar exhibiting periodontal bone loss involving the mesial root. **B,** A horizontal root resection that maintains the crown. **C,** A vertical resection removing the mesial root and associated portion of the crown.

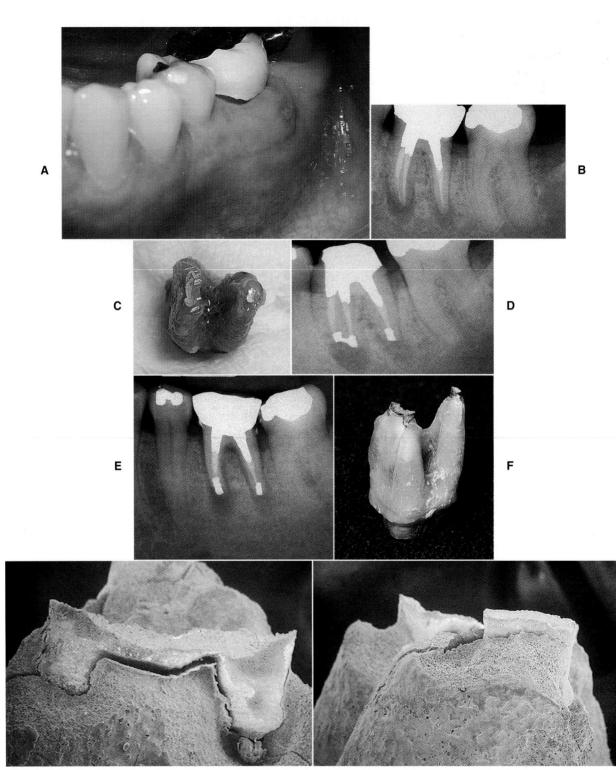

FIGURE 10-25   **A,** A clinical photograph of a mandibular first molar with a history of previous root canal treatment, retreatment, and restoration with an amalgam core and crown. Note the buccal area of inflammation. **B,** A preoperative radiograph displays radiolucent areas associated with the mesial and distal roots. **C,** Intentional replantation was selected as the treatment of choice because of the thickness of the buccal cortical bone. Root end resection was accomplished using a high-speed handpiece and water coolant. Root end fillings were placed in each root. **D,** A postoperative radiograph of the tooth. Note that the crown was dislodged during extraction. **E,** A 3-year recall radiograph. A deep mesial-buccal periodontal pocket was evident clinically. **F,** Examination on extraction revealed a vertical root fracture and external apical resorption. **G** and **H,** Scanning electron microscopic examination of the apical resorption.

should move independent of the crown. The area is irrigated and inspected after root removal to ensure the absence of overhangs or sharp edges and establish that the area is cleanable. Both the tooth and bone can be shaped to provide a cleanable area. Regardless of the technique employed, the clinician must exercise care to ensure that no overhanging tooth structure is left in the furcation and that 3 mm of circumferential tooth structure remains coronal to the osseous crest.

Success rates for root resection are 60% to 70%.[60-62] Failures tend to occur for a variety of reasons after extended periods of time. Root resection is a predictable treatment option that may offer the opportunity to maintain a portion of a strategic tooth.[63]

INTENTIONAL REPLANTATION

Intentional replantation is a procedure that offers the clinician the opportunity to maintain a tooth that cannot be managed nonsurgically. It can also be used in cases where root end surgery is not a viable option (Figure 10-25). Although intentional replantation is a treatment alternative, it should be used as a last resort because extraction of the tooth may lead to fracture, which renders replantation impossible. Success rates vary from 70% to 80%, with case selection being crucial.[64,65] Teeth with flared roots may fracture during extraction and must be evaluated closely when they are being considered for this type of procedure.

The success of intentional replantation primarily depends on the amount of time the tooth is out of the socket. Another factor is management of the root surface. After atraumatic extraction the periodontal tissue on the root or roots should be maintained in a moist environment. This can be accomplished by holding the tooth by the crown in a gauze soaked in physiologic saline or Hank's balanced salt solution. The root is kept moist with frequent saline irrigation.

If endodontic treatment is possible, the clinician should clean, shape, and fill the canal or canals and restore access before extraction and replantation. In cases where previous endodontic treatment has been undertaken or where the canals are calcified, the root end should be resected, a root end preparation performed, and a root end filling placed extraorally.

Immediately before replantation the socket should be irrigated with saline to remove the clot. The tooth is then replanted and stabilized if necessary. In posterior areas, splinting is often not necessary. If a tooth requires stabilization, an acid-etch physiologic splint or sutures can be used.

Success depends on precise and efficient performance of the procedure. Damage to the root surface during extraction and the length of time the tooth is out of the socket affect the prognosis. Maintaining the viability of the periodontal membrane reduces the incidence of replacement resorption and enhances healing.

References

1. Bergenholtz G et al: Retreatment of endodontic fillings, *Scand J Dent Res* 87:217, 1979.
2. Hartley F et al: The success rate of apicoectomy–a retrospective study of 1,016 cases, *Br Dent J* 129:407, 1970.
3. Milzman DP, Milzman JB: Patient assessment and preventive measures for medical emergencies in the dental office, *Dent Clin North Am* 43:383, 1999.
4. Morris WO: Informed consent and assault and battery. In Morris WO, editor: *The dentist's legal advisor,* St Louis, 1995, Mosby.
5. Denio D, Torabinejad M, Bakland LK: Anatomical relationship of the mandibular canal to its surrounding structures in mature mandibles, *J Endodon* 18:161, 1992.
6. Squier CA, Nanny D: Measurement of blood flow in the oral mucosa and skin of the Rhesus monkey using radiolabeled microspheres, *Arch Oral Biol* 30:313, 1985.
7. Canady JW, Johnson GK, Squier CA: Measurement of blood flow in the skin and oral mucosa of the rhesus monkey *(Macaca mulatta)* using laser Doppler flowmetry, *Comp Biochem & Physiol* 106:61, 1993.
8. Johnson GK et al: Blood flow and epithelial thickness in different regions of feline oral mucosa and skin, *J Oral Path* 16:317, 1987.
9. Johnson WT et al: Measurement of blood flow to osseous tissue in dogs using the radiolabeled microsphere method, *Comp Biochem & Physiol* 106:649, 1993.
10. Cutright DE, Hunsuck EE: Microcirculation of the perioral regions in the *Macaca rhesus* part I, *Oral Surg* 29:776, 1970.
11. Cutright DE, Hunsuck EE: Microcirculation of the perioral regions in the *Macaca rhesus* part II, *Oral Surg* 29:926, 1970.
12. Kim S: Hemostasis in endodontic microsurgery, *Dent Clin North Am* 41:499, 1997.
13. Buckley JA, Ciancio SG, McMullen JA: Efficacy of epinephrine concentration on local anesthesia during periodontal surgery, *J Periodontol* 55:653, 1984.
14. Grung B: Healing of gingival mucoperiosteal flaps after marginal incision in apicoectomy procedures, *Int J Oral Surg* 2:20, 1973.
15. Harrison JW, Jurosky KA: Wound healing in the tissues of the periodontium following periradicular surgery. I. The incisional wound, *J Endodon* 17:425, 1991.
16. Gutmann JL, Harrison JW: Posterior endodontic surgery: anatomical considerations and clinical techniques, *Int Endod J* 18:8, 1985.
17. Lang NP, Loe H: The relationship between the width of keratinized gingiva and gingival health, *J Periodontol* 43:623, 1972.
18. Kamper BJ, Kaminski EJ, Osetek EM: A comparative study of the wound healing of three types of flap design used in periradicular surgery, *J Endodon* 10:17, 1984.
19. Sanz M et al: Clinical enhancement of post-periodontal surgical therapy by a 0.12% chlorhexidine gluconate mouthrinse, *J Periodontol* 60:570, 1989.
20. Soulti A, Torbinejad M: Histologic study of healing periradicular lesions with and without curettage, *J Endodon* 20:188, 1994.
21. Lin LM, Gaengler P, Langeland K: Periradicular curettage, *Int Endod J* 29:220, 1996.
22. Rud J, Andreasen JO: Operative procedures in periapical surgery with contemporaneous root filling, *Int J Oral Surg* 1:297, 1972.
23. Rubenstein R: The anatomy of the surgical operating microscope and operating positions, *Dent Clin North Am* 41:391, 1997.
24. Carr GB: Ultrasonic root end preparations, *Dent Clin North Am* 41:541, 1997.
25. Gagliani M, Taschieri S, Molinari R: Ultrasonic root-end preparation: influence of cutting angle on the apical seal, *J Endodon* 24:626, 1998.
26. Hsu Y, Kim S: The resected root surface. The issue of canal isthmuses, *Dent Clin North Am* 41:529, 1997.
27. Gutmann JL et al: Ultrasonic root-end preparation. Part 1. SEM analysis, *Int Endod J* 27:318, 1994.

28. Gorman MC, Steiman HR, Gartner AH: Scanning electron microscopic evaluation of root-end preparations, *J Endodon* 21:113, 1995.

29. Engel TK, Steiman HR: Preliminary investigation of ultrasonic root end preparation, *J Endodon* 21:443, 1995.

30. Lin CP et al: The quality of ultrasonic root-end preparation: a quantitative study, *J Endodon* 24:666, 1998.

31. Mehlhaff DS, Marshall JG, Baumgartner JC: Comparison of ultrasonic and high-speed-bur root-end preparations using bilaterally matched teeth, *J Endodon* 23:448, 1997.

32. Saunders WP, Saunders EM, Gutrmann JL: Ultrasonic root-end preparation. Part 2. Microleakage of EBA root end fillings, *Int Endod J* 27:325, 1994.

33. von Arx T, Walker WA: Microsurgical instruments for root-end cavity preparation following apicoectomy: a literature review, *Endod Dent Traumatol* 16:47, 2000.

34. Layton CA et al: Evaluation of cracks associated with ultrasonic root-end preparation, *J Endodon* 22:157, 1996.

35. Abedi HR et al: Effects of ultrasonic root end cavity preparation on the root apex, *Oral Surg Oral Med Oral Pathol Oral Radiol Endod* 80:207, 1995.

36. Bader G, Lejeune S: Prospective study of two retrograde endodontic apical preparations with and without the use of CO_2 laser, *Endod Dent Traumatol* 14:75, 1998.

37. von Arx T, Kurt B: Root-end cavity preparation after apicoectomy using a new type sonic and diamond-surfaced retrotip: a 1 year follow-up study, *J Oral Maxillofac Surg* 57:656, 1999.

38. Withespoon DE, Gutmann JL: Haemostasis in periradicular surgery, *Int Endod J* 29:135, 1996.

39. Sauveur G et al: The control of haemorrhage at the operative site during periradicular surgery, *Int Endod J* 32:225, 1999.

40. Kim S, Rethnam S: Hemostasis in endodontic microsurgery, *Dent Clin North Am* 41:499, 1997.

41. Besner E: Systemic effects of racemic epinephrine when applied to the bone cavity during periapical surgery, *Va Dent J* 49:9, 1972.

42. Jeansonne BG, Boggs WS, Lemon RR: Ferric sulfate hemostasis: effect on osseous wound healing. II. With curettage and irrigation, *J Endodon* 19:174, 1993.

43. Ibarrola JL et al: Osseous reactions to three hemostatic agents, *J Endodon* 11:75, 1985.

44. Selden HS: Bone wax as an effective hemostat in periapical surgery, *Oral Surg Oral Med Oral Pathol Oral Radiol Endod* 29:262, 1970.

45. Craig K, Harrison JW: Wound healing following demineralization of resected root ends in periradicular surgery, *J Endodon* 19:339, 1993.

46. Pantschev A, Carlsson AP, Andersson L: Retrograde root filling with EBA cement or amalgam. A comparative clinical study, *Oral Surg Oral Med Oral Pathol Oral Radiol Endod* 78:101, 1994.

47. Williams SS, Gutmann JL: Periradicular healing in response to Diaket root-end filling material with and without tricalcium phosphate, *Int Endod J* 29:84, 1996.

48. Dorn SO, Gartner AH: Retrograde filling materials a retrospective success-failure study of amalgam, EBA IRM, *J Endodon* 16:391, 1990.

49. Torabinejad M, Chivian N: Clinical applications of mineral trioxide aggregate, *J Endodon* 25:197, 1999.

50. Frank AL, Glick DH, Patterson SS: Long-term evaluation of surgically placed amalgam fillings, *J Endodon* 18:391, 1992.

51. Torabinejad M et al: Histologic assessment of mineral trioxide aggregate as a root-end filling in monkeys, *J Endodon* 23:225, 1997.

52. Saad AY, Clem WH: The use of radiographs in periapical surgery, *Oral Surg Oral Med Oral Pathol Oral Radiol Endod* 69:361, 1990.

53. Selim HA, El Deeb ME, Messer HH: Blood loss during endodontic surgery, *Endod Dent Traumatol* 3:33, 1987.

54. Harrison JW, Jurosky KA: Wound healing in the tissues of the periodontium following periradicular surgery. 2. The dissectional wound, *J Endodon* 17:544, 1991.

55. Pecora G et al: The guided tissue regeneration principle in endodontic surgery: one-year postoperative results of large periapical lesions, *Int Endod J* 28:41, 1995.

56. Bohning BP, Davenport WD, Jeansonne BG: The effect of guided tissue regeneration on the healing of osseous defects in rat calvaria, *J Endodon* 25:81, 1999.

57. Seymour RA, Meechan JG, Blair GS: Postoperative pain after apicoectomy. A clinical investigation, *Int Endod J* 19:242, 1986.

58. Sumi Y et al: Ultrasonic root-end preparation: clinical and radiographic evaluation of results, *J Oral Maxillofac Surg* 54:590, 1996.

59. Rubenstein RA, Kim S: Short-term observation of the results of endodontic surgery with the use of a surgical operation microscope and Super-EBA as a root end filling material, *J Endodon* 25:43, 1999.

60. Langer B, Stein SD, Wagenberg B: An evaluation of root resections: a ten year study, *J Periodontol* 52:719, 1981.

61. Erpenstein H: 3-year study of hemisectioned molars, *J Clin Periodontol* 10:1, 1983.

62. Buhler H: Evaluation of root resected teeth, results after 10 years, *J Periodontol* 59:805, 1988.

63. Buhler H: Survival rates of hemisected teeth; an attempt to compare them with survival rates of alloplastic implants, *J Perio Rest Dent* 14:537, 1994.

64. Bender IB, Rossman LE: Intentional replantation of endodontically treated teeth, *Oral Surg Oral Med Oral Pathol Oral Radiol Endod* 76:623, 1993.

65. Ragboebar GM, Vissink A: Results of intentional replantation of molars, *J Oral Maxillofac Surg* 57:240, 1999.

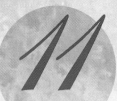

TRAUMATIC INJURIES TO THE PERMANENT DENTITION

WILLIAM T. JOHNSON

Traumatic injuries to the teeth and supporting structures can occur at any age. Although treatment may be necessary on an urgent or emergent basis, the sequelae to a traumatic episode may not become apparent or require treatment for many years.

The majority of traumatic injuries to the dentition occur in children and adolescents, but adults also often require treatment for injuries to the teeth and supporting structures. Maxillary and mandibular anterior teeth are the most vulnerable, with crown fractures being the most common injury.[1] More severe injuries include crown fractures with pulp exposure, crown root fractures, root fractures, luxation injuries, and tooth avulsion.

Unfortunately, injuries to the head and neck often result from physical abuse.[2] Signs of abuse include a delay between the time of injury and the time the patient seeks treatment, a vague story of the accident, repeated injuries to the face and neck, unusual or suspicious parental or child behavior, differences between the histories given by the parent and the child, and a marked discrepancy between the history and the extent of injury noted on examination.[3] Abuse is not limited to children. Spousal abuse and abuse of the elderly also can occur. Dental practitioners as well as physicians have a moral, ethical, and legal responsibility to report suspected cases of child and dependent abuse.[4]

HISTORY

Obtaining an adequate history is essential to the diagnosis and treatment planning process. A complete medical and dental history is essential. Often the treatment of a traumatic episode requires the administration of prophylactic tetanus toxoid. Other medical conditions may affect patient management. The dental history should include when the injury occurred, where the trauma took place, and the way the injury occurred.

CLINICAL EXAMINATION

The clinical examination should include an assessment of the extraoral and intraoral tissues. Lacerations, abrasions, and contusions may be present. Osseous fractures may be detected by visualization of a deviation on opening and closing or by tenderness to palpation. In addition, a neurologic assessment should be performed.

Intraoral examination provides visualization of the hard and soft tissues. The examination permits the clinician to assess damage to the mucosal and gingival tissues and observe coronal structures, displaced teeth, and tooth discoloration. Palpation should be performed in conjunction with the visual examination to assess for root fractures, tooth mobility, fractures to the osseous tissues, and objects that might be embedded in the soft tissues.

Pulp testing at the initial visit provides baseline data for establishing a diagnosis as well as comparative data for future reference.[5] Although pulp tests stimulate only the neural components of the pulp, the results can be extrapolated to indicate pulp vitality. Responsiveness to testing immediately after traumatic injury indicates pulp vitality.[6] If teeth that initially test positive are unresponsive on recall examination, necrosis has most likely occurred. Teeth that are not responsive on initial testing are not necessarily nonvital. Damage to the neural tissues may have occurred, with the vascular elements remaining intact. Evaluation and recall examination of these teeth may reveal that they have become responsive to testing over time.[7] Teeth that remain unresponsive may not be necrotic, and the astute clinician will wait for signs and symptoms such as pain, swelling, tooth discoloration, the development of an apical radiolucent area, or the formation of a sinus tract before initiating root canal treatment.[8]

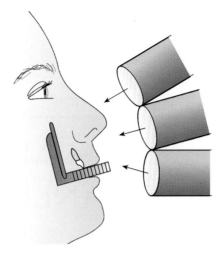

FIGURE 11-1 Detection of a horizontal root fracture may require increasing or decreasing the vertical angulation of the beam.

RADIOGRAPHIC EXAMINATION

Radiographs taken after traumatic injury may reveal tooth displacement, root fractures, osseous fractures, and foreign objects present in soft tissues. In cases of suspected root fractures, films exposed from several vertical angles may be required to reveal the fracture line[9] (Figure 11-1). In lacerated areas a film of the soft tissues may reveal an embedded object.[10] Radiographs are also helpful in assessing the degree of apical root development in teeth exhibiting crown fractures. A pantomograph may be indicated in cases of suspected osseous fractures.

DOCUMENTATION

Documentation of findings from the history, clinical examination, and radiographic examination is important for an accurate diagnosis, justification of treatment, future diagnostic considerations, insurance issues, and defense against potential litigation.[11]

CROWN FRACTURES
Uncomplicated Fractures

Infraction is a term used to designate an incomplete fracture in enamel without loss of structure (see Figure 11-4, *A*). Enamel infractions result from direct impact, are best visualized with transillumination, and may be the only visible evidence that trauma has occurred.

Crown fractures result from a high-velocity impact. Fracture of the crown dissipates the force and minimizes injury to the supporting periodontal structures and bone. Coronal fractures can involve enamel or enamel and dentin. The primary symptom associated with fractures involving enamel and dentin is thermal sensitivity. Although a fracture involving enamel often appears insignificant and can be managed by selective grinding or placement of an acid-etched composite restoration, the potential for pulpal damage exists. Pulp testing should be performed to assess vitality. The most severe pulp response is often seen in teeth exhibiting little or no physical damage.[12] In general, however, the pulpal prognosis for uncomplicated fractures of enamel and dentin is favorable.[13,14]

Crown fractures involving both enamel and dentin expose dentinal tubules to saliva and bacteria (Figure 11-2). The treatment of choice involves placing a protective base and an acid-etch composite restoration. Recent advances in enamel-dentin bonding have enhanced the bonding of fractured segments.[15] In cases with extensive damage, laminate veneers, porcelain-fused-to-metal crowns, or all-ceramic crowns may be required to restore form, function, and esthetics. With coronal fractures of enamel or enamel and dentin, recall evaluation is required to assess pulp vitality.

Complicated Crown Fractures

Fractures of enamel and dentin have the potential for pulp exposure. When a coronal fracture is complicated by pulp exposure in young patients, the extent of apical development must be determined. Teeth with incomplete root formation require apexogenesis for continued root development. Teeth that become nonvital before complete root formation require apexification.

Crown fractures that expose the dental pulp exhibit the best prognosis when treated immediately. The longer the pulp is exposed, the greater the bacterial contamination. This is especially important in teeth with incomplete apical development where maintaining vitality is

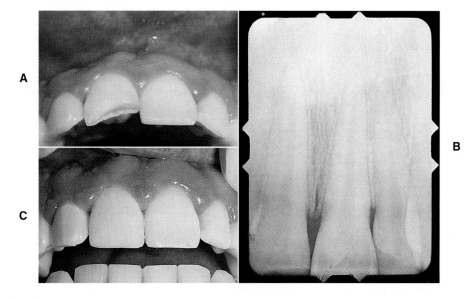

FIGURE 11-2 A, An uncomplicated crown fracture involving enamel and dentin. The patient was asymptomatic with the exception of sensitivity to cold. **B,** A periapical radiograph demonstrates the normal periradicular structures. **C,** Treatment consisted of placing a Class IV acid-etch composite restoration.

essential for continued root formation. If necrosis occurs, root development may cease.

APEXOGENESIS. Treatment procedures for teeth with exposed pulp include pulp capping, pulpotomy (Figure 11-3), and root canal treatment (Figure 11-4). Pulp capping is indicated for teeth with small exposures that can be treated soon after the injury. Capping can be accomplished with calcium hydroxide or a new material, mineral trioxide aggregate (MTA). Pulpotomy is indicated for more severe fractures or teeth in which treatment is delayed. Removal of several millimeters of pulp tissue provides space for placement of calcium hydroxide or MTA and is adequate to remove superficial inflamed tissue in cases where treatment is delayed. Removal of coronal pulp tissue is best accomplished with an abrasive diamond in a high-speed handpiece using a water coolant.[16] The amputation site should be clean of debris and tissue tags. Bleeding can be controlled with the application of a cotton pellet soaked with sterile saline. If calcium hydroxide is used, a glass ionomer or intermediate restorative material (IRM) base can be placed before restoration with composite resin. If MTA is used, the material should set for 1 week before the permanent restoration is placed.[17] An acid-etch composite restoration is placed to provide a coronal seal and restore esthetics and function.

With both pulp capping and pulpotomy, treatment consists of débridement of the wound and placement of calcium hydroxide or MTA. Although calcium hydroxide has been shown to be clinically effective over time, it pro-

duces a superficial layer of coagulation necrosis. The low-grade irritation of this layer induces the formation of a hard tissue barrier.[18] MTA, however, has been shown to induce a hard tissue barrier without inflammation.[19]

The time interval between exposure and treatment does not appear to be a significant factor affecting prognosis as long as the coronal inflamed tissue can be removed. Success rates for pulp capping and pulpotomy procedures after traumatic injury are high.[20] This is probably because of the acute nature of the injury and minimal bacterial contamination.

Recall evaluation should be performed after pulp capping and pulpotomy to assess the patient's response to treatment. Evaluation is often based on clinical and radiographic findings because pulp testing may not produce accurate information. In cases where root development is incomplete, verification of continued growth is evidence of successful treatment. Clinical studies indicate that successful pulpotomy procedures correlate with normal histopathologic findings in the pulp tissue.[20] Removal of the pulp after complete root development is contraindicated unless a post is required for coronal restoration. In cases where root development is complete and extensive coronal destruction has occurred, nonsurgical root canal treatment can be performed to facilitate placement of a post, core, and crown.

APEXIFICATION. In cases where necrosis occurs before complete root formation, apexification procedures are indicated to establish an apical barrier before obturation of the canal space with gutta-percha (Figure 11-5). In these

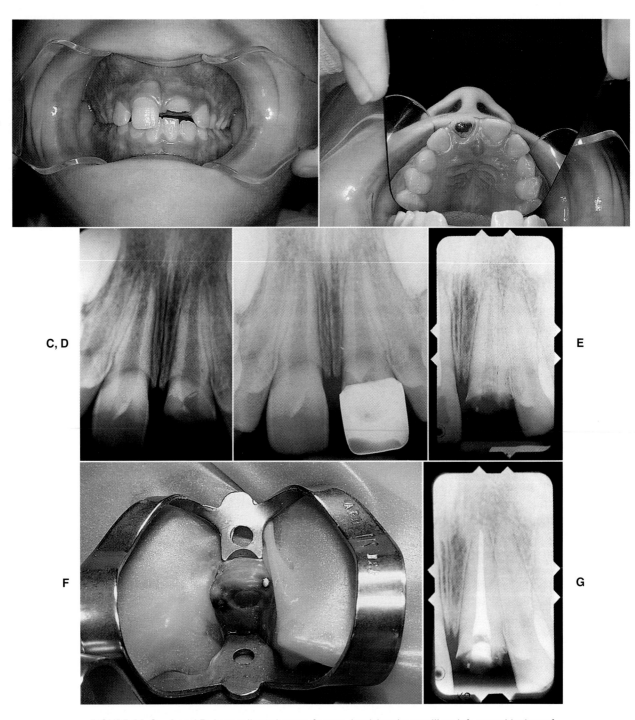

FIGURE 11-3 **A** and **B,** A complicated crown fracture involving the maxillary left central incisor of an 8-year-old child. **C,** A periapical radiograph revealed incomplete root formation. **D,** Postoperative film after a calcium hydroxide pulpotomy and placement of a stainless steel crown. **E,** A 2-year re-call film demonstrates complete root formation. Note the dentin bridge that has formed coronally. **F,** A clinical view of the dentin bridge. **G,** Postoperative film taken after nonsurgical root canal treatment to facilitate placement of a post and core.

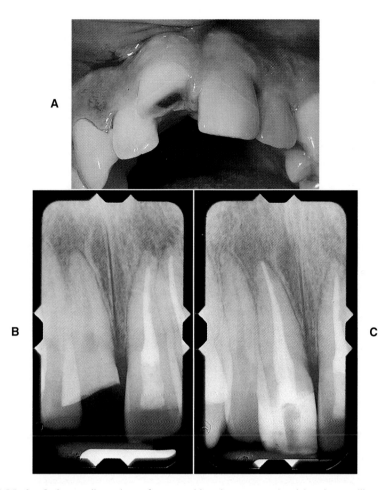

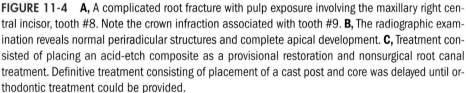

FIGURE 11-4 **A,** A complicated root fracture with pulp exposure involving the maxillary right central incisor, tooth #8. Note the crown infraction associated with tooth #9. **B,** The radiographic examination reveals normal periradicular structures and complete apical development. **C,** Treatment consisted of placing an acid-etch composite as a provisional restoration and nonsurgical root canal treatment. Definitive treatment consisting of placement of a cast post and core was delayed until orthodontic treatment could be provided.

cases the clinician débrides the necrotic tissue remnants from the canal walls using traditional endodontic procedures. The canal is then packed with calcium hydroxide powder or a proprietary paste, which is left in place for 2 to 3 months. The location of the barrier depends on the level at which the calcium hydroxide contacts vital tissue, so it is important to place the material to the apex.

During the recall examination the calcium hydroxide is removed and the apical area is assessed radiographically and clinically for the development of a barrier. If no barrier is present, the procedure is repeated. The average time for barrier development is 6 to 12 months.[21, 22] The success rates for apexification are high.[21-23]

CROWN ROOT FRACTURES

Crown root fractures involve enamel, dentin, and cementum and account for 5% of all injuries involving the permanent dentition.[24] Because the fracture extends onto the root, esthetics and restorability are concerns in treatment planning (Figure 11-6). The fractures generally are oblique and extend into the gingival sulcus on either the buccal or lingual surface. Forces impacting on the tooth from a facial direction result in fractures that extend onto the lingual tooth surface. Forces from a lingual direction result in fractures that extend onto the facial surface of the tooth. Clinically the fractured segment is often held in place by the periodontal attachment apparatus. Symptoms are related to movement of the fractured segment. The fractures can be uncomplicated or complicated depending on whether the pulp is exposed. To assess restorability, the clinician must remove the fractured segment. Radiographic evidence regarding the extent of the fracture is often inconclusive.

Treatment options include crown lengthening and orthodontic extrusion to reestablish the biologic width in

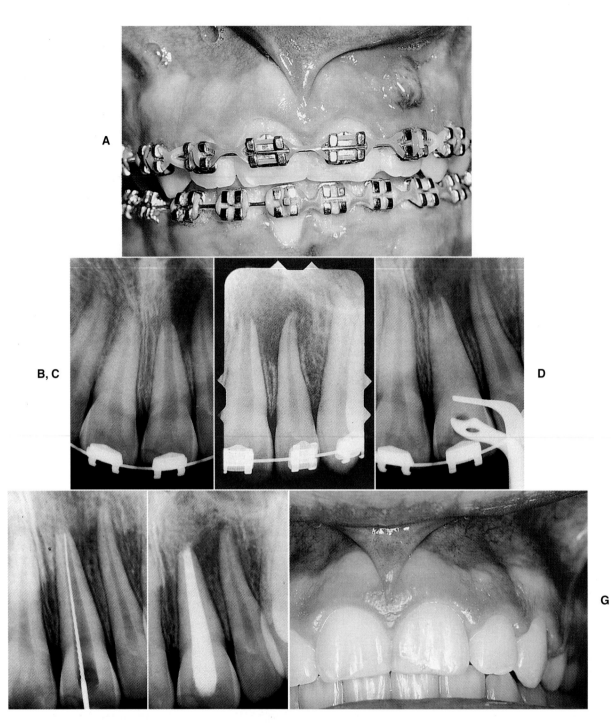

FIGURE 11-5 **A,** A clinical photograph of a patient with a history of a trauma (coronal fracture) to the maxillary left central incisor. The patient developed an apical abscess secondary to pulp necrosis while undergoing orthodontic treatment. **B,** A periapical radiograph demonstrating incomplete root development. Note the difference in canal size and root formation between #8 and #9. **C,** Although the radiolucent area appears to involve the maxillary left lateral incisor, this tooth was responsive to pulp testing. **D,** After initiating root canal treatment, the clinician packed the canal with dry calcium hydroxide powder. **E,** A calcific bridge could be detected with a file at the 3-month recall examination. **F,** Postoperative radiograph demonstrating apical bridge formation and osseous regeneration. **G,** A clinical photograph after treatment.

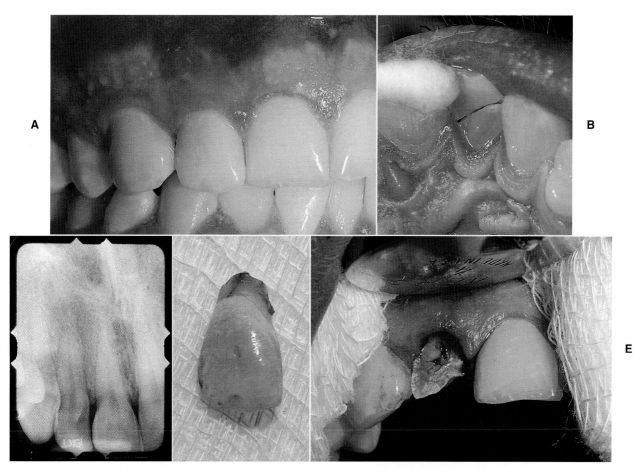

FIGURE 11-6   A and **B,** Clinical photographs of a maxillary right lateral incisor exhibiting a crown root fracture. **C,** Radiographic examination reveals normal structures, and the fracture is not apparent. **D** and **E,** Removal of the fractured segment permits evaluation of the tooth for restorability.

conjunction with required endodontic and restorative procedures; extraction also may be considered.[25,26] Because most of these fractures involve anterior teeth, esthetics is a major concern. Extrusion may result in a tooth that exhibits a smaller mesial-distal dimension and decreased crown-root ratio. Crown lengthening results in elongation of the tooth with diminished bone support.

An alternative treatment technique is surgical extrusion.[27] This technique is only appropriate for teeth with complete apical development. After administering local anesthesia, the clinician gently luxates the apical segment, moves it in a coronal direction, and stabilizes it with sutures or a splint. Root canal treatment can be performed after initial healing takes place, and restorative treatment can begin within 6 to 8 weeks after periodontal healing.

ROOT FRACTURES

Horizontal root fractures frequently occur as the result of facial trauma to the anterior teeth (Figure 11-7). They are frequently oblique and therefore often difficult to detect.

Clinical features that suggest root fracture are tenderness to percussion and palpation, tooth mobility, displacement, and bleeding from the gingival sulcus. Teeth with root fractures often do not respond to pulp testing. Recent evidence suggests that a negative initial response is significantly related to later pulp necrosis.[28] Several radiographic projections may be required to identify the fracture line (see Figure 11-1).[29] If the initial parallel film does not demonstrate a fracture, occlusal films may be required. Variation of the vertical angle may also be useful.

The pulp of the majority of teeth with intact root structure remains vital. Treatment procedures are designed to enhance the healing of osseous and supporting periodontal structures. Four types of healing responses have been described for root fractures[30]:

1. Calcific healing with callus formation between the closely approximated segments (Figure 11-8)
2. Connective tissue healing whereby the segments are separated by a fibrous attachment (see Figure 11-7)
3. A combination of bone and connective tissue healing in which bone grows between the segments

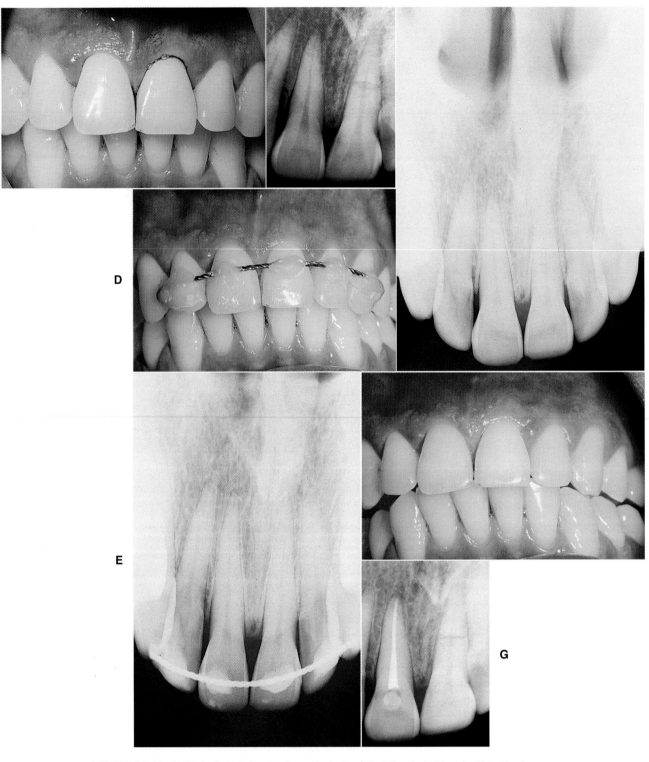

FIGURE 11-7   A, Clinical photograph of a patient who fell while playing tennis. Note the hemorrhage from the gingival sulcus of the maxillary left central incisor. **B,** A parallel periapical radiograph demonstrates a horizontal root fracture **C,** The fracture is less apparent on a maxillary occlusal film. **D,** A postoperative photograph of a rigid wire and composite splint. **E,** Postoperative film taken after splint placement. **F,** A photograph of the dentition after splint removal. **G,** On recall examination the tooth was responsive and exhibited normal mobility. Note that during the recall interval, tooth #8 required endodontic treatment because of pulp necrosis.

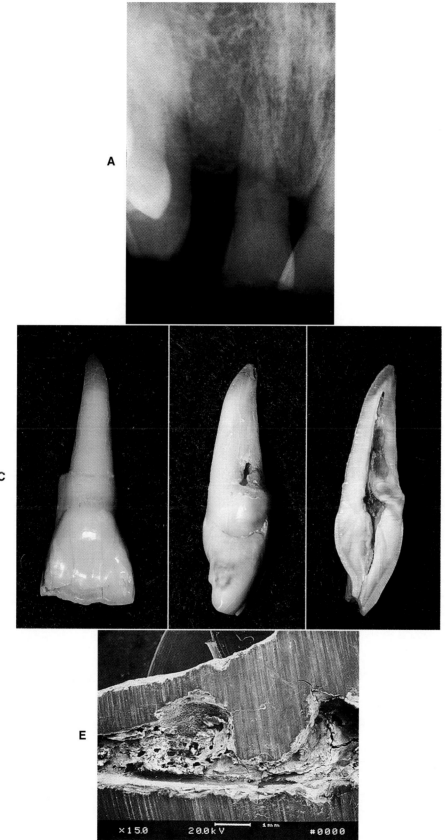

FIGURE 11-8 **A,** A radiograph of a patient who related having his maxillary right central incisor fractured in World War II. **B,** Healing of the fracture site was noted on extraction. **C,** Note the resorptive lesion on the external surface of the root below the fracture site. **D,** A vertical section reveals the resorptive lesion to be internal and demonstrates destruction of the facial canal wall. As the resorption progressed, external perforation occurred. **E,** Scanning electron microscopy of the resorptive defect.

and periodontal ligament formation occurs between the osseous tissues and the root segments (Figure 11-9)

4. Nonunion, with granulation tissue formation at the fracture site resulting from necrosis of the coronal pulp tissue, which initiates an inflammatory reaction at the fracture line (Figure 11-10); the inflammation then spreads laterally into the alveolar bone, inducing resorption and formation of a "butterfly" radiolucent area

Treatment procedures for teeth exhibiting root fracture should enhance the potential for union of the fractured segments. In cases of root fracture in which no displacement has occurred and the tooth exhibits normal mobility, treatment may not be required. In

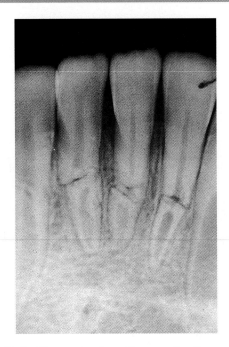

FIGURE 11-9   Fracture healing with connective tissue and bone.

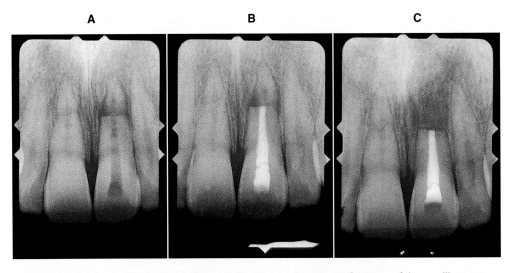

FIGURE 11-10   **A,** A periapical radiograph depicting horizontal root fractures of the maxillary central incisors. The left maxillary central incisor became necrotic and was opened for drainage. The maxillary right central incisor is responsive to pulp testing. **B,** The coronal segment was treated and the apical segment, which exhibited resorption, was surgically removed. **C,** A recall radiograph exhibits osseous regeneration. The maxillary right central incisor remains responsive to testing.

cases where the tooth exhibits displacement or mobility, the clinician should reduce the fracture immediately and place a rigid splint to immobilize the segments. Radiographic verification of the tooth position after splinting should be obtained.

Fractures that have a vertical component or extend near the gingival sulcus have a poor prognosis because of bacterial contamination from the oral environment and subsequent periodontal breakdown. Options for treatment of these teeth include removal of the coronal segment and crown lengthening, orthodontic extrusion, and extraction.

The splint should remain in place for 8 to 12 weeks to permit the calcified tissues to heal. The clinical recall evaluations should assess the pulpal status, tooth mobility, and periodontal probing depths. A lack of response to pulp testing does not indicate that necrosis has occurred as long as no other signs or symptoms are associated with the tooth. The pulp remains vital in the majority of cases.[31] Signs of necrosis include discoloration, sensitivity to percussion and palpation, and radiographic evidence of resorption or a radiolucent lesion. When necrosis occurs it generally affects only the coronal segment, with the apical segment remaining vital.[32] Mobility after 8 to 12 weeks of splinting may require continued splinting.

If pulp necrosis develops, the coronal segment can be treated with nonsurgical endodontic techniques as long as no radiolucent area is associated with the apical segment, the apical segment exhibits hemorrhage, and an adequate constricted area is available in the coronal segment for instrumentation and obturation with gutta-percha (see Figure 11-10). If the apical segment exhibits signs of necrosis, both segments can be treated nonsurgically or the coronal segment can be treated and the apical segment removed surgically (see Figure 11-10). If a constriction cannot be detected or created, apexification of the coronal segment is indicated before obturation.

A common finding on recall examination of teeth with root fractures is canal obliteration and discoloration resulting from calcification. The majority of teeth with canal obliteration do not become necrotic.[33] Endodontic treatment of teeth exhibiting calcification is not warranted unless evidence of necrosis exists.

LUXATION INJURIES

Concussion

Concussion is defined as traumatic injury to a tooth that does not result in mobility or displacement from the socket (Figure 11-11). The primary clinical finding is tenderness to biting pressure and percussion resulting from injury to the supporting structures. An additional clinical finding is discoloration, although this is not common. Pulp testing may reveal responsiveness, but the pulp also may not be responsive to initial testing. Radiographic findings reveal normal structures.

Treatment is generally palliative. Recall examination is essential to assess pulpal status. If a tooth that is initially responsive becomes unresponsive over time, necrosis has most likely occurred. A tooth that is initially unresponsive can become responsive after the injury, indicating a positive pulpal response.[34] Of the luxation injuries, concussion has the best pulpal prognosis, with only 3% becoming necrotic.[35]

Subluxation

Subluxation is defined as a tooth that is slightly mobile after a traumatic episode but not displaced from the socket (Figure 11-12). On clinical examination, bleeding from the gingival sulcus may be observed and the tooth may be unresponsive to pulp testing. Radiography may reveal widening of the periodontal ligament.

Treatment is palliative, although the mobility may require splinting. Because the injury is primarily to the attachment apparatus, a physiologic splint of monofilament fishing line and composite resin should be placed for 7 to 14 days when needed.

Recall examination is performed to assess pulpal status. Pulpal necrosis occurs in approximately 6% of all cases.[35]

Lateral and Extrusive Luxation

Lateral and extrusive luxation is a traumatic injury that results in a tooth being displaced from its socket (Figure 11-13). Because the tooth is moved from the socket, fracture of the alveolar process is a common finding. Often numerous teeth are involved. Pulp testing is unreliable. Displacement disrupts the vascular and neural elements, frequently resulting in pulp necrosis. Occlusal radiographs are often valuable in demonstrating tooth displacement.[9]

Teeth that are displaced without damage to the socket can be repositioned and stabilized with a physiologic splint consisting of monofilament fishing line or orthodontic wire and composite for a period of 7 to 14 days. If a fracture of the alveolar process has occurred, the tooth should be repositioned and a rigid splint placed for 4 to 6 weeks. Because the incidence of pulp necrosis is high and often remains undetected, root canal treatment should be initiated after initial stabilization.[35,36]

Intrusive Luxation

The intruded tooth is displaced centrally into bone (Figure 11-14). Clinical examination reveals a short clinical crown with gingival hemorrhage. Because the tooth is displaced into the bone, mobility is absent. Radiographic examination demonstrates the tooth position. Because of the crushing injury, the periodontal ligament space may not be evident. Treatment of teeth that are intruded depends on the extent of apical development. In cases where root formation is incomplete, the teeth may reerupt. If the roots are completely formed, the clinician

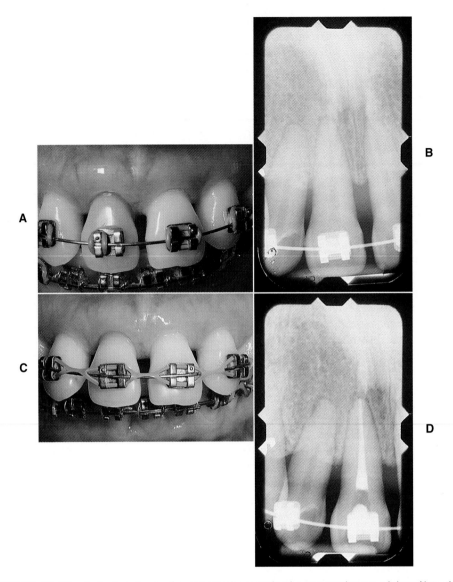

FIGURE 11-11   **A,** A photograph of a patient who sustained a concussion-type injury. Note the hemorrhage into the dentin. **B,** A periapical radiograph reveals horizontal bone loss consistent with previous periodontal disease and normal apical structures. **C,** Clinical photograph taken after non-surgical root canal treatment and internal bleaching. **D,** A postoperative radiograph.

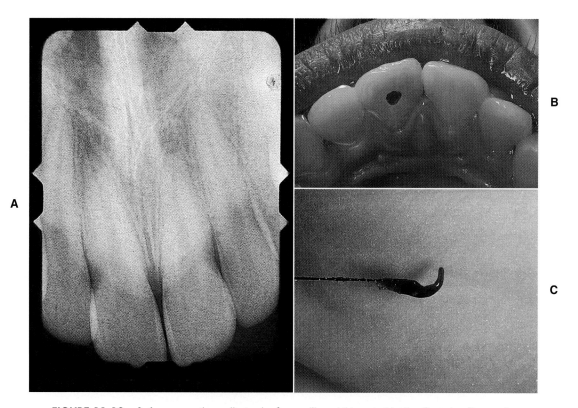

FIGURE 11-12 **A,** A preoperative radiograph of a maxillary right central incisor 2 weeks after a subluxation injury. The tooth is tender to biting pressure and unresponsive to testing. **B,** A test cavity reveals bleeding into the dentin. **C,** Photograph of the hemorrhagic pulp after extirpation.

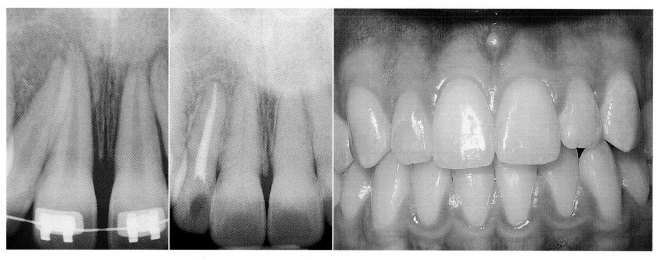

FIGURE 11-13 **A,** A preoperative radiograph of a maxillary right lateral incisor after a lateral extrusive luxation injury. **B,** A recall radiograph taken after endodontic treatment and orthodontic repositioning. Note the calcification present in the maxillary central incisors. **C,** Clinical examination reveals normal tissues and tooth coloration.

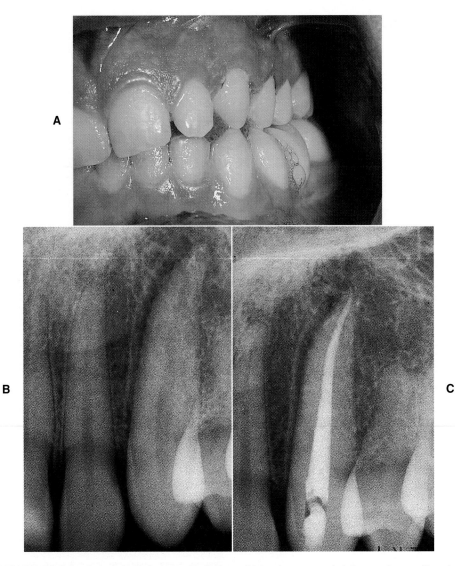

FIGURE 11-14   A, A clinical photograph of a lateral intrusive traumatic injury to the maxillary left canine. **B,** A preoperative radiograph demonstrates a widened mesial periodontal ligament space. **C,** A postoperative radiograph taken after endodontic treatment.

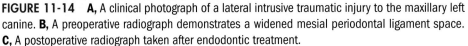

must reposition the tooth surgically with forceps or through orthodontic movement. If surgical repositioning is performed, the tooth should be splinted. Orthodontic treatment is recommended because it produces decreased resorption and preserves the crestal bone.[38] Orthodontic treatment should be initiated promptly because the development of replacement resorption or ankylosis may prevent tooth movement.

Root canal treatment should also be initiated because of the poor pulpal prognosis with this type of injury.[35,37] Although the placement of calcium hydroxide is recommended to prevent root resorption, it should take place only after initial healing is complete because calcium hydroxide has been shown to increase resorption when placed immediately after injury.[39]

AVULSION

Avulsion is defined as complete displacement of a tooth from the socket (Figure 11-15). Although time is of the essence in treating an avulsed tooth, obtaining a complete medical and dental history and performing a clinical and radiographic examination are essential. Treatment procedures are directed toward management of the pulp and the more significant periodontal reactions to injury.

Periodontal Reactions to Avulsion

After replantation a coagulum forms between the root and alveolar bone. After 1 week the epithelial attachment is reestablished at the cementoenamel junction and the gingival collagen fibers become spliced.[40] This limits bacterial invasion and permits healing to continue. Four

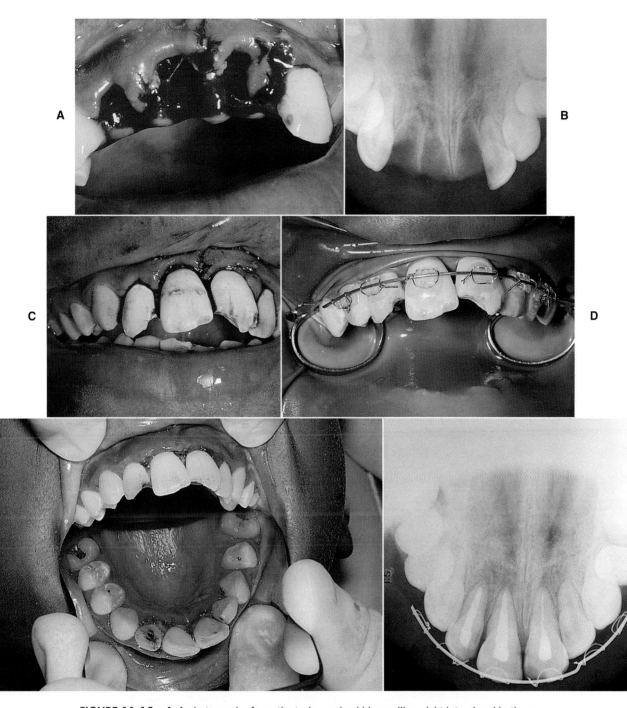

FIGURE 11-15   A, A photograph of a patient who avulsed his maxillary right lateral and both central incisors while playing baseball. **B,** A preoperative radiograph demonstrating complete avulsion with intact socket walls. **C,** A photograph of the teeth after replantation. **D,** An orthodontic appliance and wire splint in place. **E,** Splint removal after the initiation of nonsurgical root canal treatment at 2 weeks. **F,** Calcium hydroxide placement.

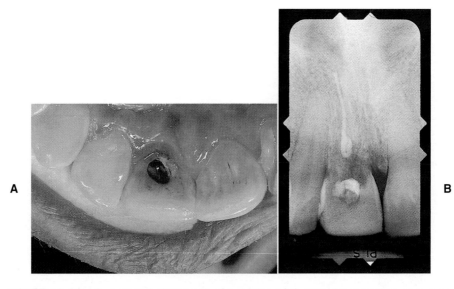

FIGURE 11-16   A, A clinical photograph of a maxillary left central incisor that was previously avulsed. **B,** A radiograph of the involved tooth demonstrating replacement resorption.

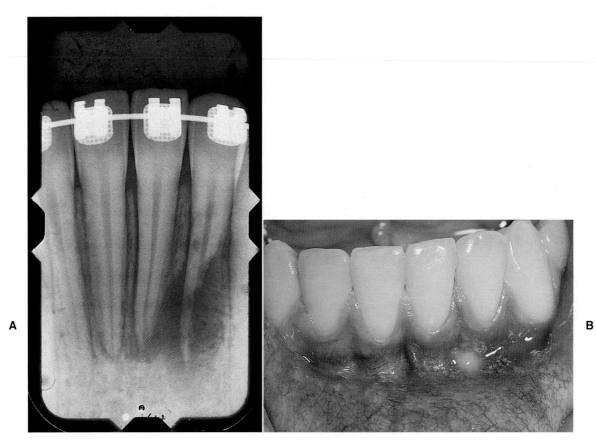

FIGURE 11-17   A, A radiograph of a mandibular left central incisor with a history of lateral luxation and a lateral incisor that was avulsed and demonstrates inflammatory resorption. **B,** Clinical view of a sinus tract that developed as a result of pulp necrosis.

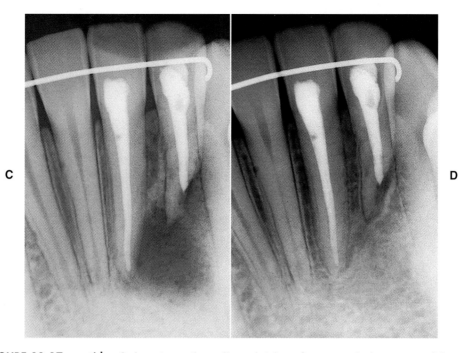

FIGURE 11-17, cont'd   C, A postoperative radiograph taken after nonsurgical treatment of the central and lateral incisors and surgical removal of the apex of the lateral incisor. **D,** A 6-month recall radiograph demonstrates osseous regeneration.

types of periodontal healing have been described.[41] The first is healing with a normal periodontal ligament. Clinically the tooth exhibits a normal position and mobility. Radiographically the periodontal ligament space is evident and displays no signs of bone or root resorption. The second type of healing has been described as healing with surface resorption. Histologically this response is characterized by localized areas of superficial resorption that are repaired by the deposition of new cementum. The resorptive process is self-limiting, and clinically the tooth is normal. The resorptive defects are usually not evident radiographically. The third type of periodontal response is described as healing with ankylosis or replacement resorption (Figure 11-16). This type of resorption is related to loss of vitality of the periodontal ligament on the root surface.[42] It can be transient with minimal damage or progressive with extensive damage. It is characterized by osteoclastic activity and resorption of the root followed by deposition of bone into the defect. Clinically the tooth is immobile and percussion elicits a clearly different sound compared with normal teeth. The radiographic appearance is consistent with the replacement of root structure by bone and the loss of a visible periodontal membrane. No known treatment is available for replacement resorption. The fourth type of periodontal response is healing with inflammatory resorption (Figure 11-17). Resorptive areas in both the root and adjacent alveolar bone characterize this process. Inflammatory resorption occurs when the external resorption of cementum and dentin exposes the dentinal tubules. Necrotic tissue elements from the pulp, as well as bacteria and their by-products, penetrate to the tubules to induce an inflammatory reaction in the periodontal tissues.[43] Clinical evaluation may detect signs and symptoms of inflammation, infection, and mobility. Radiography reveals radiolucent areas in the root and adjacent bone. Endodontic treatment may arrest inflammatory resorption.

Pulpal Reaction to Avulsion

With mature apical development the pulpal reaction is necrosis resulting from the severed vascular elements. In teeth with incomplete apical development the reaction is also necrotic, although revascularization is possible if the tooth is replanted within 3 hours (Figure 11-18).[44]

Treatment of Avulsion

Factors affecting the prognosis after replantation include time out of the socket, treatment of the root surface, the storage or transport medium, splinting, and endodontic treatment. Of these factors, the time out of the socket is the most important. The incidence of replacement resorption increases with the extraoral time interval before replantation because of loss of viability of the periodontal ligament cells on the root. Teeth replanted within 30 minutes of avulsion exhibit the best prognosis.[45] For this

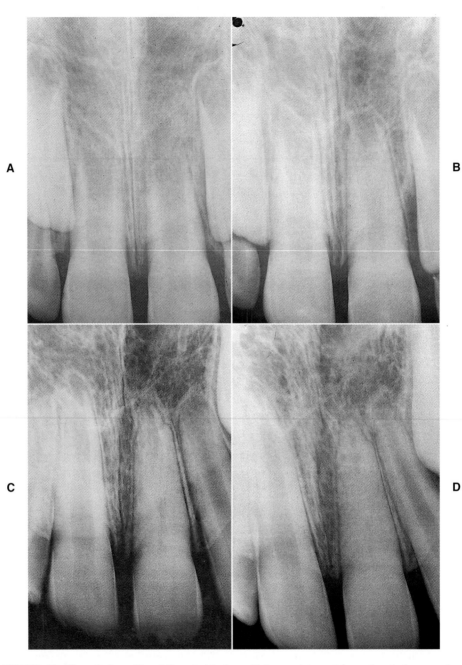

FIGURE 11-18 **A,** A maxillary left central incisor with incomplete root formation that was avulsed 1 month previously and replanted immediately by the patient's mother. **B,** A 6-month recall radiograph reveals continued root formation. Clinical testing elicited a slow response to cold but none to electric pulp testing (EPT). **C,** An 18-month recall radiograph reveals calcific metamorphosis and nearly complete root formation. The tooth remained responsive to cold but not to EPT. **D,** A 30-month recall radiograph reveals complete root formation, apical closure, and continuing calcification. The tooth exhibited a slight yellowish discoloration and was responsive to EPT but not to cold. (A and D from Johnson WT, Goodrich JL, James GA: Replantation of teeth with immature root development, *Oral Surg Oral Med Oral Path Oral Radiol Endod* 60:420, 1985.)

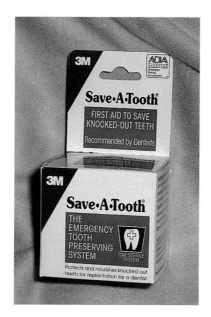

FIGURE 11-19   The Save-A-Tooth emergency tooth-preserving system is sold through Life-Assist, Inc., in Rancho Cordova, CA.

reason, immediate replantation by the patient or parent is recommended.

Treatment of the root surface is a factor that affects healing. The root should not be scraped or scrubbed.[46] If debris is present on the tooth, it should be gently removed with saline solution, milk, saliva, or Hank's balanced salt solution. Tap water is to be avoided whenever possible.

If a tooth cannot be replanted immediately, it should be placed in an appropriate storage medium for transportation to a dental setting. Air drying is to be avoided and storage in tap water is damaging to the cellular elements because of differences in osmolarity.[47,48] Maintaining viability of the periodontal ligament cells is crucial because loss of these cells leads to replacement resorption. Saliva, milk, saline solution, Hank's balanced salt solution, and Viaspan (Barr Laboratories, Inc., Pomona, NY) are acceptable storage media.[49-52] Milk has the advantages of being readily available and acceptable for 6 hours of extraoral storage. Saliva is also readily available, but it is effective for only 2 hours. The superiority of milk may be related to osmolarity, nutritional factors, and bacteria present. Hank's balanced salt solution has been used to maintain tissue cultures. It has been shown to be superior to milk and comparable to Viaspan, an organ transplant storage medium. Although it is not readily available, Hank's balanced salt solution is available as Save-A-Tooth (Life-Assist, Inc., Rancho Cordova, CA), an emergency tooth-preserving system (Figure 11-19).

Maintaining intact and viable periodontal ligament cells on the root surface is the single most important factor in preventing replacement resorption.[53] The presence of an intact periodontal ligament inhibits the invasion of osteoclasts and subsequent osteoblasts.

In cases where an avulsed tooth experiences a prolonged extra-alveolar period without an appropriate storage medium, the clinician can assume that the periodontal ligament is necrotic. In these cases the root should be treated with sodium fluoride because the incorporation of fluoride ions into the cementum produces a tissue more resistant to resorption.[54] The tooth can be placed in sodium fluoride for 20 minutes before replantation. Because the presence of a necrotic periodontal ligament retards the resorptive process, it should not be removed after prolonged periods of extraoral dry time.[55]

Although much attention has been given to managing the avulsed tooth, the socket also appears to play a role in the prognosis for maintenance of the avulsed tooth.[56] Teeth maintained in an appropriate storage medium had more resorption as the time out of the socket increased.[57] Before replantation the clinician should inspect the socket for alveolar fractures and take care not to curette the socket. If a blood clot is present, removal of the coagulum should be accomplished by irrigation with sterile saline. Because removal of the coagulum does not appear to affect the prognosis, the clinician should not risk damaging the remaining periodontal ligament fibers and osseous tissues by attempting to remove the entire clot.[58]

Splinting of the avulsed tooth is designed to immobilize the tooth during the healing process. Because the injury primarily involves the connective tissues of the periodontal ligament, hygienic and passive splinting techniques that permit physiologic movement are advocated to permit regeneration of the attachment apparatus. Although rigid splinting increases the incidence of resorption (as does prolonged splinting), the type of splint does not seem to be as crucial as the maintenance of a short splinting period.[59-61]

The use of a monofilament nylon fishing line or a 0.015- or 0.030-mm orthodontic wire with acid-etch composite permits placement of a passive splint that allows for physiologic movement.[62,63] An additional technique employs bonded orthodontic brackets and an orthodontic wire. If a fracture of the alveolar process occurs in conjunction with avulsion, a more rigid splint should be used for 4 to 6 weeks.

In teeth exhibiting immature apical development, revascularization may occur if the tooth is replanted within 3 hours. Endodontic treatment is not required unless signs and symptoms of necrosis are present. Patients with teeth exhibiting immature apical development should be followed weekly for the first 4 weeks and then monthly to evaluate continued root formation and pulp necrosis. Pulp testing is of questionable value in these cases because of the type of injury. Moreover, teeth with immature apical development do not always respond to pulp testing. In addition, canal obliteration, which is a common occurrence with revascularization, may give a false negative test result. If necrosis occurs, apexification procedures are indicated if the tooth is to be maintained.

Revascularization is rare in teeth with complete root formation, and therefore endodontic treatment is indicated. Periradicular inflammation occurs when the pulp tissue is not removed.[64] Inflammation results when bacteria and toxic tissue by-products enter the periodontal ligament through the apical foramen and dentinal tubules that communicate with resorptive defects on the surface of the root. Early root canal intervention and removal of the necrotic pulp prevent this process.

Endodontic treatment should not be initiated at the time of replantation. It delays replacement of the tooth in the socket and may damage or contaminate the root surface. Root canal treatment should only be initiated after initial healing takes place. Pulp extirpation at 7 to 14 days is adequate to prevent periapical inflammation and resorption.[64] Endodontic procedures should be performed before splint removal when possible. Rubber dam isolation is achieved by clamping adjacent healthy teeth. The placement of calcium hydroxide is indicated after initial healing. Calcium hydroxide placement at the replantation visit is contraindicated because of the increased incidence of replacement resorption.[65] After performing complete cleaning and shaping procedures, the clinician can place calcium hydroxide powder or paste. Barium sulfate can be added to give radiopacity to the material. The powder can be placed in the canal with a Messing gun (Produits Dentaires, S.A., Vevey, Switzerland) and

packed with pluggers. Proprietary injectable calcium hydroxide–containing pastes are easy to use and convenient. An interim restoration is placed and the calcium hydroxide left in place for 2 weeks. Evidence suggests that long-term use of calcium hydroxide does not enhance the prognosis.[66,67] Obturation of the canal can be accomplished after short-term calcium hydroxide treatment, usually within 7 to 14 days. This is especially important for the treatment of patients who are not compliant.

Although long-term use of calcium hydroxide is not effective in preventing inflammatory resorption, it is effective in treating the process.[68] If inflammatory resorption is evident, calcium hydroxide should be placed for 6 to 24 months.[69]

Treatment Sequence for Avulsion

The following treatment plan should be followed for teeth with complete apical development that are placed in an acceptable transport medium (e.g., Hank's balanced salt solution, milk, saline solution, saliva) *or* those that have had less than 2 hours of dry extraoral time:

1. Replant immediately.
2. Splint for 7 to 10 days.
3. Initiate root canal treatment within 7 to 14 days.
4. Place calcium hydroxide for 7 to 14 days.
5. Obturate with gutta-percha.

The following treatment plan should be followed for teeth that have had more than 2 hours of dry extraoral time:

1. Soak in topical fluoride for 5 to 20 minutes, rinse with saline, and replant.
2. Perform either intraoral or extraoral root canal treatment (if extraoral treatment is selected, avoid chemical or mechanical damage to root).
3. Splint for 7 to 10 days.
4. Place calcium hydroxide for 7 to 14 days if endodontic treatment is intraoral.
5. Obturate with gutta-percha.

The following treatment plan should be followed for teeth with immature root formation that have had less than 3 hours of dry extraoral time:

1. Splint.
2. Remove the splint in 7 to 14 days.
3. Perform a weekly evaluation for signs of pulpal necrosis.
4. If revascularization occurs, perform a 6-month recall evaluation.
5. If the pulp does not revascularize, débride the canal, provide calcium hydroxide therapy, and perform 3-month recall evaluations (apexification).

References

1. Jarvinen S: Fractured and avulsed permanent incisors in Finnish children: a retrospective study, *Acta Odontol Scand* 37:47, 1979.

2. Naidoo S: A profile of the oro-facial injuries in child physical abuse at a children's hospital, *Child Abuse & Neglect* 24:521, 2000.

3. Becker D, Needleman HL, Kotelchuck M: Child abuse and dentistry: orofacial trauma and its recognition by dentists, *JADA* 97:24, 1978.

4. Sfikas PM: Reporting abuse and neglect, *JADA* 130:1797, 1999.

5. Zadik D, Chosack A, Eidelman E: The prognosis of traumatized permanent anterior teeth with fracture of enamel and dentin, *Oral Surg Oral Med Oral Pathol Oral Radiol Endod* 47:173, 1979.

6. Teitler D et al: A clinical evaluation of vitality tests in anterior teeth following fracture of enamel and dentin, *Oral Surg Oral Med Oral Path Oral Radiol Endod* 34:649, 1972.

7. Skieller V: The prognosis for young teeth loosened after mechanical injuries, *Acta Odontol Scand* 18:171, 1960.

8. Bhaskar SN, Rappaport HM: Dental vitality tests and pulp status, *JADA* 86:409, 1973.

9. Andreasen FM, Andreasen JO: Diagnosis of luxation injuries: the importance of standardized clinical, radiographic and photographic techniques in clinical investigations, *Endod Dent Traumatol* 1:160, 1985.

10. Jostell SD, Abrams RG: Traumatic injuries to the dentition and its supporting structures, *Pediatr Clin North Am* 29:717, 1982.

11. DeVore DT: Legal considerations for treatment following trauma to teeth, *Dent Clin North Am* 39:203, 1995.

12. Andreasen JO: Luxation of permanent teeth due to trauma. A clinical and radiographic follow-up study of 189 injured teeth, *Scand J Dent Res* 78:273, 1970.

13. Ravn JJ: Follow-up study of permanent incisors with enamel fractures after acute trauma, *Scand J Dent Res* 89:213, 1981.

14. Ravn JJ: Follow-up study of permanent incisors with enamel-dentin fractures after acute trauma, *Scand J Dent Res* 89:355, 1981.

15. Andreasen FM et al: Long-term survival of fragment bonding in the treatment of fractured crowns: a multicenter clinical study, *Quintessence Int* 26:669, 1995.

16. Granath L-E, Hagman G: Experimental pulpotomy in human bicuspids with reference to cutting technique, *Acta Odontol Scand* 29:155, 1971.

17. Torabinejad M, Chivian N: Clinical applications of mineral trioxide aggregate, *J Endodon* 25:197, 1999.

18. Schröder U, Granath L-E: Early reaction of intact human teeth to calcium hydroxide following experimental pulpotomy and its significance to the development of hard tissue barrier, *Odont Rev* 22:379, 1971.

19. Ford TR et al: Using mineral trioxide aggregate as a pulp-capping material, *JADA* 127:1491, 1996.

20. Cvek M, Lundberg M: Histological appearance of pulps after exposure by a crown fracture, partial pulpotomy, and clinical diagnosis of healing, *J Endodon* 9:8, 1983.

21. Ghose LJ, Baghdady VS, Hikmat YM: Apexification of immature apices of pulpless permanent anterior teeth with calcium hydroxide, *J Endodon* 13:285, 1987.

22. Kleier DJ, Barr ES: A study of endodontically apexified teeth, *Endod Dent Traumatol* 7:112, 1991.

23. Finucane D, Kinirons MJ: Non-vital immature permanent incisors: factors that may influence treatment outcome, *Endod Dent Traumatol* 15:273, 1999.

24. Andreasen JO: Etiology and pathogenesis of traumatic dental injuries. A clinical study of 1,298 cases, *Scand J Dent Res* 78:329, 1979.

25. Heithersay GS: Combined endodontic-orthodontic treatment of transverse root fractures in the region of the alveolar crest, *Oral Surg Oral Med Oral Pathol Oral Radiol Endod* 36:404, 1973.

26. Ingber JS, Rose LF, Coslet JG: The "biologic width"-a concept in periodontics and restorative dentistry, *Alpha Omegan* 70:62, 1977.

27. Kahnberg K-E: Surgical extrusion of root-fractured teeth–a follow-up study of two surgical methods, *Endod Dent Traumatol* 4:85, 1988.

28. Andreasen FM, Andreasen JO, Bayer T: Prognosis of root-fractured permanent incisors—prediction of healing modalities, *Endod Dent Traumatol* 5:11, 1989.

29. Bender IB, Freedland JB: Clinical considerations in the diagnosis and treatment of intra-alveolar root fractures, *JADA* 107:595, 1983.

30. Andreasen JO, Hjorting-Hansen E: Intraalveolar root fractures: radiographic and histologic study of 50 cases, *J Oral Surg* 25:414, 1967.

31. Zachrisson BV, Jacobsen I: Long term prognosis of 66 permanent anterior teeth with root fracture, *Scand J Dent Res* 83:345, 1975.

32. Jacobsen I, Kerekes K: Diagnosis and treatment of pulp necrosis in permanent anterior teeth with root fracture, *Scand J Dent Res* 88:370, 1980.

33. Jacobsen I, Zachrisson BU: Repair characteristics of root fractures in permanent anterior teeth, *Scand J Dent Res* 83:355, 1975.

34. Pileggi R, Dumsha TC, Myslinksi NR: The reliability of electric pulp test after concussion injury, *Endod Dent Traumatol* 12:16, 1996.

35. Andreasen FM, Vestergaard Perersen B: Prognosis of luxated permanent teeth–the development of pulp necrosis, *Endod Dent Traumatol* 1:207, 1985.

36. Dumsha T, Hovland EJ: Pulpal prognosis following extrusive luxation injuries in permanent teeth with closed apexes, *J Endodon* 8:410, 1982.

37. Andreasen JO: Luxation of permanent teeth due to trauma. A clinical and radiographic follow-up study of 189 injured teeth, *Scand J Dent Res* 78:273, 1970.

38. Andreasen JO, Andreasen FM: *Textbook and color atlas of traumatic injuries to the teeth*, ed 3, St Louis, 1994, Mosby.

39. Cvek M; Prognosis of luxated non-vital maxillary incisors treated with calcium hydroxide and filled with gutta-percha. A retrospective clinical study, *Endod Dent Traumatol* 8(2):45, 1992.

40. Andreasen JO: A time related study of root resorption activity after replantation of mature permanent incisors in monkeys, *Swed Dent J* 4:101, 1980.

41. Andreasen JO: Treatment of fractured and avulsed teeth, *ASDC J Dent Child* 38:29, 1971.

42. Andreasen JO: Relationship between cell damage in the periodontal ligament after replantation and subsequent development of root resorption. A time-related study in monkeys, *Acta Odontol Scand* 39:15, 1981.

43. Andreasen JO: Relationship between surface and inflammatory resorption and changes in the pulp after replantation of permanent incisors in monkeys, *J Endodon* 7:294, 1981.

44. Andreasen JO et al: Replantation of 400 avulsed permanent incisors. 2. Factors related to pulpal healing, *Endod Dent Traumatol* 11:59, 1995.

45. Andreasen JO, Hjorting-Hansen E: Replantation of teeth. I. Radiographic and clinical study of 110 human teeth replanted after accidental loss, *Acta Odontol Scand* 24:263, 1966.

46. Andreasen JO, Kristerson L: The effect of limited drying or removal of the periodontal ligament. Periodontal healing after replantation of mature permanent incisors in monkeys, *Acta Odontol Scand* 39:1, 1981.

47. Blomlof L et al: Periodontal healing of replanted monkey teeth prevented from drying, *Acta Odontol Scand* 41:117, 1983.

48. Andreasen JO et al: Replantation of 400 avulsed permanent incisors. 4. Factors related to periodontal ligament healing, *Endod Dent Traumatol* 11:76, 1995.

49. Andreasen JO: Effect of extra-alveolar period and storage media upon periodontal and pulpal healing after replantation of mature permanent incisors in monkeys, *Int J Oral Surg* 10:43, 1981.

50. Blomlof L et al: Storage of experimentally avulsed teeth in milk prior to replantation, *J Dent Res* 62:912, 1983.

51. Krasner P, Person P: Preserving avulsed teeth for replantation, *JADA* 123:80, 1992.

52. Trope M, Friedman S: Periodontal healing of replanted dog teeth stored in Viaspan, milk and Hank's balanced salt solution, *Endod Dent Traumatol* 8:183, 1992.

53. Andreasen JO: Relationship between cell damage in the periodontal ligament after replantation and subsequent development of root resorption. A time-related study in monkeys, *Acta Odontol Scand* 39:15, 1981.

54. Coccia CT: A clinical investigation of root resorption rates in reimplanted young permanent incisors: a five year study, *J Endodon* 6:413, 1980.

55. Loe H, Warhaug J: Experimental replantation of teeth in dogs and monkeys, *Arch Oral Biol* 3:176, 1961.

56. Morris ML et al: Factors affecting healing after experimentally delayed tooth transplantation, *J Endodon* 7:80, 1981.

57. Trope M, Hupp JG, Mesaros SV: The role of the socket in the periodontal healing of replanted dogs' teeth stored in ViaSpan for extended periods, *Endod Dent Traumatol* 13:171, 1997.

58. Andreasen JO: The effect of removal of the coagulum in the alveolus before replantation upon periodontal and pulpal healing of mature permanent incisors in monkeys, *Int J Oral Surg* 9:458, 1980.

59. Andreasen JO: Effect of splinting upon periodontal healing after replantation of permanent incisors in monkeys, *Acta Odontol Scand* 33:313, 1975.

60. Nasjleti CE et al: The effects of different splinting times on replantation of teeth in monkeys, *Oral Surg Oral Med Oral Path Oral Radiol Endod* 53:557, 1982.

61. Berude JA et al: Resorption after physiologic and rigid splinting of replanted permanent incisors in monkeys, *J Endodon* 14:592, 1988.

62. Antrim DD, Ostrowski JS: A functional splint for traumatized teeth, *J Endodon* 8:328, 1982.

63. Oikarinen K: Comparison of the flexibility of various splinting methods for tooth fixation, *Int J Oral Maxillofac Surg* 17:125, 1988.

64. Barbakow FH, Austin JC, Cleaton-Jones PE: Experimental replantation of root-canal-filled and untreated teeth in the vervet monkey, *J Endodon* 3:89, 1977.

65. Andreasen JO, Kristerson L: The effect of extra-alveolar root filling with calcium hydroxide on periodontal healing after replantation of permanent incisors in monkeys, *J Endodon* 7:349, 1981.

66. Dumsha T, Hovland EJ: Evaluation of long-term calcium hydroxide treatment in avulsed teeth—an in vivo study, *Int Endod J* 28:7, 1995.

67. Trope M et al: Effect of different endodontic treatment protocols on periodontal repair and root resorption of replanted dog teeth, *J Endodon* 18:492, 1992.

68. Trope M et al: Short vs. long-term calcium hydroxide treatment of established inflammatory root resorption in replanted dog teeth, *Endod Dent Traumatol* 11:124, 1995.

69. Trope M: Clinical management of the avulsed tooth, *Dent Clin North Am* 39:93, 1995.

LEGAL CONSIDERATIONS IN ENDODONTIC TREATMENT

G. GARO CHALIAN

Technologic advances in dentistry have not only improved the quality and prognosis of endodontic treatment, they have also provided an avenue, albeit a sometimes uncontrolled one, for patient education. Patients can easily obtain information from commercial institutions and the Internet regarding their dental and legal rights. Because of this, claims involving dental malpractice, including the practice of endodontics, are on the rise.

Risk management and prevention are crucial to limiting malpractice claims. The best defense in dental malpractice litigation is a thorough examination, an accurate diagnosis, a comprehensive treatment plan, patient education and informed consent, and appropriate endodontic treatment. Moreover, complete dental treatment records, including a properly administered written informed consent, document the quality of treatment provided. The risk management tools of consistent patient education and accurate record keeping greatly reduce the legal exposure of dentists performing endodontic procedures.

Every state provides guidelines establishing the minimum requirements dentists must meet. Many states provide sample documents such as written informed consent forms that have been approved for use in the state. Dentists have a responsibility to seek and obtain this information if it is available in the states where they provide dental care.

TREATMENT RECORDS

Clearly, the most important tools in the prevention and/or defense of a dental malpractice claim are the patient/plaintiff treatment record and signed informed consent. Each state has its own unique Dental Practice Act that usually contains minimum requirements for in-

formation to be included in the patient record. Licensed practitioners have the responsibility of knowing what their individual state Dental Practice Acts dictate regarding treatment documentation. Nevertheless, some basic recommendations should be considered in any treatment record.

As a prelude to the aforementioned recommendations, each practitioner should establish a standardized protocol regarding procedures required for the diagnosis and treatment of pulpal and periapical pathosis. For example, after evaluating the patient's chief complaint, the clinician must complete a thorough review of the patient's medical and dental history. Subjective information should include the patient's description of symptoms associated with the chief complaint. The clinician can then perform a series of objective tests as part of the clinical examination. These include not only pulpal and periapical tests, but also a localized periodontal examination of the area of the suspect tooth or teeth. In addition, appropriate diagnostic radiographs are made and interpreted. Finally, the clinician comprehensively evaluates all the gathered information to establish a pulpal and periapical diagnosis. At the conclusion of the diagnostic process, all treatment options are explained and the patient is given an opportunity to ask questions. Depending on the patient's desires, one of the suggested treatment plans may be initiated.

In addition to establishing a standardized approach to diagnosis and treatment, the practitioner should develop a systematic approach to written documentation of the treatment provided:

1. A detailed written medical history identifying predisposing conditions that may affect prognosis or patient management is essential. If medical consultation with an appropriate health care provider is

indicated, the results of that consultation should be recorded.

2. The patient's chief complaint and dental history should be reviewed and recorded in his or her own words. Analysis and evaluation of previous treatment records and radiographs should be noted.

3. An extraoral examination should be conducted and the results, including medical and dental referrals, should be recorded.

4. An intraoral examination should be conducted and the results, including medical and dental referrals, should be recorded.

5. An examination of the affected tooth or teeth should be completed. Both subjective and objective tests should be completed and recorded. If necessary, a timely referral to a dental specialist may be indicated and recorded.

6. Current radiographs of diagnostic quality should be made and interpreted. The radiographs provide information regarding the particular tooth or teeth and allow the clinician to make and record observations regarding the periradicular structures. Again, a timely referral to a dental specialist may be indicated and recorded.

7. A periodontal examination should be conducted and the results, including dental specialty recommendations and medical referrals, should be recorded.

8. Based on the systematic evaluation of the examination results, a pulpal and periapical diagnosis should be ascertained and recorded.

9. A proposed treatment plan and options presented to the patient should be recorded. This record should include the prognosis for treatment.

10. Informed consent should be obtained and included in the patient's treatment record. A written document is preferred to oral consent.

11. The treatment rendered, including any medications prescribed, should be detailed in the patient treatment record.

12. A statement indicating that postoperative instructions and requirements for future visits were reviewed with the patient or legal guardian should be included in the record.

13. The provider should always sign the record.

In addition to the importance of providing a complete and accurate account of treatment provided to patients, written dental records should be maintained with the following recommendations in mind:

1. Clinicians should know their state mandates regarding record keeping and retention of dental records as defined in each state's Dental Practice Act.

2. Entries may become public record. Therefore subjective commentary is inappropriate. Financial details should not be listed with the chronologic record of treatment. In addition, documentation of conversations with attorneys and insurance carriers has no place in the treatment record.

3. Always keep the original record, radiographs, consultation reports, and any other documents related to patient care.

4. All records should be typed or written in black or blue ink.

5. All records must be legible.

6. Avoid using abbreviations or codes that are not generally accepted in the profession.

7. Never destroy a record, rewrite information, or use correction fluid or paper. The mere appearance of alteration of the record creates an aura of impropriety. If an entry must be corrected, put a single line through the unwanted verbiage and continue recording the findings. If information is inadvertently left out of the treatment record, make an additional entry entitled *Addendum*. The addendum should be signed and reflect the date the data were entered.

8. Ensure that patients sign and date informed consent documents for every procedure.

In addition to the requirement of maintaining accurate treatment records, dentists have a legal obligation to review the diagnosis and treatment options with their patients and obtain informed consent to continue with or refuse endodontic treatment.

INFORMED CONSENT

The doctrine of informed consent is based on the legal maxim that every human being of adult years and sound mind has a right to determine what shall be done with his or her own body. A provider who performs a procedure without the consent of the patient commits an assault and incurs liability. The informed consent document is an agreement by the patient, after full disclosure of facts needed to make an informed and intelligent decision, to allow a specific treatment to be performed. The courts have established that providers have a duty to disclose information that a reasonably prudent practitioner would disclose to patients regarding any grave risks of injury resulting from a proposed course of treatment.[1] Moreover, the courts clearly state that health care providers, as an "integral part" of their responsibilities to their patients, have a duty of reasonable disclosure regarding available alternatives to proposed treatment options as well as the potential complications inherent in each treatment option.[2]

With respect to informed consent regarding endodontic care provided to a patient, the American Association of Endodontists (AAE) is consistent with the courts in its recommendations. As a general rule, the AAE advises that the informed consent requirement is fulfilled after the practitioner "has discussed with his or her patient all relevant information so as to assist the patient in making an informed decision with respect to undergoing that proposed procedure."[3]

As a general rule the information presented to a patient must be presented in terminology that can be easily understood. At the very least, the written informed consent should include the following[3]:

1. The date the informed consent document was presented and signed by the patient or legal guardian
2. The diagnosis for each tooth involved, including both a pulpal and a periapical component
3. A description of the treatment recommended
4. A review of potential complications and postoperative risks associated with the proposed treatments
5. The prognosis regarding the success of each of the treatment options
6. Alternative treatment options, including no treatment or extraction
7. A review of potential complications associated with proposed alternative treatment options
8. The prognosis regarding the success of alternative treatment options
9. A general acknowledgment that the patient or legal guardian was given an opportunity to ask questions and that all questions were answered to the patient's or legal guardian's satisfaction
10. Signature and date spaces for the patient or legal guardian to sign

No specific form can be used for every case. Furthermore, each practitioner should develop an informed consent form that is consistent with the requirements outlined in their individual state's Dental Practice Act. The AAE has developed a sample written informed consent that is to be used solely as an example; it is not to be considered a standard or accepted example of a written informed consent for every state (Figure 12-1). Moreover, the use of a written informed consent form in no way substitutes for a personal review by the practitioner of proposed treatment options or alternatives, including their potential risks.

ABANDONMENT

By initiating endodontic treatment, the dentist has accepted the legal responsibility to follow the case to completion or until the case can be referred to a specialist. This responsibility includes not only completing endodontic therapy, but also being available for subsequent inter-appointment and postoperative emergency care. If the dentist fails to comply with his or her obligations to complete treatment and provide adequate emergency care, he or she is exposed to liability on the grounds of abandonment. Therefore the treating dentist should al-

ways have adequate ways for a patient to access him or her in the event of an after-hours emergency.

This is not to say that the treating practitioner does not have the power to sever the doctor/patient relationship unilaterally. A treating dentist may have various reasons for wanting to end his or her treatment obligations with a particular patient. The dentist may argue that the patient failed to cooperate with recommended dental care, failed to keep appointments, or failed to meet financial obligations. Regardless of the justification for treatment cessation, a dentist who fails to follow the proper procedures may incur liability for abandonment litigation.

The best defense to an abandonment claim is preparation based on the concept of reasonable notice. Successful endodontic care is based on mutual trust between the treating dentist and the patient. The treating dentist should have a prepared procedural template to dismiss a patient unilaterally from the practice in situations in which this trust has been compromised.

The clinician should take into account the following considerations when developing a letter to provide reasonable notice of termination of endodontic care for a particular patient. Termination should only be considered if no immediate threat to the patient's dental or subsequent medical health is evident.

1. The letter should be firm, clearly stating the dentist's plan to terminate the professional relationship.
2. The letter should detail the reasons for the proposed severance. For example, if the patient has failed to keep scheduled treatment appointments, the letter should include the dates of the missed appointments.
3. The clinician should volunteer to provide copies of the treatment record and the appropriate radiographs to the new endodontic care provider.
4. The clinician should allow the patient a reasonable time to locate a new practitioner. Reasonable time may be influenced by different factors. For instance, a reasonable time in a heavily populated metropolitan area with an abundance of dental care practitioners may be less than a reasonable time in a rural or secluded area with a limited number of dentists.
5. The clinician should volunteer to provide emergency care limited to the treatment already provided while the patient locates a new provider.
6. The letter should provide an opportunity for the patient to respond. The clinician should specify a telephone number and a contact person (either the providing dentist or an office employee).
7. The letter should be sent by certified mail with return receipt requested.

SUMMARY

Clearly, the best defense against litigation associated with endodontic treatment is adequate preparation.

In today's volatile professional liability environment, litigation involving informed consent issues is more common than ever. Corresponding to the increase in litigation is a similar increase in the rate of malpractice premiums.

While the endodontist may conform to applicable standards of care in the performance of his or her procedures, that alone will not prevent him or her from being subjected to a claim by the patient for an untoward result. Failure to inform the patient of the risk of an untoward result prior to the performance of that procedure will just as likely result in a claim by the patient for failing to obtain his or her consent.

As a general rule, informed consent is satisfied after the endodontist has discussed with his or her patient all relevant information so as to assist the patient in making an informed decision with respect to undergoing that proposed procedure.

History

Informed consent originally developed from common law principles of negligent non-disclosure. It has since evolved from repeated interpretations by the courts and state legislatures into the patient's right to participate in the decision-making process regarding the type of treatment he or she is about to undergo. Because of the confusion created by various interpretations of the doctrine of informed consent by the courts and state legislatures, it is difficult to formulate a single, simple statement on the legal requirements of informed consent.

General guidelines

Despite these various interpretations of informed consent, it is generally accepted that to obtain the informed consent of the patient, the endodontist needs to:

1. Disclose the following information in understandable lay language:
    *   Diagnosis of the existing problem
    *   Nature of the proposed treatment or procedure
    *   Inherent risks associated with the proposed treatment or procedure
    *   Prognosis
    *   Feasible alternatives to the proposed treatment or procedure
    *   Inherent risks associated with the alternative treatments or procedures
    *   Prognosis of alternative treatments or procedures

2. Provide a generalized opportunity to question the doctor about any of the above.

Diagnosis

It is required before treatment is rendered that there be a diagnosis of the existing condition and that this diagnosis be given in a manner that is readily understood by the patient.

No treatment

Keep in mind that choosing no treatment at all is always an alternative to every treatment or procedure. However, the likely results of no treatment must also be explained.

Lay language

It is important to note that the discussion regarding the proposed procedure and alternatives and their prognoses must be presented in language and terms understandable by each individual patient.

Doctor must discuss

The practitioner who is to perform the procedure must personally present the details of the case, and the patient must be able to question the provider regarding treatment or alternatives. The office staff does not have the power to obtain consent. **A written consent form, while imperative for accurate record keeping, CANNOT be used as a substitute for the doctor's discussion with each individual patient.**

A thoughtful, well documented dialogue between the doctor and the patient can reduce misunderstandings and incidence of claims and suits alleging a lack of informed consent.

Signatures

Your consent form must be signed and dated by the patient (legal guardian if under 18 years of age) and should be signed and dated by the practitioner as testimony to the fact that the endodontist did discuss the elements of the consent form. The signature of a witness is also recommended.

Consent is limited to procedures discussed

It is important to note that consent is limited to the procedures discussed and is not open ended. Therefore, informed consent should be thought of as an ongoing process that may have to be modified if procedures change (i.e., nonsurgical to surgical, unexpected results, or procedural mishaps).

Designing a form

The form should:
*   Document the date and time of the consent process
*   Include a statement that the patient was given the opportunity to question the provider regarding treatment or alternatives
*   Provide space for signatures by the patient, parent or guardian, the provider, and a witness.

It should be clearly understood that no particular form could possibly be suggested for use on a uniform basis. The form provided is a sample and should not be considered a standard form.

Consult with an attorney and check your state statutes

These guidelines are not to be considered legal advice. Members should consider their own particular needs and on the basis of those needs, draft forms and procedures for use in their own offices.

Recognizing that state statutes regarding informed consent vary, it is recommended that members consult their state statutes when developing their own informed consent forms. A copy of your state statute can be obtained from your attorney or by writing to the local county bar association where you practice or reside.

FIGURE 12-1   AAE sample informed consent form. (Courtesy of the American Association of Endodontists, Chicago, IL.)

Sample Statement of Consent for Endodontic Treatment

1. I hereby authorize Dr. _____ and any other

   agents or employees of _____ and such

   assistants as may be selected by any of them to treat the condition(s) described below:

   _____

   _____

2. The procedure(s) necessary to treat the condition(s) have been explained to me, and I understand the

   nature of the procedure(s) to be: _____

   _____

3. The prognosis for this(these) procedure(s) was described as: _____

   _____

4. I have been informed of possible alternative methods of treatment including no treatment at all.

5. The doctor has explained to me that there are certain inherent and potential risks in any treatment plan or procedure. I understand that the following may be inherent or potential risks for the treatment I will receive:
   swelling; sensitivity; bleeding; pain; infection; numbness and/or tingling sensation in the lip, tongue, chin, gums, cheeks, and teeth, which is transient but on infrequent occasions may be permanent; reactions to injections; changes in occlusion (biting); jaw muscle cramps and spasm; temporomandibular joint difficulty; loosening of teeth, crowns, or bridges; referred pain to ear, neck, and head; delayed healing; sinus perforations; treatment failure; complications resulting from the use of dental instruments (broken instruments—perforation of tooth, root, sinus), medications, anesthetics, and injections; discoloration of the face; reactions to medications causing drowsiness and lack of coordination; and antibiotics may inhibit the effectiveness of birth control pills.

6. It has been explained to me and I understand that a perfect result is not guaranteed or warranted and cannot be guaranteed or warranted.

7. I have been given the opportunity to question the doctor concerning the nature of treatment, the inherent risks of the treatment, and the alternatives to this treatment.

8. This consent form does not encompass the entire discussion I had with the doctor regarding the proposed treatment.

Patient's signature _____ Date/time _____

Doctor's signature _____ Date/time _____

Witness's signature_____ Date/time _____

FIGURE 12-1, cont'd   For legend, see opposite page.

Practitioners have an obligation to practice within the guidelines established by the Dental Practice Acts of their particular states. Copies of particular Dental Practice Acts can be obtained from the individual State Board of Dental Examiners or the local dental society. The information provided in this chapter is not intended to provide legal advice or substitute for legal counsel. In fact, every practitioner who develops written and procedural record templates is strongly encouraged to seek legal counsel regarding record-keeping policies, preparation of informed consent forms, and abandonment issues. The dental record is the eyewitness in any litigation proceedings a dentist may face.

References

1. *Ze Barth v Swedish Hospital Medical Center,* 81 Wash 2d 12, 499 P.2d 1, 8.
2. *Cobbs v Grant,* 8 Cal 3d 229, 502 P.2d 1, 104 Cal.Rptr. 505.
3. American Association of Endodontists: *Informed consent guidelines,* Chicago, American Association of Endodontists.

INDEX*

*Page numbers followed by f indicate figures; t, tables; b, boxes.